D0794070

ORGANIZATION RESEARCH
ON HEALTH INSTITUTIONS

ORGANIZATION RESEARCH ON HEALTH INSTITUTIONS

Basil S. Georgopoulos
Editor

 INSTITUTE FOR SOCIAL RESEARCH
THE UNIVERSITY OF MICHIGAN

ISR Code No. 3437

The Project on which this book is based was performed pursuant to Research Contract No. HSM 110-69-207 with the Public Health Service, U.S. Department of Health, Education, and Welfare. The Project Director, and Editor, expresses his sincere thanks. He wishes also to acknowledge the support provided by the Survey Research Center, Institute for Social Research, The University of Michigan, in partial underwriting of publication costs. And, finally, with appreciation, he acknowledges the contributions made to the book by his collaborating colleagues.

International Standard Book Number: 0-87944-125-9
Library of Congress Catalog Card Number: 72-619554

The Institute for Social Research,
The University of Michigan, Ann Arbor, Michigan 48106

PREFACE

This volume embodies the contributions of a group of researchers and scholars who were invited to examine the state of organizational research in the hospital field, to review the product of such research during the decade of the 1960's, and to present their current thinking on research needs for the 1970's. It offers a timely account of the panorama and implications of this body of knowledge as it identifies significant trends, examines promising concepts and developing models, and, in the process, explores not only important theoretical issues but also the question of practical applications. It thus represents both a critical review and a meaningful though partial synthesis of existing knowledge, and is addressed as much to students of complex organizations and the social science community as to health care professionals and organization practitioners.

The book grew out of concern over the lack of a systematic examination of the scattered but sizable research literature of the 1960's, as well as out of concern for a better understanding of the problem-ridden health care delivery system. The number of organizational studies and cumulated mass of data in this area have risen phenomenally during this period, as have the costs of research, and still continue to increase, but with little effort at meaningful scrutiny or integration. At the same time the needs of researchers and practitioners alike for evaluation and utilization of available findings have become correspondingly great. Taking into account also the ever more rapid obsolescence of scientific knowledge—both social-psychological and technical-professional—attempts to take stock of the situation are all the more imperative if society is to insist upon a reasonable return from the research effort it has subsidized.

More directly, however, the present work grew out of a research project which is still in progress, and which is aimed at an appraisal of the state of dependable knowledge in the area by carrying out a uniform review and evaluation of the empirical literature. In the initial phase of this project, as principal investigator, and in cooperation with the National Center for Health Services Research and Development, the Editor invited the contributors to prepare working papers on topics related to their professional interests and the substantive areas covered by the study (see Appendix). Writers undertook to examine and synthesize current knowledge on their particular topic, and also to present their own views and theoretical frameworks. The resulting papers were distributed among the writers and certain other colleagues, and then presented at an invitational conference convened exclusively for their discussion and critique by the authors and other participants.

A two-day research conference was held at the Institute May 22-23, 1970, with the Editor serving as chairman. In the succeeding months contributors revised their formal papers in light of the interaction at the symposium, and submitted new drafts. The revised drafts were then edited for uniformity of format, clarity and consistency, organization, and precision of documentation (bibliographic references are shown at the end of each chapter). Throughout this process, however, the data and concepts presented, the theoretical exposition, and the ideas and conclusions of individual contributors were left intact, so that the integrity of the manuscripts was scrupulously maintained in all cases. Individual contributors, therefore, bear primary responsibility for their respective papers, while the Editor assumes all responsibility for the editorial modifications that he made and for the volume as a whole.

Presented here are all of the formal papers, as revised and edited, together with edited but comprehensive summaries of the critiques and discussion which they elicited. The Editor is grateful to his collaborators—both authors and other participants—without whose assistance this work would have not come to light, and pleased to bring together their insightful contributions. The outcome, it is hoped, should facilitate not only teaching and research but also organizational problem-solving in health care institutions.

The research which provided the impetus for the book is being conducted at the Institute for Social Research, in the Organizational Behavior Program of the Survey Research Center, under the direction of the Editor. It is supported by the National Center for Health Services Research and Development, under Research Contract HSM 110-69-207. Special thanks are due to Sherman R. Williams, Director of the Social and Economic Analysis Division, and to Dennis F. Siebert and Dr. Daniel C. Walden, also of the National Center, for their active support of the project. Locally, at the University of Michigan, the Editor is fortunate to have the valued support of his colleagues at the Institute, particularly Drs. Robert L. Kahn, Stanley E. Seashore, and Arnold S. Tannenbaum, and of the Director of the Institute, Dr. Angus Campbell. The project is also able to draw on the counsel of an advisory committee consisting of Edward J. Connors, Director of the University Hospital; John R. Griffith, Director of the Program and Bureau of Hospital Administration; Dr. Wanda E. McDowell, Associate Dean for Research, School of Nursing; Dr. Fred C. Munson, Professor of Hospital Administration; and Dr. Lewis E. Weeks, Managing Director of the Cooperative Information Center, Hospital Management Studies. To all these people, to my understanding family, to Linda Ozzello who typed the manuscript, and to Bill Haney and Ed Surovell for their editorial assistance, I wish to express my thanks and appreciation.

B.S.G.

Ann Arbor, Michigan
December 1971

Authors and Other Contributors

Contributing Authors

Ronald Andersen, Ph.D. — *The University of Chicago*

Basil S. Georgopoulos, Ph.D. — *The University of Michigan*

Robert H. Guest, Ph.D. — *Dartmouth College*

Feather D. Hair, Ph.D. — *Washington, D.C.*

E. Gartly Jaco, Ph.D. — *University of California, Riverside*

Anthony R. Kovner, Ph.D. — *University of Pennsylvania*

Hans O. Mauksch, Ph.D. — *University of Missouri*

Duncan Neuhauser, Ph.D. — *Harvard University*

Edmund D. Pellegrino, M.D. — *State University of New York, Stony Brook*

W. Richard Scott, Ph.D. — *Stanford University*

Robert Straus, Ph.D. — *University of Kentucky*

Mayer N. Zald, Ph.D. — *Vanderbilt University*

Other Contributors

Bertha Bryant, R.N.
*National Center for Health Services
Research and Development*

Luther Christman, R.N., Ph.D.
Vanderbilt University

John R. Griffith, M.B.A.
The University of Michigan

Sandra M. Morter, M.A.
The University of Michigan

Fred C. Munson, Ph.D.
The University of Michigan

Donald V. Nightingale, Ph.D.
*University of Ottawa
Canada*

Fredric A. Powell, Ph.D.
State University College at Brockport

Dennis F. Siebert
*National Center for Health Services
Research and Development*

Daniel C. Walden, Ph.D.
*National Center for Health Services
Research and Development*

Paul E. White, Ph.D.
The Johns Hopkins University

CONTENTS

Preface

PART ONE

Part One

1

INTRODUCTION

*Basil S. Georgopoulos**

In recent years the health care system in the United States has come under
sharp and sustained attack from many quarters, being persistently criticized
for inability to meet society's health needs and goals and for the staggering
costs of patient care to the public. This past decade hospitalization costs have
been increasing at an unprecedented rate, both absolutely and in comparison
to the rise in the cost of living (average per diem charges by hospitals are
about two and a half times as high as they were ten years ago). At the same
time public expectations for improved service and better performance in
terms of coverage, quality, and cost have been growing very significantly, and
pressures by community groups and consumers for better health care
delivery at more reasonable cost have been mounting as never before.

It is widely acknowledged, moreover, not only by interest groups and public officials but also by health care professionals and social scientists, that
these pressures and expectations have been rising much faster than the organizational capabilities and effectiveness level of the system in its present
shape. At a time when access to health care services by all has come to be
considered a national goal and a right, the stark recognition that the health
care delivery system is not functioning effectively, even allowing for economic
inflation and the cost of genuine improvements, has been producing heavy
demands for change. In turn the major components of the system,
particularly the nation's hospitals, have been experiencing correspondingly
serious difficulties under the impact of these forces, as all concerned have
been debating the issues and seeking solutions without much success.

All health care institutions, but especially hospitals and medicine, have
been charged with the crisis that pervades the present system. Increasingly,
hospitals have been unable to cope with the spiraling costs of care and to perform in accordance with social expectations. Institutional medicine has been
challenged to reform conventional practice and be more responsive to the
health problems and needs of the nation, being assailed even from within for
its shortcomings (the vigorous criticism of the profession by graduating
medical students of the class of 1971 witnessed recently in a number of
campuses is but one case in point). And the relative efficiency of the total

---

*Program Director and Coordinator of Research, Organizational Behavior Program of the
Survey Research Center, Institute for Social Research, and Professor of Psychology, The University of Michigan.

health care system has been judged seriously wanting within and outside the field, for the gap between expectations and performance has been widening rather than decreasing. In the process, economic, political, and social pressures for large-scale improvements, controls, and organizational solutions that would "rationalize" the system and make it more effective have grown to the point that major changes appear necessary and inevitable.

Currently, various solutions are being proposed at all levels by responsible parties, and care programs of different kinds are being formulated and occasionally even implemented in some communities, but the basic problems still persist on a massive scale throughout the system. Yet medical knowledge and clinical capability, health care technology, and the scientific base of the system have never been higher, more promising, or more dependable than they are today. Obviously, the solution of the basic problems must lie largely elsewhere, and mainly in the organization of the system and its subsystems and components.

Better understanding and adequate knowledge of organization at all levels of the system may hold the key to effective approaches and successful solutions. Knowledge from the social, behavioral, and management sciences, in particular, could well prove crucial in this respect and infinitely more important than knowledge from the health sciences themselves. The so-called $70 billion a year health industry (current annual health care expenditures by the American people amount to about $75 billion) apparently requires, and could benefit very substantially from, careful and intensive scrutiny of the organization problems on whose resolution effective hospital functioning and medical practice and, hence also, the effectiveness of the total system depend most. It is this area and this kind of knowledge and understanding with which this book is concerned and to which it aspires to contribute.

Much of the necessary knowledge already exists but is neither well integrated nor readily available in convenient form, being widely scattered in the massive research literature of the last two decades. At first glance, this happenstance leaves an overwhelming impression of futility for the organizational practitioner and policy maker who is a potential user, as well as an impression of either intelligible chaos or unintelligible order for the uninitiated student. But much of the relevant knowledge is there for those who are sufficiently motivated to seek it through diligent search and perseverance. More important, a good part of it can be made intelligible and understandable and communicated in useful form with books of this kind.

This volume presents a critical review, together with an attempt at meaningful, though partial, synthesis of recent social-psychological research on hospital organization and current thinking about the health care field. It presents the contributions of a group of knowledgeable researchers, scholars, and practitioners who undertook to summarize and then discuss the key issues and unfolding contributions of organization theory and knowledge relating to the crisis and major problems of health care institutions.

The Problem of Hospital Organization

One of the most critical concerns of modern society is how to create and maintain organizations which are rational and adaptive (so as to minimize unpredictability of behavior and uncertainty of outcomes while taking full advantage of the benefits of an advanced technology), economically efficient, and satisfying to their members, clients, and communities. This, broadly conceived, is essentially the pervasive and challenging problem of organizational effectiveness. It is also the central underlying theme of this book.

A key aspect of the problem is how to organize and manage human efforts most effectively in complex formal organizations, and how to accomplish this in socially responsible ways under prevailing conditions of rapid change and increasing uncertainty in the environment. Clearly, once-and-for-all solutions are not feasible, and the outcomes of attempts at solution through traditional means are typically unproductive. The problem of organizational effectiveness is extremely difficult and its solution elusive, partly because of its magnitude and complexity and partly because conventional problem-solving mechisms no longer work. Successful solutions now demand both a great deal of dependable social-psychological knowledge (available, at least in principle) and a more systematic application of such knowledge (a highly complicated and generally poorly performed task) than in the past.

In most cases, for hospitals as well as for other complex organizations, acceptable and relatively lasting solutions require greater social-psychological sophistication rather than a more sophisticated technology. In all likelihood they require social innovations, organizational experimentation, and the testing of new forms and patterns of organization, or at least significantly modified structures than those now in operation. They cannot be achieved satisfactorily simply with more money or an even more perfect technology.

As an organization the contemporary hospital is a specialized community institution functioning under the constraints of a problem-ridden health care delivery system and within a turbulent social environment to which it must constantly relate and adapt. Moreover, it is a highly complex organization that is based on the mutual cooperation of a large and heterogeneous number of interdependent professional, semiprofessional, and nonprofessional members. These participants possess different levels of education and skill, belong to different socioeconomic strata, and represent different values and orientations. Yet all must work in close proximity and constantly deal with human problems in the interest of health care goals and service to the community.

Sound economics and technological achievements are extremely useful and important to the modern hospital, but of themselves they cannot ensure organizational effectiveness. These must be accompanied by sound "politics," internally as well as in relation to the outside community, and by commensurate levels of social efficiency, if the problem-solving capacity of the system is to be maximized. For its social efficiency the hospital depends upon its human assets. Constantly it must rely very heavily on the psychological commitment, the motivations, the cooperation, and voluntary adjustments that its members are prepared and willing to make in relation to one another and their respective roles and work groups, in relation to the total hospital as an organization and a work place, and in relation to the patients and the external community. However useful or necessary technological progress might be, it is not a substitute for social efficiency; technological innovations and improvements cannot compensate for obsolescence in the social-psychological sector and organizational arrangements on which the system relies.

The American hospital now is under heavy and continuous pressure for modernization, both physical and organizational, and for a major reorientation of its goals and operations via-à-vis community interests and consumer demands, governmental involvement, and medical-scientific capabilities. A highly advanced health care technology, continuous progress in medicine, increasing specialization in medicine, nursing, and allied health occupations, the professionalization of hospital administration, and the general explosion of knowledge inside and outside the health field have combined to render the traditional, and still prevalent, social organization of this system visibly ineffective.

There is also in evidence a gradual redefinition of the institutional role of the hospital as a health care center within the more encompassing care delivery system. This redefinition is taking place in the context of major societal trends relating to community demands, national health priorities and goals, and health care conceptions on the part of the public and its representatives. These include Medicare and Medicaid, the development of regional medical programs, the emphasis on comprehensive health planning and health maintenance organizations (HMOs), the support and expansion of health manpower training programs and the recent development of continuing education programs, the promulgation of a national goal of adequate health care for all, and the organization of consumer groups and community interests.

All of these changes, and the forces which they generate, have a strong impact on the hospital and concrete implications for shaping the kind of social structure and organization that would be most appropriate or more effective for the system. In combination and in interaction, they are forcing the hospital to alter, now and in the future, many aspects of its traditional character and organizational functioning. Most of the current major problems of hospitals and of the total health care system relate directly to these contemporary forces.

The hospital is becoming increasingly, but probably too slowly, more responsive to the interests, expectations, and health care needs of the entire outside community, as well as more sensitive to the interests and contributions of all of its various groups of members at all levels, and not just those of the medical staff. It is becoming a more open system that is more community oriented and less inner-directed than ever before. But today's hospital is still ruled by three dominant decision-making elites—physicians, administrators, and trustees—which guide the organization and define the action framework for its numerous other groups. Current trends indicate, however, that a broader base of decision-making is slowly developing, with an interaction-influence structure that transcends the conventional tripartite arrangement, and that is gradually expanding to encompass more and more of the participants, regardless of their professional affiliation or hierarchical position, and to accommodate the community's inputs and wishes much more fully than in the past.

Increasingly less and less effective are the traditional maintenance and control mechanisms of the organization: hierarchical authority and formal rule enforcement, unquestioned medical dominance and control of clinical decision-making by physicians, member identification with the organization primarily on the basis of service values, distribution of influence and rewards according to professional status and position. Inside and outside the system, the premises of the conventional structure no longer remain unchallenged, and new bases of organizational stability are required and sought by all concerned.

The internal institutional arrangements of hospitals for decision-making, optimal manpower utilization and task allocation, and role performance and its evaluation are generally considered deficient, outdated, and questionable. External relations arrangements and interorganizational cooperation remain largely unexplored. The supply of properly trained doctors, nurses, and technicians to meet existing and future health needs and expectations also is deemed insufficient by many and poorly utilized by most. On the other hand, the quantity and quality of relevant technical and organizational knowledge available to hospitals and the health professions are constantly growing and improving through modern research. And they are growing much faster than they are utilized. This lag between available and utilized knowledge is perhaps nowhere greater than in the case of health care institutions.

Some alternative models of hospital organization, based on current organizational research and social-behavioral science thinking, are presented here (e.g. Georgopoulos, Pellegrino, Straus) not only for the purpose of examining the present state of knowledge in this field and its implications for research and action, but also for the purpose of defining major existing problems and suggesting the character that the system might assume in the future. The form and magnitude of social-organizational restructuring needed for greater hospital effectiveness, at any rate, in large part will depend upon the kind of organizational system today's hospital is. They will depend upon the major social-psychological characteristics and prevailing interaction-influence patterns which distinguish contemporary hospitals. Organization restructuring and new institutional patterns in part will be determined by past experience and future choice. But they will also be determined by the objectives and problems of the system, the composition and characteristics of organizational groups and subsystems, the type of work to be done, the patterns of professional relationships and behavior in the system, the nature of prevailing organization-member and organization-community relations, and other similar features of the system now in existence. It is these important determinants, among others, which interest us here.

The Contributions

Nine original contributions are presented in the various chapters, preceded by this introduction and an overall integrative piece (Chapter 2) by the Editor. To facilitate transition and maximize integration, the contributions are arrayed roughly in the order in which they were discussed. The exact order at the three sessions of the symposium was as follows: the papers presented in Chapters 3, 4, and 9; those in Chapters 6, 7, and 10; and those in Chapters 12, 13, and 15. Interspersed among these are chapters presenting the discussion and critique of the formal contributions.

The rationale behind the sequence was, first, to look at hospitals from without, in terms of their social environment (Chapter 3); next, to examine hospitals comparatively, using an environment-structure-process-outcome model and focusing on the total institution as the main unit of analysis (Chapter 4); and then to consider certain major aspects of the internal system—the work of professionals in relation to technology, the organization, and patient care factors (Chapters 6, 7, and 9), and the physical-ecological structure at the patient unit level (Chapter 10). And, finally, to present contributions on the role of the doctor in institutional management (Chapter 12), on clinical and organizational decision-making and control (Chapter 13), and on hospital administration and organizational effectiveness (Chapter 15)—these all using the total organization as the unit of analysis and looking at it both from within and in terms of the external environment.

The book is organized into six parts. Part One consists of the present introduction and the integrative chapter, "The Hospital as an Organization and Problem-Solving System." Part Two includes two of the formal papers and their discussion. The Zald-Hair paper on the social control of general hospitals is presented in Chapter 3. Drs. Zald and Hair consider certain major societal trends (technological, legal, professional, economic) that impinge on the organization, and significant changes in the area of social control of the institution as they affect its structure, authority arrangements, and internal decision-making. Next, Drs. Neuhauser and Andersen, using a structural-comparative study framework, examine and integrate a number of important environmental, structural, and outcome variables, and their interrelationships (Chapter 4). The contributions of Zald and Hair and Neuhauser and Andersen are both discussed in Chapter 5.

Part Three shifts attention to the internal situation of the organization. In Chapter 6, Dr. Scott presents a stimulating analysis of research trends and of the relation of technology to organizational structure, and offers a model for the study of the work of professionals in relation to the technology and the organization of the system. In the process, he examines much of the pertinent research literature, and related issues, and suggests promising avenues for future study. Scott's contribution is discussed in Chapter 8, along with that of Dr. Mauksch which is presented in Chapter 7. Mauksch, using patient care as a perspective and an interactionist, "negotiated-order" type of orientation, introduces the concepts of hospital "worlds," "stages," and "process systems" (cure, care, and core), in an effort to view hospital organization from a fresh vantage point. He also considers certain task models and their characteristics, and the importance of these to the study of behavior within the system.

Part Four contains the contributions of Dr. Straus (Chapter 9) and Dr. Jaco (Chapter 10), and their critique at the conference (Chapter 11). First, Straus presents a conceptual framework and a unified concept of behavior for the study of hospital organization in terms of patient needs and patient-centered goals. Then, Jaco reviews the research literature, including a study of his own, on the physical structure of patient units, and considers various ecological aspects in relation to nursing performance, hospital organization, and physician reactions.

Part Five focuses on medicine. In Chapter 12, Dr. Guest examines the physician's role in institutional management, as distinguished from his clinical-professional role, and illustrates the problems with reference to historical trends and in the light of recent studies in the area, paying special attention to policy-making matters and doctor-trustee-administrator relationships. In the following chapter (13), Dr. Pellegrino offers a sweeping and instructive account of the changing matrix of clinical decision-making in health care institutions. Emphasis is placed here on the problems and character of the health care delivery system, on external and internal forces which influence the physician's role, on the need for institutional controls, on the role of the consumer in relation to the governing authority and decision-making structure of the hospital, and on the subject of community participation. The contributions by Guest and Pellegrino are discussed in Chapter 14.

Part Six consists of the final three chapters of the book. Chapter 15 presents Dr. Kovner's extensive review of research on hospital administration and organizational effectiveness. Kovner provides an account of substantive problem areas, including those of organizational leadership, policy making power sharing among doctors, trustees, administrators, and nonmedical employees, the problem of costs and financing, the role of unions, consumer representation and participation, and the problems of manpower utilization, performance, and goal achievement. Chapter 16 contains the discussion of these problems and related issues. The next, and last, contribution (Chapter 17) brings together the closing remarks of the collaborators. It includes some further observations by Dr. Pellegrino on the need for social-behavioral science research into the clinical decision-making process, remarks by Dean Luther Christman on nursing and hospital organization and on certain innovative efforts for restructuring professional role arrangements to improve patient care, and observations by Dr. Paul White on inter-organizational research in health and on the themes emerging from the preceding discussions. These observations are accompanied by the discussion that ensued in each case and followed by the closing comments of participants.

2

THE HOSPITAL AS AN ORGANIZATION AND PROBLEM-SOLVING SYSTEM*

Basil S. Georgopoulos

A hospital is not merely a place where people with health problems go, where doctors, nurses, and others can perform their professional activities, where teaching and research in the fields of health are carried out, or where a segment of the community's population finds employment. It is not just an impressive physical plant or gigantic laboratory with a complicated technology and sophisticated equipment operated by a collection of people with appropriate skills and talents. It is not only an essential community facility representing a major and important investment of labor, capital, and other resources for the provision of critical services to the public. Nor is it merely a complex structure where people are placed to do certain work for financial compensation according to the particular demands of a work plan, and in terms of specific rules, regulations, and procedures based upon bureaucratic requirements and formal authority dictates.

A general hospital is all of these, but much more. Like other large-scale organizations, a hospital consists of many different, but interlocking and interdependent, parts—departments, staffs, positions, work roles; it possesses certain human and material resources and facilities and is designed to pursue certain objectives. It is a highly specialized and internally differentiated system which is intended to do certain work in order to solve particular human problems. It is a work-performing sociotechnical system that can generate certain outcomes through the proper utilization of human energy and knowledge, the careful use of physical resources and technical facilities, and the collective coordination, regulation, and integration of the functions and activities of its many human and nonhuman components. The problem-solving capacity and outcomes of the system are, as this book shows, determined by the work technology and economic parameters of the organization, internal and external "political" considerations, i.e. control-power-

---

*The integrative statement in this chapter is intended, first, to serve as a general introduction both to the field of hospital organization research and the contributions of my collaborators presented in the chapters which follow and, second, to provide a statment of the research framework used in my studies of hospital organization. To a substantial extent, the theoretical analysis is adopted from several previous publications reporting on this work and referred to in the text, especially from "An Open-System Theory Model for Organizational Research" (Georgopoulos, 1970), and is based in large measure on findings from this work.

influence factors, and social-psychological factors. All of these jointly determine the overall effectiveness of the system.

The hospital is also an adaptive system. It is a dynamic, self-regulating system which is in constant interchange with the external social and organizational environment. It imports a variety of personnel, equipment, supplies, funds, information, and patients, transforms some of these through the organizational processes of work and resource allocation, coordination of effort, social-psychological integration, and management, and then exports "finished" outputs back into the environment, while maintaining its own identity and integrity as a system at all times. This input-transformation-output cycle, comprised of numerous smaller and overlapping work subcycles, is a recurring problem-solving cycle which the system begins and completes on a continuing basis, so long as it functions as an ongoing organization and remains adapted to the external environment. In order to do its work, the system must find solutions to a variety of recurring major problems along its entire work cycle.

Equally important, as an organization the hospital is a complex social system. Its most important "raw" inputs (patients and staff) are human; its principal outputs (patient care and health) consist of personal service and information to people; most of its work is done directly by human means; and its major objectives—direct, individualized aid and professional attention to people who need or request it, research and training in the interests of such aid, and high quality service to the community—are all social objectives. The hospital is a problem-solving system whose principal components are purposive human beings who have the ability to act, interact, and communicate at will, to think and feel in both conscious and unconscious ways, to reason and solve problems, and to make decisions that may be rational or nonrational, correct or incorrect, self-oriented or altruistic, and organizationally relevant or irrelevant. It is a "living" system consisting of the patterned and orderly activities and interactions of numerous professional and nonprofessional persons in interrelated organizational roles. These persons carry out an extensive variety of specialized and interdependent tasks and functions, and their combined and converging work performances enable the organization to deal with particular problems and pursue specific objectives within its particular environment.

Organizations as Open Systems

One of the major current, and probably also most promising, trends in organizational research can be traced to the recent contributions of open-system theory (see Chapter 6 herein by Scott). According to modern open-system theory (Miller, 1965; Schein, 1965; Katz and Kahn, 1966; Pugh, 1966; Stagner, 1966; Emery, 1967; Gross, 1967; Thompson, 1967; Buckley, 1968; Georgopoulos, 1970), organizations such as the hospital are best viewed as open, living systems (Miller, 1965); as complex social systems (Parsons 1960, 1966) or sociotechnical systems (Emery and Trist, 1960) that are capable of problem-solving and of internal self-regulation, including restructuring of their parts without serious loss of continuity; and as adaptive systems (Miller, 1965; Schein, 1965; Buckley, 1968), i.e. capable of interchange with and adjustment to the external environment. Human organizations are always subject to external forces, pressures, and stimuli that have significant consequences for behavior within the system, and vice versa. In the process of mutual stimulation and response they are influenced by the environment and in turn affect the environment; and, through continuous interchange and negotiation with the environment they can maintain their basic integrity and internal adjustment while coping with external change. Human organizations, in short, are dynamic, open systems. They are systems whose boundaries are relatively elastic and permeable rather than fixed, or sufficiently open to permit all those input-output transactions of matter, energy, and information with the relevant environment that are necessary to the existence and functioning of the system.

On the input side, organizations import a great variety of material and nonmaterial resources and facilities from the environment. They import raw materials, supplies, equipment, funds, labor, and information with which to minimize uncertainty (J. Thompson, 1967, regards uncertainty as the central problem of organizations) and combat "entrophy"—the generic tendency of open systems to become unorganized and disorganized, to break down and disintegrate (see Katz and Kahn, 1966). Of these, those of highest interest to social, behavioral, and management research are the human and informational inputs that organizations obtain and utilize in order to do the work. The personnel, and the skills, attitudes, and knowhow they bring to the system, and the utilization and management of these, are of greater concern to organizational research than are the physical and material inputs that the technology demands and members use at work. The latter are also important to consider, of course, but they are not as critical, as complex, or as variable as the human assets and social organization of the system. As we will see, this is especially true for hospitals.

In terms of output, organizations may be classified into those whose primary output is some physical product, as in the case of industrial and manufacturing firms; those whose primary output is some service, as in the case of hospitals and government agencies; and those whose primary output is information, as in the case of educational institutions and research organizations. These three types of systems, of course, tend to show characteristically different forms of social organization, e.g. in terms of control and member compliance requirements (see Etzioni, 1964), but also tend to share a number of important features and problems in common. Organizations of a particular type are more alike in comparison to those of another type. But even within the same type, organizations can and do differ significantly. The prevailing patterns of task control, for example, are considerably different among organizations whose primary output is a physical product depending upon, among other things, whether production is organized on a unit, batch, or continuous processing basis (see Woodward, 1970). In addition, of course, many complex organizations produce and export all three of the above kinds of output, though rarely to the same degree or in equivalent amount.

In the case of complex human organizations, however, simple input-output models do not suffice. Even if the outputs of the oganization were precisely specified and our knowledge of its inputs complete, we would still be unable to assess the problem-solving capacity and effectiveness of the system. Between inputs and output there are the critical processes of resource allocation and control, of coordination of effort, of social and psychological integration, and of organizational strain and its management, all of which intervene to modify very substantially any zero-order relationships that one might find between input variables and outcomes. An organization may have excellent inputs in terms of quality, cost, and amount, but very poor output because these social-psychological processes may be generating dysfunctions and problematic outcomes for the system, or may be taking place in ways which do not optimize efficient performance. As the various contributions to the present volume show, many of the enduring and most critical organizational problems of hospitals are associated with these intervening processes and their outcomes.

Hospitals are complex work-performing and problem-solving systems. They are social systems which exhibit a high degree of structural, informational, and social-psychological complexity. They are task-oriented socio-technical systems which are rationally structured and organized, typically on the basis of hierarchical authority principles, bureaucratic rules and impersonal controls, functional positions, and formal work roles, and significantly but less obviously in terms dictated by the clinical decision-making process (see Pellegrino, Chapter 13). Their highly complex structure constitutes the basic problem-solving framework of the system, and the system's social structure, no less than its work technology, contrains and regulates behavior and interaction within the organization and between it and the environment.

Like other complex organizations, hospitals are structured so as to do a certain kind of work. To do this work, however, they must provide satisfactory solutions to a number of system-wide problems. Basically, they must import various resources from the environment and acquire and process information regularly, and then handle, along their characteristic input-conversion-output cycle, certain major problems which they encounter in relation to the processes that are required in order to do the work. As mentioned above, they include the internal problems of organizational allocations, coordination, integration, and strain, the problem of adaptation to the environment, and the problems of output and system maintenance.

It is precisely these problems that hospitals and other organizations, as complex social systems, constantly face and resolve at various levels; it is these major problems with which the management-control-authority subsystem of organizations is primarily concerned; and it is these problems, for the most part, that this books seeks to illuminate. Organizations, in short, face not only input and output problems, but problems along the entire input-conversion-output cycle, and they are structured so as to deal with problems at every stage and phase along their work cycle. Some of these problems are internal system problems while others concern the relationships of the system to the environment. All are related to the basic properties of the system.

It would be possible, of course, to study any organization in terms of input-output variables and relationships, and to compare and contrast organizations of the same general type on the basis of simple input-output differences and similarities. From the standpoint of open-system theory, however, this would not be an adequate research model, unless we were also able to take into account the internal structure and major intervening problems and processes of the system. What is required is not an input-output model, but rather an input-transformation-output model (for a concrete application of such a model to hospital research, see chapter by Neuhauser and Andersen), and this implies knowledge of the internal organization of the system. What is required in addition to considering input-output variables is consideration of organizational structure and process—an understanding of the concept of "organization" per se, along with an understanding of the properties of the organization as a system and of the problems which it encounters along its entire work cycle.

"Organization" and the System Properties of Organizations

To understand fully the hospital, or any other complex organization, as a work-performing and problem-solving system that is a dynamic and adaptive social entity, it would be necessary (1) to employ an input-transformation-output research model, such as outlined above, and (2) to ascertain the basic properties and problems of the system, understand the interrelationships of these properties and of these problems, and examine the consequences of each property for each problem, and vice versa. Only then could the problem-solving capacity and overall organizational effectiveness of the system be assessed adequately and the behavior of participants meaningfully explained. In this section we shall briefly consider the basic system properties of organizations in relation to the concept of "organization" and in the context of open-system theory.

Underlying all organizational research, though often not as explicitly as its importance warrants, is the basic and crucial question of what "organization" is. What is the meaning of the concept of *organization*—not *an* organization but "organization" per se. An organization is a system, and a system is a set of elements with relationships among them, as Ashby (1960), Hall and Fagen (1956), Miller (1965), von Bertalanffy (1956, 1969), and other systems theorists have pointed out. In the case of large-scale human organizations, moreover, the basic elements of the system are behaviors, social activities, and work roles defined in terms of human activities or, more precisely, patterned and regulated human activities. Briefly, then, an organization such as the hospital is a particular kind of system. But what is "organization"? Essentially this concept subsumes certain core aspects all of which are necessary to define it explicitly and meaningfully.

In the first place "organization" presupposes a set of elements or component units. Unconnected elements or events that are unrelated do not constitute organization, even though each may carry important information or other qualifications. Organization involves information, but it also involves order and coupling, or interconnectedness, among elements; it implies structure and form. Each of a number of elements carrying certain information or qualifications is connected to other elements, and the various elements involved are arranged in some particular order according to some controlling or "organizing" principle (e.g. the principle of rationality or hierarchical authority in the case of most complex organizations, or the principle of clinical decision-making in the case of hospitals). The resulting configuration represents "organization" and necessarily entails information, coupling, and ordering, which together make individual elements into components of a particular *set* of elements possessing a certain recognizable form and structure of its own. This is the essential meaning of the concept of organization in its most rudimentary but also most fundamental level.

Order plus information constitutes *patterning*, and patterning is a core aspect of "organization," as well as a basic system property of organizations. Organizations are systems of human activities, and specifically patterned human activities which are organized into social roles and clusters of roles, i.e. subsystems. By patterned we mean that the activities are nonrandom. They show certain order and underlying regularity. Each has certain meaning in relation to the other activities subsumed by a particular role, just as every role has certain meaning in relation to other roles in a system.

The property of patterning reflects the level of structurance within an organization and is related to the relative openness of the system (the less open a system is, or the more fixed the boundaries, the more rigid its internal structure is likely to be) and to the problem of entropy mentioned earlier. Increased uncertainty levels undermine patterning. In every social system, moreover, the rate of entropy production is always greater than zero (see Miller, 1965), and this demands that the system constantly act to contain or reduce its entropy. This is accomplished in various ways, but primarily with additional or different information, with the acquisition of new components or the rearrangement of existing elements, and with increased patterning of activities and behavior within the system. In complex organizations the authority structure serves to combat entropy and reduce uncertainty, though uncertainty always represents an important problem (J. Thompson, 1967).

Another basic system property of organizations such as the hospital is that of *interdependence*. The organization's work roles are carried out by members, and groups of members, who interact with one another, in both planned and unplanned ways, and who relate themselves in various ways to their respective roles and groups, to each other, and to the total system. There can be no organization, nor an organization, without interdependence among the component elements—subsystems, roles, or members.

Perhaps the most critical as well as most distinguishing characteristic of organizations is that their members do not act as separate individuals or in parallel ways. They behave conditionally, and carry out their roles in ways which are contingent upon each other's inputs, relationships, and outputs, and so as to maintain the structural arrangements of the system. (For a discussion of different types of interdependence and their relationship to the problem of organizational coordination of efforts, see J. Thompson, 1967.) Activities in the system always are more or less patterned and interrelated, and the paticipants function more or less interdependently, though not always jointly or cooperatively. Organizational members, moreover, are interdependent not only in the functional sense, but also in the social-psychological sense.

A third basic system property of organizations is that of *wholeness*. The numerous components of the system together form a unique totality or overall configuration—a distinctive entity which is something different than the sum of its parts. The sum of the parts is not equal to the whole. This is due to the fact—which can be shown mathematically—that in human organizations and open systems the articulation of parts follows not an additive but a "superadditive" composition rule (Miller, 1965). It can also be shown descriptively and analytically, with specific reference to hospitals, as in the case of Dr. Pellegrino's contribution (Chapter 13).

In any event, the organization as a total system possesses a certain character and uniqueness of its own—a particular identity (but one whose boundaries are not fixed)—and its overall problem-solving capacity and ability cannot be computed by simple summation of the problem-solving capacities and abilities of individual parts. Correspondingly, the system performs organization-wide functions and solves certain problems that can be resolved successfully only at the level of the total system (e.g. the problem of organizational adaptation to the environment). The property of wholeness, which differentiates a system from the environment and renders it a distinctive and recognizable social entity with its own identity and boundaries, obviously is affected by the openness of the system, and vice versa, as well as by patterning.

Organizations are also characterized by two coordinate system properties not yet mentioned. These are the important properties of *constancy* and *continuity*. Within certain limits, ongoing human organizations are relatively stable systems internally, but also dynamic, changing, and adaptive systems. External constancy serves to define the system for the environment, and internal continuity serves to define the system for its members.

Internally, organizations are characterized by a certain degree of *continuity*; the patterns of articulation and interdependence among subsystems and components are not transient or ephemeral patterns; they exhibit a certain continuity in time and space, and their relationships are more or less stable and predictable. Moreover, as pointed out earlier, unlike both other living systems and mechanical systems, human organizations have the ability to restructure themselves internally without serious loss to their continuity. Internal organizational continuity depends on the social psychological integration of the different participants and on the coordination and regulation of their specialized efforts.

Similarly, in relation to the external environment, during their life span, organizations always exhibit a certain degree of *constancy* (Weiss, 1959).

Without such constancy, an organization could not retain its character and identity. Internal continuity could not be achieved and maintained in the absence of some such constancy. Likewise, adaptation would not be possible, and the system could not remain viable for long if it were not able to count upon regular and more or less predictable interchance with the environment upon which it depends for its existence and functioning. The property of constancy, then, is intimately related to the problem of organizational adaptation and, therefore, also to the openness of the system.

The last basic system property of complex social organizations and other open living systems to be indicated here (for other interesting properties, see: Miller, 1965; Katz and Kahn, 1966; J. Thompson, 1967; and Buckley, 1968) is that of *equifinality* (von Bertalanffy, 1956). This important property simply means that from different initial conditions, e.g. different inputs or different patterns of organization, the same final outcome, e.g. role performance of a certain kind or a particular organizational outcome or output, can be attained. Different kinds of management behavior or styles of leadership, for example, may lead to the same outcome. And, conversely, identical outcomes may be the result of different structural arrangements or internal system conditions.

Because of the property of equifinality, human efforts may be organized and managed in a great variety of ways, even in the case of organizations such as hospitals which are intended to accomplish very similar, if not identical, objectives. Equifinality is also related to the property of patterning—low equifinality correlates with organizational rigidity, and probably also tight internal controls, while high equifinality correlates with relative lack of organization.

Distinguishing Organizational Features of Hospitals

The basic system properties of organizations discussed above are complexly interrelated, affect behavior within the system, and have important implications for the problems that organizations face, both internally and in relation to the environment. An important task of modern organization research and theory is to deal adequately and explicitly with these properties, their interrelationships, and their consequences for organizational behavior. Of particular importance in this connection, for both hospitals and other organizations, would be research efforts to relate these properties to the structural, social-psychological, and informational complexities of the system, and to the major problems which the system encounters along its characteristic input-transformation-output work cycle.

But with reference to specific types of organizations such as hospitals, which are likely to present relatively distinctive organizational problem and system property profiles, the major problems and basic properties of the organization could be more adequately understood if the more peculiar, specific, and unique characteristics of the system were also taken into account. In common with other complex social organizations, hospitals exhibit to some degree all of the above system properties. But at the same time, and unlike a great many other organizations, they also have distinguishing organizational features of their own—features not unrelated to the basic system properties described above, or to the major problems to be discussed subsequently, but sufficiently characteristic of the hospital as an organization to warrant special attention. Before discussing the major organizational problems of hospitals, therefore, we shall briefly deal with some of the distinctive characteristics of hospital organization (for more detailed accounts and related research findings, see Georgopoulos and Mann, 1962; Georgopoulos and Wieland, 1964; Georgopoulos, 1966; Georgopoulos and Matejko, 1967; and Georgopoulos and Christman, 1970; and the various contributions in subsequent chapters of this book).

First, the main objective of the general hospital, though currently under redefinition, is still to render personalized care and professional treatment to individual patients. This treatment is provided according to their particular problems and needs and is based upon what is considered medically appropriate within the constraints of facilities and medical-nursing skills available, and in the context of organizational and financial limitations which society deems proper or prevailing circumstances dictate. This objective has not been modified to any substantial degree by the current trends toward hospital-based but out-reaching community health medicine with comprehensive coverage, toward more home care and outpatient treatment and minimal in-hospital stay in place of the traditional emphasis on in-patient hospitalization arrangements, and toward health care, preventive medicine (or preventicare) rather than conventional patient care. However, it is virtually certain that such progress will be seen in the future (see the chapters by Zald and Hair, Pellegrino, and Kovner). In the future, the community's wishes will undoubtedly be taken into account much more fully than is now the case for the vast majority of hospitals.

Until very recently there was little ambiguity about the primary organizational objective of the hospital, about society's acceptance and support of it, or about the legitimacy and importance of the institution within the larger community in which it is embedded. Moreover, within the system (which has such additional objectives to attain as research and experimentation, teaching and training, employment), there was relatively high agreement among all concerned about the principal purpose of the organization (Georgopoulos and Mann, 1962, and Georgopoulos and Matejko, 1967). Conflicts and disagreements concerning means were, of course, not lacking. Nor did the harmony extend to encompass all of the objectives of the institution, either in terms of emphasis and priority or in terms of commitment by the various participants. Now, however, this picture is changing, moving from consensus and becoming considerably more ambiguous even in relation to the overall objectives of the organization.

Because the main objective of the hospital is professional individualized care and treatment rendered directly to the client by medical, nursing, and other specialists, according to the needs and requirements of each case, much of the work in the system cannot be mechanized, standardized, or preplanned. Thus the work problems of the organization and its members tend to be more variable and more uneven than is the case for industrial and other complex organizations whose principal output is a physical product, with the result that the hospital has relatively little control over the volume or makeup of its work load at any given time. In addition, the demands of work are frequently of an emergency nature and nondeferable, and this demands readiness which places a heavy burden of both functional and moral responsibility upon the organization and its members.

Moreover, the nondeferrable character of work and the relative inability to anticipate some of its demands often lead administrators and supervisors to adopt a management-by-crisis, instead of management-by-objectives, approach in running the organization. Similarly, the emergency nature of the work invites certain exploitation of ambiguity by physicians, some of whom do not hesitate to make unreasonable demands upon organizational facilities and resources on the grounds of "emergency" which they alone so define (see chapters by Guest, Straus, and Pellegrino). Except for a few hospitals having a salaried staff, the organization has little effective control over its most influential group, the medical staff—which by controlling the clinical decision-making process—affects the functioning of the total organization to a degree far larger than patient care requirements necessitate (see Chapter 13 by Pellegrino.) Thus, it is not difficult to explain some of the inter-group tensions and friction in the system.

Because of the nature of its work, moreover, the hospital shows great concern for favorable outcomes and for clarity of responsibility and accountability, with little tolerance for ambiguity or errors. Correspondingly, even at the risk of dysfunctional rigidity, it frowns upon deviation from existing rules and procedures. The familiar emphasis on traditionally close supervision in nursing, leading to frequent "checking and correcting" of the work of subordinates, for example, is not accidental. These organizational concerns often result not only in exacting performance expectations and associated pressures upon many of the members, but also in organizational inflexibility, aversion toward social and organizational innovation, and even economic inefficiency, while failing to reduce the very social-psychological uncertainty and informational complexity that the organization attempts to combat and make manageable for its members.

In the hospital, people with extremely different skills and abilities and very unlike backgrounds are in frequent interaction, within a work structure whose requirements for functional interdependence and close cooperation are unmatched when compared to the great majority of complex human organizations of similar size. Work in the system is highly specialized and divided among a great variety of roles and numerous members with heterogeneous attitudes, needs, orientations, and values. When compared with organizations of similar size, the hospital has a remarkable division of labor; specialization of roles and functions therein reach extremely high levels both in intensity and extensiveness. In an organization such as this, the sources and possibilities of stress, friction, and misunderstanding are numerous, while the impact of errors and difficulties can readily generalize throughout the entire system. The fact that the system can contain and resolve conflicts and contradictions to the extent that it does is an important result of member adjustment, voluntary cooperation, and involvement, more than it is an outcome of formal authority sanctions, high professional standards, or monetary rewards to complying participants.

As unlike as they may be in their organizational roles and professional-occupational skills and characteristics, the numerous participants do not merely perform as separate individuals who carry out their respective roles independently of one another, in a parallel or unilateral fashion. On the contrary, they can only work interdependently, because their inputs and outputs are highly interrelated and the performance of each is always contingent on the performance of others. No single group or individual in the hospital can escape for long the pervasive interdependence of activities in which members engage. One's tasks, role performance requirements, and the problems to whose solutions one contributes are all contingent upon those of other organizational groups and members. The efforts and contributions of all the participants, therefore, would be ineffective if not coordinated and made to converge toward the solution of organizational problems and system outcomes which promote the collective objectives of patient care and service to the public. But convergence presupposes adequate coordination and requires partial subordination of personal interests to collective concerns, mutual trust and understanding, and continuous voluntary cooperation, adjustment, and readjustment by all involved.

As an organization, the hospital formally defines the roles of its members, constrained only by its own sociotechnical limitations and limitations associated with prevailing societal definitions of the major professional roles of physicians and nurses. It sets limits to the amount and kinds of interaction, communication, responsibility, and discretion that are appropriate for different role incumbents. To a certain extent it also constrains the work and performances of participants by insisting upon particular approaches and not others. For example, it may favor the "team approach" in preference to "functional assignment" in nursing, or it may support an individual practice approach as against various forms of group practice for its medical staff. It may resist or promote the introduction of computer aids not only for its administrative, personnel, financial, and record-keeping functions, but also for computer-assisted medical and nursing practice. It may actively foster an interdisciplinary approach to solving problems of all kinds and at all levels, or continue the older separation-of-disciplines, divide-and-rule philosophy. It may foster professional collaboration among physicians, nurses, and others, consistent with the requirements of their work interdependence, and irrespective of authority considerations or traditional status distinctions, or may reinforce the conventional dependence of other groups upon medicine. It may emphasize group problem-solving or individual problem-solving confined to superior-subordinate channels and mechanisms. Behavior in the system is, in turn, correspondingly affected and constrained, with certain patterns of relationships being more likely or prominent and others absent.

Hospitals typically tend to prescribe and expect of their members relationships which are task-relevant, impersonal, and authority oriented, i.e. contractual or secondary relations. Yet patient care, which is both the main objective of the organization and the principal product of medicine and nursing, presumably must be individualized and personalized, rendered according to the specific requirements of the patient and his condition rather than on the basis of generally applied organizational rules and standards. In effect, members are likely to refrain from innovative and spontaneous behavior. They participate in the system primarily in terms of fragmented and impersonal relationships, rather than on the basis of a more encompassing psychological involvement which is possible only where a substantial volume of primary relations and informal interchange among the participants occurs. Patient participation in the care process is similarly constrained, partly for the same reasons and partly as a result of traditional medical and nursing practices, possibly prolonging the patient's health impairment. Observers of the health scene are beginning to suggest the introduction of the concept of "patient's advocates" (see Chapters 9 and 13 by Straus and Pellegrino), pointing out that the patient should have someone in the system to represent all of his interests so long as doctors, nurses, and others continue to relate to him not only with professional detachment but also in highly specialized, partial, and discontinuous ways. More generally, for most people it is the primary kind of social relations that is psychologically most gratifying.

Still, a hospital in its present organizational form cannot function effectively without a good deal of compliance by members with existing rules, regulations, and prescriptions for role performance that result in regimentation of behavior. In turn, members cannot satisfy important personal needs and goals that are met through work without subjecting themselves to such organizational regimentation and behavioral constraints. At the same time, however, some of the more important psychological needs of the participants, including the need for primary relations, are so potent that when the organization fails to meet them the members may create an informal organization with which to offset or attenuate some of the work requirements imposed by the formal system.

Moreover, professionals, including physicians and nurses, have strong needs for personal independence, prefer maximum freedom and autonomy in their work, and are averse to the regimentation to which organizational prescriptions tend to lead (see Chapters 6 and 12 by Scott and Guest). On the other hand, even though organizational regimentation and constraints could be minimized through more prudent management and administration, they could not be eliminated altogether. This would not be possible because of the specialization of work and the high functional interdependence among organizational groups and members, and also because current trends are in the direction of greater involvement in decision making by nonphysicians and broadening of the base of the control-influence structure of the organization (see Chapter 13 by Pellegrino). However, organizational regimentation and administratively imposed requirements can be minimized as doctors, nurses, and others learn to accept their interdependence and function both according to the demands of their respective roles and according to each other's work problems and needs.

Effective role performance in the hospital seems to require a balance between primary and secondary relations (in most cases at the expense of the
latter). This can be brought about only by system-wide efforts which minimize unneeded organizational requirements and constraints, on the one
hand, and maximize opportunities for sufficient professional autonomy and
self-expression for all participants (not just doctors), on the other. Yet these
efforts must be consistent with the patterns of functional interdependence
which characterize work in the system. It is basically the responsibility of
organizational leadership, both administrative and medical, to achieve and
maintain such a balance, provided however, that members accept their interdependence and behave accordingly, and provided also that the distribution
of influence and rewards among organizational groups and members in the
system itself is generally acceptable to all concerned. Authoritarian leadership does not promote excellent and reliable role performance in the hospital,
just as the pure human-relations approach with its one-sided emphasis on
primary and informal relations is unworkable. The best solution is to be
found in a combined emphasis on broad member participation in the decision-making processes of the system at all levels, in the context of a
structured yet not rigid work framework, and upon task-oriented behavior
which does not disregard the personal needs and goals of members (see e.g.
Searles, 1961; Georgopoulos and Mann, 1962; and Georgopoulos, 1966).

The fact that the principal workers in the hospital—physicians and
nurses—are professional specialists raises additional issues, which are
further complicated by the coexistence of multiple authority lines in the system. These authority lines are the administrative line, extending from the
patient's physician, and the quasi-professional, quasi-administrative line
encountered in the nursing service. Specialists and professionals tend to be
committed to their profession more than to the organization where they
work, and this generates both administrative and motivational difficulties.
For example, research by the author shows that nurses in general hospitals
are more strongly identified with their profession than with the team which
treats the patients, and only then with the hospital and with the outside
community, in that order (Georgopoulos and Matejko, 1967). Other obvious
reasons for the complex personnel and management problems that a hospital
faces include: (1) the professional nursing shortages experienced in recent
years, (2) approximately forty percent of hospital-employed registered nurses
are working only part-time, (3) nurses constitute both the largest and the
most unstable organizational group in the system. It should be noted that
this instability is in terms of length of employment, turnover, mobility,
extraorganizational female role obligations, and other characteristics.

Furthermore, specialists and professionals presumably have the expert
knowledge and technical competence required to perform their roles relatively autonomously, but many organizational decisions which affect them and
their work often are made by administrators who have legitimate organizational authority to do so. The latter ordinarily have good knowledge of
hospital organization, but very limited technical, medical, or nursing exper-

tise; the former usually are organizationally naive, having a very narrow conception of the total system and its problems and needs. These circumstances can readily lead to serious conflicts, or at least raise important authority issues revolving around the question of right balance between power and knowledge for the various groups of organizational participants (see chapters by Kovner, Guest, and Pellegrino). As the "explosion of knowledge" continues and specialization increases further in all fields, hospitals and other complex organizations will be forced to devise and use more satisfactory mechanisms than they now employ for handling this problem.

A certain degree of specialization among and within organizations, and professions and occupations, is indispensable to efficient role performance, individual adaptiveness, and organizational effectiveness. In the hospital field, over the years medical and nursing specialization have undoubtedly led to improved patient care, just as administrative professionalization has led to improved hospital functioning. The basic advantage of specialization is that it makes possible the utilization and assimilation of available human knowledge, as well as the generation of new knowledge, while itself being the most powerful social invention available with which to handle the great complexity engendered by man's vast and growing knowledge. But increased specialization also makes it more difficult for the individual to relate effectively to his coworkers or to understand satisfactorily the relationship between his activity and the organization's total effort. Specialization makes interaction more demanding for all involved, frequently leading to excessive fragmentation of organizational tasks and member functions with the result that a great many of the members find their work uninteresting and psychologically meaningless or unrewarding.

Increasing specialization, moreover, results in higher interdependence at work among the participants, and excessive specialization tends to engender problems of professional allegiance and organizational identification, and even problems of competition and conflict. The disadvantages of specialization can be minimized, but only through elaborate coordination, effective communication, and member cooperativeness in all parts of the system. At optimal levels, specialization (particularly professional specialization and specialization by skill rather than by task) makes for efficiency and adaptability. Underspecialization and overspecialization may be equally detrimental (the former by impeding efficiency, and the latter by generating unnecessary complexity and conflicts in the system) to an organization and its members. Regrettably, research to date has not provided satisfactory answers as to the levels of specialization that would be optimal for hospitals and other organizations. What is clear, however, is that properly regulated specialization in organizations with high internal social integration need not be dysfunctional (Georgopoulos and Christman, 1970; Georgopoulos and Jackson, 1970; Georgopoulos and Sana, 1971).

In any case, the nature of work in the hospital, along with the high levels of professionalization and specialization among its members, and accompanying functional interdependence for all involved, necessitates the development and maintenance of complementary expectations and mutual understanding among the participants about one another's roles and work problems and needs. Member compliance with formal rules and requirements is not enough if members are to perform their roles effectively. The same conditions necessitate elaborate provisions for adequate coordination of work efforts throughout the organization, and particularly at points where diverse and specialized activities converge, e.g. the patient. Good coordination is essential because it is a necessary though not sufficient condition for work efficiency and good patient care. But, again, much of the required coordination must be achieved directly by human means and through voluntary efforts and spontaneous adjustments by the members; it cannot be effected through departmental routines, work schedules, and work plans alone. This entails further difficulties.

The issue of balance between the performance of clinical and coordinative functions by nurses, for example, continues to be a thorny one in hospitals. Nurses are the only major professional group whose members are present at work at all times, thus being capable of ensuring continuity of effort. But the more nurses assume coordinative functions, the less time and energy they have to devote to patient care functions. Traditionally, nursing has served as repository of residual and supportive functions in the system—functions that are essential to coordination but not necessarily to professional nursing practice. As nursing specializes further (very likely in the manner and pattern of medicine), however, it will no longer be willing or able to carry out coordinative activities and still discharge its professional responsibilities to the patient and the organization. New ways of handling coordination problems will have to be sought out, for such problems will become even more acute rather than diminish.

It must also be pointed out that both nursing and medicine today face a twofold and somewhat paradoxical problem, which is also a hospital problem. On the one hand, the supply of adequately trained professional manpower to meet existing and future health needs and demands is deemed insufficient and unsatisfactory by all concerned (although in significant part the problem may be one of proper manpower utilization). On the other hand, as in most other fields, the amount of relevant knowledge and expertise available to the health professions is constantly growing through research, and growing much faster than utilized to raise the levels of clinical competence and professional excellence in actual practice. Moreover, all available evidence and discernible trends indicate that the needs for more and better trained doctors and nurses, and also administrators and technical personnel, in the years to come will increase futher, becoming even more pressing than at present.

Among the major factors and trends which are combining to assure even higher levels of need for well-trained physicians, nurses, and allied health professionals in clinical, administrative, teaching, and research roles in the field of health are:

1. population increases, longevity, rising living standards, higher public aspirations and expectations (in part brought about by improvements in

medicine), and staggeringly rising hospital, medical, and health care costs;

2. the nationwide emphasis on comprehensive planning and far-reaching national and regional organization (e.g. Medicare, Regional Medical Programs, Community Health Planning, Health Maintenance Organization programs) for comprehensive and high-quality health care for all;

3. continuing improvements in medicine, nursing, and other health-related fields, as well as better management and organizational knowledge based on social-psychological and behavioral research;

4. the ever more rapid obsolescence of scientific, technical and professional knowledge transmitted to medical, nursing, and other professional students in formal education settings, with accompanying greater needs and demands for continuing education and training throughout one's professional career; and

5. the increasing specialization and interdependence among all health workers inside and outside the hospital.

The preceding characteristics of hospital organization make it clear that in a social system such as they portray no organizational work plan, however rational, can be mechanistically or routinely implemented. Even a perfect work plan could not be effectively implemented without consideration for the social efficiency of the system (including both social-psychological and "political" efficiency), or without taking into account the complex human factors and powerful social-psychological forces at work, in addition to economic and technological efficiency.

For hospitals, organizational effectiveness depends upon social efficiency more than it does upon technical-economic efficiency, and the same may be said of reliable and high-level performance on the part of the members. Stated differently, a high level of commitment, loyalty, and involvement, as well as a genuine sense of satisfaction on the part of its numerous groups and members, are critical to the functioning of this organization (Dalton, 1970; Georgopoulos, 1971). In general, social efficiency entails personal goal-attainment for the participants at all levels, and this includes meaningful participation in the decision-making process, identification with the organization, opportunities for expressive behavior and satisfaction of intrinsic motives, and psychological rewards. The social-psychological efficiency of an organization, of course, in the short run may be low while its technical-economic efficiency is high, and vice versa. In the long run, however, high technical-economic efficiency in the absence of substantial social efficiency would be extremely unlikely for hospitals in this country. At any rate, organizational effectiveness in the case of the hospital requires a high level of both.

Economy of operation is obviously a critical factor in hospital effectiveness (see Chapter 15 by Kovner). Technological efficiency is likewise critical, not only from the standpoint of having and using up-to-date equipment, but also and more significantly, from the standpoint of how the work technology, broadly defined (for example as treated in the chapter by Scott rather than in the more narrow sense used by Woodward, 1970), is perceived and used by the participants. The importance of work technology for organizational behavior and hospital effectiveness has been emphasized by Perrow (1965), and is here insightfully elaborated by Scott in relation to the work of professionals in hospitals.

Less obvious, perhaps, may be the critical role of social efficiency in hospital effectiveness. This will be further clarified in this chapter, and more convincingly shown throughout the book. Here, we shall confine ourselves to only a few further observations. To reiterate, the organizational effectiveness of the hospital depends both upon technical and social efficiency. For its social efficiency, the hospital must rely on its members and their behaviors and contributions. Formal authority principles and hierarchical arrangements have their place in the hospital, as in any complex large-scale organization, and the same is true of formal work plans, rules, regulations, and procedures. These serve to minimize uncertainty, to enable the participants to cope with complexity, to ensure certain continuity and uniformity of action and its outcomes, and to maximize reliability and predictability of role performance and organizational functioning along the entire input-transformation-output cycle of the system. But concerted effort and organizational effectiveness cannot be attained by means of impersonal controls, standardized work routines, explicitly detailed job prescriptions, and rational activity programs alone.

Adequate organizational coordination, which is a necessary condition for effective functioning by the total system, for example, cannot be achieved and maintained on the basis of hierarchical authority and rational controls, or on the principle of planned means and programmed activity for all involved. It also depends very greatly, according to much recent research (Georgopoulos and Mann, 1962, especially chapters 6 and 7; Heydebrand, 1965; Wieland, 1965) upon the voluntary and spontaneous adjustments which organizational groups and members are able and willing to make in order to accommodate one another and mutually facilitate their role performance in the daily work. A great deal depends upon the extent to which the various groups and members understand each other's work problems and needs; the degree to which the work-relevant expectations, attitudes, motivations, and values of members in related jobs are congruent or complementary; the degree to which interacting groups and individuals are guided by informal norms of reciprocity, trust, and mutual helpfulness; the degree to which members can satisfy important personal needs and goals within the system rather than outside; and the extent to which the participants, regardless of their professional role and formal status, are willing to cooperate and promote organizationally relevant behavior on the basis of self-discipline, professional self-control, self-regulation of individualistic activity, and internalized altruistic motivation.

It is these and other similar social-psychological forces which make possible not only the coordination of diverse and specialized efforts of numerous members of the hospital, but also the integration of members into the organization and the social integration of the system itself. Concepts such as those of hierarchical authority, formal executive power, delegation and decentralization, administrative discretion, work standardization and simplification, industrial engineering, task control, and cost accounting are useful, but inadequate from the standpoint of total system effectiveness. The same may be said of technological innovations, including improvements in equipment design, work techniques and procedures, automation of routine activities, and other technological innovations which are frequently introduced in hospitals. Even sophisticated PPBS ("planning, programming, budgeting 'systems' ") are not exempt from serious limitations, and the same may be expected regarding the much talked about computer-assisted professional practice by the medical and nursing staffs of hospitals in the foreseeable future. These improvements and innovations are all very useful work means to the modern hospital, but of themselves they cannot ensure high organizational effectiveness if not accompanied by commensurate levels of social efficiency. As stated earlier, for its social efficiency, the hospital depends upon its human assets and resources.

Major Problems of Hospital Organization

Hospitals, like other complex human organizations, it was pointed out, are dynamic, adaptive, work-performing, and problem-solving sociotechnical systems. As such, in common with other organizations, they are characterized by a set of basic system properties—openness, patterning, interdependence, wholeness, continuity, constancy, and equifinality. But in addition, as indicated above, unlike other types of organizations, they have certain distinctive characteristics of their own, which suggest that the social efficiency of the system may be a more critical determinant in organizational functioning than technical efficiency. To understand hospital organization and the behavior of participants in the system, it is necessary to take into account these characteristics and study the basic properties of the system, both in relation to one another and in relation to the major problems which the system encounters along the entire input-transformation-output work cycle. It is similarly necessary to study the interrelationships of these problems, both at the collectivity level (i.e. the system and subsystem or institutional and group level) and at the individual level.

If, indeed, the hospital can be best viewed as a problem-solving system, it is essential for organizational research to specify and understand the substantive problems that the system faces and resolves, the mechanisms and problem-solving processes involved, and their outcomes, and ultimately also the relative success with which the system handles each particular problem and all of the problems combined. As briefly noted earlier, the problems in question include those of adaptation to the environment, the internal problems of resource allocation and utilization, coordination of diverse but interdependent efforts, social-psychological integration, strain and its management, and the problems of output and system maintenance. Only by taking into account the problem-solving performance of the organization and its members in relation to these problems would it be possible to assess the effectiveness of the system satisfactorily.

More concretely, the technical and social efficiency of the system alike, which together determine overall organizational effectiveness, depend upon the solutions that the hospital as an organization provides to certain major problems. These concern: procurement, deployment, allocation, and utilization of human and material resources; the fit between the social structure of the system and the organization's work technology, and between formal and informal behavior patterns; intergroup communication and influence; interdepartmental coordination and cooperation; interpersonal and intergroup tensions or conflict relationships with the community and other relevant outside publics or interest groups. As an ongoing social system the hospital encounters important problems on a recurring basis in a number of areas. These include: integrating organizational requirements with the needs and goals of members; developing and maintaining appropriate leadership practices and supervisory skills for each organizational level; devising means for the management of tensions and strain; developing suitable reward distribution mechanisms and providing adequate incentives; maintaining sufficient structural flexibility and preparedness for meeting unanticipated contingencies; and facilitating social-psychological integration on an organization-wide basis.

Both the viability and effectiveness of the hospital are basically determined by the problem-solving capacity of the system in these important areas. The same may be said regarding the attainment of the organization's major objectives, including the kind of health care which the institution provides, and the performance of the system in relation to such objectives. The crucial question underlying effectiveness is how well the hospital is functioning in its totality as a unified system—how all parts and members of the organization perform together and jointly contribute to the solution of major problems and attainment of major objectives.

In the light of these propositions, in recent years the focus of organizational research inside and outside the hospital field has shifted. Attention has moved from the question of whether the hospital (or any other complex organization) can meet specific minimal requirements, or whether the separate contributions of particular groups and individual units are sufficient in each case to accomplish specified goals, to more encompassing and more significant issues (see, e.g. Etzioni, 1964, and Georgopoulos and Matejko, 1967). It has begun to focus, instead, on the more fundamental task of specifying the patterns of interrelationships among the various elements of the organizational system which would make it most effective from the standpoint of its overall problem-solving capacity and ability, and not merely efficient in the service of some particular goal. The simpler but also less fruitful goal-oriented approaches used in earlier research gradually have given way to more promising system-oriented approaches, and earlier "survival models" of organization have gradually been replaced by "effectiveness models" (for these distinctions, see Etzioni, 1964). The crucial issue regarding organizational effectiveness is no longer merely one of viability, whether an organization can maintain and perpetuate itself in a specific environment, given its particular structure, resources, and problems. Organizational survival reflects organizational effectiveness only at the simplest and most primitive level. To be effective as a system, the hospital at least must be able to maintain itself and function at a level past the threshhold of viability. But beyond self-maintenance and survival there are many possible levels of organizational effectiveness that a hospital can reach, depending upon the solutions to its major problems that the system can provide.

More specifically, effective hospital functioning depends upon the problem-solving capacity and performance of the entire organizational system, and is determined jointly (though not necessarily linearly or to equal degrees) by:

1. The ability of the organization to adapt to the external environment and carry on an effective interchange with it at all times. This includes ability to respond successfully to relevant changes in the outside world; to obtain resources and personnel; to maintain advantageous relationships with the community; and generally to influence the environment in ways that benefit the system and its members in relation to all aspects of organization-environment articulation. This is the problem of *organizational adaptation.*

2. The ability of the organization to deploy, allocate, and utilize available resources, facilities, funds, and personnel in the most appropriate manner; to handle related problems of access to, and distribution of, authority, rewards, and information among the participants; to ensure participation by all concerned in the decision-making process; and to solve problems concerning work specialization and the allocation of tasks and functions among departments, groups, and members. This is the problem of *organizational allocation.*

3. The ability to articulate, interrelate, and regulate—to constantly coordinate, in time and space—the many diverse but related roles and interdependent activities of its many different staffs and members, and to regulate and synchronize different functions, so that the energies and efforts of all the participants always converge toward the solution of system problems and the attainment of organizational objectives. This is the problem of *organizational coordination.*

4. The ability of the system to integrate itself. This includes all necessary functions associated with the problem of integrating individual members into the organization and securing their cooperation and compliance, and the problem of integrating all parts of the social system with one another so that the total organization can achieve a certain overall social-psychological

unity and coherence. Development of common organizational values and shared norms, attitudes, and mutual understandings, which can serve to provide a common universe of discourse for the different groups and members, and to socialize and bind the members securely into the system, are all important in this area. This is the problem of *organizational integragration.*

5. The ability to resolve or minimize and manage the tensions and conflicts which arise within the organization, particularly frictions and confrontations among key groups (e.g. trustees, doctors, and administrators), among highly interdependent groups and members, and among unequal status participants, and to control stress and strain throughout the system. This is the problem of *organizational strain.*

6. The ability to reach and maintain high levels (in terms of quantity, quality, acceptability, and costs) of output, e.g. patient care or health service to the community, at all times. This involves the ability to maximize efficient and reliable performance by all departments, groups, and members, at all levels, and is in turn dependent upon maximization by the system of opportunities for personal goal attainment and job satisfaction on the part of the members. This is the problem of *organizational output* or goal attainment.

7. The ability of the organization to preserve its identity and integrity as a distinct and unified problem-solving system, or to maintain itself and its basic character and viability in the face of changes which are constantly occuring in the environment and within the system, including potential disruptions and threats to the internal continuity and to the survival and well-being of the system. This is the problem of *organizational maintenance.*

Obviously, these major substantive problems cover the total work cycle of the system—some are encountered primarily on the input side, some on the output side, and the others at intervening points. Moreover, as we shall see, they manifest themselves in the form of concrete and specific difficulties both at the collectivity level and at the individual level, that is, in relation to the behavior and activities of individual members in the organization and in terms of organization-member relations. Accordingly, it is important to examine the same problems, first, at the collectivity level, in order to ascertain their meaning for the total system and understand their consequences for the functioning of organizational groups, departments, and subsystems, and, second, at the individual level, in order to understand and explain member behaviors in the system. A portion of the difference in problem-solving capacity, organizational effectiveness, and problem-solving success in relation to each major problem of the system, within as well as across organizations, can be accounted for only by collectivity-level factors. An additional portion must be explained by individual-level factors; and, allowing for an error factor which is always present, the remaining portion is an outcome of the interaction between group forces and individual-level factors. Therefore, specification of those aspects of the above problems which are critical at the individual level, or for the behavior of individual members and organization-member relationships, constitutes another important task for modern organizational research, and we shall return to consider this matter further.

Clearly, the problems in question are complex and relatively enduring and are not amenable to a perfect or once-and-for-all solution. Their resolution requires continuous effort by the organization; there is always room for improvement. These problems are not equally pressing or acute at all times, nor are they recognized as such in every hospital by all those who control the decision-making process and thus the problem-solving priorities of the organization. However, they are problems which the hospital constantly faces and must handle at the collectivity as well as the individual level. And although hospitals may differ in the extent to which they experience specific difficulties in each problem area at any given time, and also in the amount of effort and attention which they devote to resolving such difficulties, they are never completely problem-free in these areas. Conversely, although the various problems may demand differential priority or emphasis at different times, they are never totally absent. Moreover, as complicated and multifaceted as they are, even when considered one at a time, they cannot be attacked satisfactorily and resolved in a sequential manner, or on a problem-by-problem basis, because they are highly interrelated. Figure 1 shows the relationships found among the problems concerned (except system maintenance) for a probability sample of general hospitals in a nationwide study (Georgopoulos and Matejko, 1967).

The results depicted in Figure 1 indicate how strongly each problem area was related to the rest in the hospitals studied. Briefly, relatively high interrelationships were found between: organizational coordination and patient care (strongest of all); integration and coordination; integration and adaptation; strain and coordination; and coordination and adaptation. Relatively low relationships were found between: strain and patient care; strain and allocation; allocation and integration; strain and adaptation; and allocation and adaptation. All other relationships among the six problem areas, taken two at a time, fell at an intermediate level. With respect to patient care—the principal output of the system—the obtained pattern of results indicates the following relative importance for the other problem areas; organizational coordination was more strongly related to patient care than was any of the other areas, with 76 percent of a possible 50 relevant correlations (between the five measures of care and ten coordination measures used) being positive and statistically significant at the .05 level; organizational adaptation was next most closely related to patient care, with 46

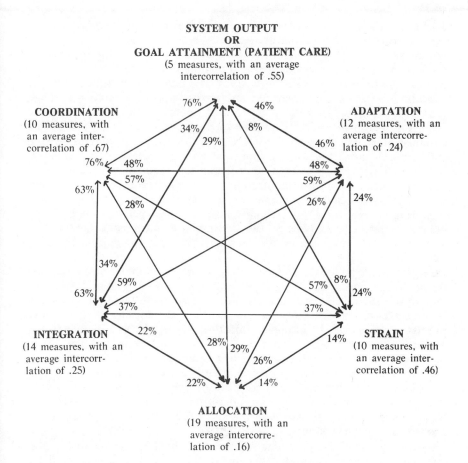

SYSTEM OUTPUT
OR
GOAL ATTAINMENT (PATIENT CARE)
(5 measures, with an average
intercorrelation of .55)

COORDINATION
(10 measures, with
an average inter-
correlation of .67)

ADAPTATION
(12 measures, with an
average intercorre-
lation of .24)

INTEGRATION
(14 measures, with an
average intercorr-
lation of .25)

STRAIN
(10 measures, with
an average inter-
correlation of .46)

ALLOCATION
(19 measures, with an
average intercorre-
lation of .16)

FIGURE 1. PROFILE OF THE SOCIAL SYSTEM OF AMERICAN GENERAL HOSPITALS
SHOWING THE OVERALL RELATIONSHIPS AMONG THE BASIC PROBLEM
AREAS OF THE SYSTEM, BASED ON A STUDY OF 41 HOSPITALS (percentage figures
indicate the level of association among the six areas, considered two at a time, or the percent
of statistically significant correlations obtained).

Source: Georgopoulos and Matejko, 1967, p. 108.

percent of a possible 60 relevant correlations being significant; social integration was third, with 34 percent of 70 relevant correlations being significant;
allocation was next, at about the same level, with 29 percent of 95 relevant
correlations being significant; and organizational strain was least strongly
related to care, with only 8 percent of a possible 50 correlations (between ten
measures of strain and five patient care measures) showing statistical significance. (N = 41 hospitals in all cases.)

Ideally, the above problems must be viewed and approached as a set, both because of the facts of pervasive interdependence which characterizes the hospital and because the solution (or lack of it) of any one problem has important consequences (sometimes positive and sometimes negative) for the solution of the rest. Moreover, it is their combined solution that counts from the standpoint of hospital effectiveness. Only decision-makers who can act according to this principle may be considered adequately equipped to make it possible for the organization to achieve a balanced overall solution to these problems. Those with major problem-solving responsibilities (trustees, the administrator, and physicians), in other words, must be capable of viewing and comprehending the hospital as a total system. Successful problem-solving in these areas is a never-ending process which requires awareness, sensitivity, and skill, a high degree of understanding of the problems and their interrelationships, and an adequate conception of the hospital as a complex organization. For maximum effectiveness, hospitals perhaps ought to be organized and managed not in the traditional departmental manner and along staff lines, but along service lines and according to the problem areas under consideration.

In any event, adequate understanding of the functioning and organizational effectiveness of the hospital presupposes satisfactory knowledge of the major problems of the system, the relationships among these problems and their solutions, and the consequences of achieved solutions for the overall problem-solving capacity of the organization. Successful performance in any one area does not necessarily correlate positively with good performance in the other problem areas (in its efforts to respond promptly to external pressures or handle its adaptation problems for example, the organization may also place the members under excessive strain or neglect internal difficulties), nor does it necessarily improve overall performance. The latter is determined by the relative success with which the whole system handles all of the major problems that it encounters.

Of course, the question of how balanced, optimal, or satisfactory is the overall solution that a hospital provides to the above problems cannot be answered at this stage in the development of organization research. It requires considerably more theoretical and empirical work than is currently available, along the lines suggested by the model here described. In spite of recent advances in organization theory and research, we still know relatively little compared to what is needed to answer this question, either for hospitals or other complex organizations. The contributions to the present volume suggest what would be needed by way of future research.

Individual Level Problems

Both the hospital, viewed as a complex social organization, and its members, viewed as psychologically organized and integrated persons, are problem-solving systems. As pointed out earlier, moreover, the major organizational problems which the hospital faces and solves manifest themselves not only at the collectivity, i.e. the system or subsystem level, but also at the individual level—at the level of individual components and in component-system relationships. The behavior of individual members in particular roles affects problem-solving performance at the collectivity level. And, conversely, each of the major problems discussed has important consequences and implications for the behavior of individual members in the organization and for organization-member relationships. Here we shall concentrate primarily on the latter.

The behavior of individual members in organizations can be fruitfully studied and in large measure explained by reference to the major problems of the system, as these involve and affect individual role performance, and to the problems and difficulties encountered by individual members at work. Members, for example, must be able to adjust to the requirements of the work technology and the physical features of the work place (see chapters by Scott, Mauksch, and Jaco). They must comply with the formal prescriptions of their roles, work group norms and professional standards, and overall policies and authority dictates, and adapt their behavior to meet the needs of the organization and their coworkers (V. Thompson, 1961, and Etzioni, 1964). In general, members must reconcile their personal needs and goals with those of the system (Georgopoulos and Matejko, 1967).

Members are called upon to perform their roles reliably and to achieve and maintain high levels of performance (Katz and Kahn, 1966). At the same time they are faced with the problem of maintaining and updating their professional skills and knowledge, even though some of these skills may remain underutilized because of the nature and definition of work roles in the system (Georgopoulos and Christman, 1970). In the process of doing their work, moreover, members are faced with the problem of how best to accomplish particular tasks or meet specific task requirements, and how to allocate their energy and time among the various tasks and functions which make up the organizational roles which they carry out. Additionally, they must coordinate their work with that of other members, because of the specialization of roles and functions and the interdependence and cooperation requirements which characterize the work, and this entails problems of communication and feedback, planning, interpersonal relations difficulties, decision-making, and authority (V. Thompson, 1961; Georgopoulos and Mann, 1962; Georgopoulos, 1966; J. Thompson, 1967). Similarly, members must cope with the complexity, uncertainties, and stresses to which they are exposed in the work situation, and handle the conflicts, frustrations, and strain that these generate (Georgopoulos and Mann, 1962; Kahn, *et al.*, 1964; and chapters by Straus, Mauksch, and Pellegrino). Finally, in the process of resolving these problems individual members must protect their own identity and psychological integrity and well-being.

The problems which an organization like the hospital faces in relation to its members are likewise numerous. These vary considerably from one category of members to another, moreover, as they do from one individual member to another in any particular personnel category. The most important of these problems, however, entail organization-wide difficulties of sufficient frequency and generality to warrant brief examination in this chapter. More detailed accounts of such problems have been offered elsewhere by Katz

(1964) and Georgopoulos (1971).

In general every complex organization, including the hospital, must be able to attract and retain sufficient and well-qualified personnel. It must be able to allocate all personnel among work roles, according to the staffing requirements of the system and the qualifications and competency of the members, and to ensure not only the physical but the psychological presence of members at work. In order to promote efficient and reliable role performance by all participants, it must be able to secure member compliance with organizational objectives and requirements at all levels. It must be able to provide opportunities for the continuous training, professional growth, and organizational socialization of participants, and make maximum use of every member's work skills and talents, whether or not these are clearly recognized by prevailing formal role definitions and job prescriptions. The organization must be flexible enough to allow for innovative and creative role performance by talented individuals, and take advantage of both the manifest and latent competencies of the members. And it must be able to provide maximum opportunities for job satisfaction and personal goal attainment at work for all the participants, and offer them appropriate and adequate incentives and rewards, so that the motivational base which sustains organizationally desirable behavior by all is strong and effective at all times.

Work behavior is motivated and goal-directed behavior, and much of the variance in role performance and job satisfaction among organizational members can be demonstrably related to or accounted for by motivational variability. Theoretically an individual's readiness to perform a particular role or activity or an individual's tendency to behave in a certain way (e.g. comply with organizational requests, cooperate with other members, produce at a high level) depends upon: (1) his expectation that performing that activity will lead to certain consequences, usually favorable outcomes such as the above, or desirable "payoff"; and (2) the relative value or attractiveness for the individual of the outcomes likely to result from performing that activity. In turn, the value of a particular outcome depends upon its instrumental utility for the attainment of other or additional favorable outcomes, and upon the individual's preferences for such other outcomes. The attractiveness of the various performance-related outcomes, together with the expectation that performance will indeed produce the anticipated outcomes, both as seen or estimated by the individual involved, are the important determinants (Georgopoulos, Mahoney, and Jones, 1957; Porter and Lawler, 1968; and Georgopoulos, 1971.)

Similarly, job satisfaction on the part of organizational members depends upon the total social-psychological return an individual can expect from the organization and his job, and not only on economic return. Generally, job satisfaction is determined by (1) the degree to which the individual feels advantaged or disadvantaged relative to others in the situation with whom he compares himself, or according to whose standards and situation he judges and evaluates his lot, and (2) the ratio of fulfilled job-related expectations on his part to the initial expectations and aspirations held by the individual (Morse, 1953; Georgopoulos, 1971).

In our society today, even in complex formal organizations such as hospitals, the dominant motives of organizational members are the motives for personal achievement and personal worth, status and social recognition, curiosity and new experience, personal independence, self-development and growth, self-actualization or for cultivating and utilizing one's capacities to the maximum degree possible, and generally ego motives and social motives (Likert, 1961, 1967; Katz and Georgopoulos, 1971). Economic and related extrinsic motives (earning more money or better fringe benefits, not having to work too hard, being able to satisfy subsistence or minimal safety and security needs), while important, especially for nonmedical employees in hospitals, are not the dominant motives of the majority of members. Correspondingly, the dominant incentives and rewards which should be provided and emphasized by the organization must be social and psychological rather than economic if organizational effectiveness is to be maximized. Member role performance is affected more by such things as challenging and interesting work, job enrichment opportunities, work group attractiveness, meaningful participation in the decision-making processes of the organization, and opportunities for personal growth and utilization of one's skills and talents, and less by economic rewards, punishment, competition, or authority-based sanctions (Bennis *et al.*, 1964; Maier, 1965; Herzberg, 1966; Fleishman, 1967; Georgopoulos, 1971).

From the point of view of its members as individual human beings with personal interests, needs, and goals, many of which must be satisfied at work, it is important that the hospital be an attractive and rewarding setting. It must be possible for the participants to influence the organization significantly, for example. At the same time, the professional autonomy of members must be respected to the extent consistent with the requirements of their work interdependence. It is important that members be protected from excessive controls and regimentation, which tend to alienate them from work and force them to seek satisfaction for their needs outside the system. Members must be able to participate in the decision-making process, and to function unconstrained from formal requirements other than those dictated by the nature of their tasks and roles, work interdependence, accepted professional norms and standards, good organizational citizenship values, and the major problems of the system.

It is also motivationally important that members be protected by the system from external interferences, unnecessary complexity and uncertainty, unreasonable work pressures or role overload, avoidable frustrations and conflicts, and organizational work requirements or expectations which demean the personal dignity and personal worth of participants or jeopardize their integrity. In short, the organization must facilitate both the role performance and personal goal attainment of its members, while removing obstacles that make work relations difficult, stifle individual freedom beyond the requirements of collective cooperation, or limit participation and involvement in the affairs of the system unduly.

In hospitals which have participated in organizational studies, all major groups (administrators, doctors, nurses, trustees) tend to place primary emphasis on patient care standards, when they consider the relative importance of various relevant goals. Improvements in administration or in medical organization, changes in professional qualifications, rights, or responsibilities, economy and finances, the adequacy of the hospital plant, expansion and bed space, and even the adequacy of employee wages and benefits are all assigned lower importance by the major groups in the organization than are patient care standards (Georgopoulos and Mann, 1962; Georgopoulos and Wieland, 1964). The subservience of personal interests to the basic goals of the institution is a widely accepted norm. The costs of such commitment to the organization, however, are by no means equally shared by the different groups of members. Physicians, the administrators, the non-medical department heads, and members in supervisory positions are all enjoying a better status (have greater access to organizational facilities and rewards, more influence and autonomy, more information about the organization, higher incomes) and are correspondingly more satisfied with their personal goal attainment than are the nurses and other employees of the organization (Georgopoulos and Matejko, 1967). Motivational problems are especially acute in relation to the latter, more disadvantaged members.

In its relations with organizational members, of course, the hospital must view each participant not only as an individual with personal needs, expectations, and values, but also as a member of some particular work group or professional-occupational group in the system. In this context the problem of satisfying the needs of all the participants and integrating their separate goals with the basic goals of the organization assumes special significance as the aspirations and expectations of nurses and nonsupervisory nonmedical employees change. As the role and organizational contributions of these groups grow further and become more visible and recognized (partly because of the inevitably higher mutual work interdependence and closer interaction in which higher and lower status members alike are thrown by increasing specialization), both within the hospital and in the larger community, doctors and administrators increasingly will have to share power and decision-making influence with them, even though they may not be eager to do so (see chapters by Guest, Kovner, and Pellegrino). Thus the traditional dominance of physicians, especially, will diminish, decreasing also because of additional factors, such as the introduction of computer-assisted practice which will make more apparent the strengths as well as weaknesses of medical practice, and the greater extrapofessional controls over medical practice which society is increasingly bent upon exercising (see chapters by Pellegrino, Scott, and Zald and Hair).

Traditionally, not unlike industrial organizations, hospitals have shown much more concern for the technology of work than for the organization's human assets. They have been concerned more with providing a safe and attractive physical work environment than with creating and maintaining an equally attractive social and psychological work climate for their members. Beyond their paramount concern for adequate patient care, they have been concerned much more with problems of recruiting and selecting members with the proper training, aptitudes, and interests for filling inflexibly defined jobs than with problems of member attitudes, needs, and values. They have been more concerned with superior-subordinate relations than with human relations. In relating to their members, moreover, hospitals have relied more on economic compensation and incentives and less on social-psychological incentives and rewards. This picture is now changing, and the conditions for effective role performance, job satisfaction, and organizational effectiveness demand different organization-member relations than in the past.

Further Aspects and Implications

Because human organizations are dynamic systems functioning within a changing and often turbulent social environment, the problem of adaptation to the environment is an incessant problem for the system (Katz and Georgopoulos, 1971). There is continuous interaction, negotiation, interchange, and interdependence between organization and environment. Adaptation encompasses all aspects of give-and-take between the hospital and its relevant outside world, at both the input and output sides. Specific difficulties in this area may include problems of cultural values and societal issues, such as those pertaining to the social control of the institution (see chapter by Zald and Hair), public pressures and community expectations (see chapters by Pellegrino and Kovner), relations with clients, suppliers, and consumers, competition for staff and resources, the introduction of technological or social innovations, resource procurement, and personnel recruitment difficulties.

In this area research shows (Georgopoulos and Matejko, 1967) that general hospitals appear to be especially weak concerning normal relationships with the immediate community; the community's knowledge of the hospital is usually low and inadequate; and public relations efforts by hospitals tend to be minimal and ineffectual. The adaptability of the organization to technological change and its success in handling unusual emergencies are relatively high, and members are likely to accept such change (P. Mott, 1961; Georgopoulos and Mann, 1962). On the other hand, hospitals are slow, if not completely resistant, concerning social innovation and structural changes that require modification of existing organizational arrangements.

Our knowledge concerning organizational adaptation, however, is still all too fragmentary and inadequate. Much more research of the kind suggested in the chapters by Pellegrino, Zald and Hair, and Neuhauser and Andersen, and in the work of Levine and White (1961), Belknap and Steinle (1963), B. Mott (1970), Reid (1970), Starkweather (1970), and Warren (1970)*, is needed. In the past few students of organizations have looked seriously at the problem of adaptation, and most have approached it rather narrowly, mainly in terms of exchange models, focusing primarily on economic and technological factors. This is a much broader problem area, however, and deserves far

---

*The papers by Mott, Reid, Starkweather, and Warren recently have been published together in P. E. White and G. J. Vlasak (Eds.), *Inter-organizational research in health*. U.S. Department of Health, Education, and Welfare, 1971.

more reserach than in the past. Every organization is a dynamic system which reacts actively, as well as responds, to the environment; it influences the environment as well as it is influenced by it at all times. There is a two-way dependence, influence, and impact between the two, and the kinds of relationships that require study are many, including exchange relations, bargaining-type relations, relations which are friendly or hostile, relations based upon cooperation, mutual accommodation, or competition and conflict. All problems and difficulties with external affairs, of course, affect internal affairs, necessitating adjustments and readjustments by the organization and its members.

The problem of organizational allocation subsumes all aspects of the deployment and distribution among subsystems and components of the organization's means of work and resources, including available human skills, funds, information and all of the various inputs acquired for use by the system. In this area, problems having to do with participation in and control of the decision-making process are especially critical in contemporary hospitals (see chapters by Pellegrino and Kovner). The same is true concerning the relationship of professional work to the technology (see chapter by Scott) and ecology (see chapter by Jaco) of the organization. Problems of centralization-decentralization, superior-subordinate relations, specialization, and work force composition are among those most frequently encountered by hospitals in this area. Difficulties concerning the distribution of organizational authority among different groups, hierarchical levels, and positions in the system, and related difficulties concerning the distribution of economic and social-psychological rewards among the participants, are typical concerns.

The prevailing distribution of organizational influence and rewards in general hospitals clearly favors the medical staffs and administrators, with opportunities and access to personal goal attainment being especially problematic for nurses and other employees (Georgopoulos and Matejko, 1967). Correspondingly, problems of goal attainment are more critical for nonphysician and nonadministrative groups. Related to this issue are also the familiar problems of staff shortages and manpower utilization. The allocation area, as the contributions to this volume show, has not been neglected in hospital research, but the issues are so pervasive, pressing, and critical for the modern hospital as to require a great deal more work.

In complex organizations, and particularly where specialization of roles and functions, professionalization of the work force, and work interdependence are high and extensive, coordination of effort presents a difficult problem for the system. Organizational coordination concerns the articulation of roles and efforts within the system, so that the activities of all interdependent groups and members converge toward the solution of system problems and the attainment of organization-relevant objectives. Planning and programming, priority setting, work scheduling and the establishment of routines, computerization and standardization of work flows, and generally problems of sequencing, timing, and synchronizing the numerous activities in the system are among the most important problems that organizations face in this area.

But programmed coordination is never sufficient in a complex social system such as the hospital. A great many of the activities cannot be preplanned, standardized, or routinized. Nor can they be precisely specified, much less predicted in a reliable manner. Much of the daily coordination of work, therefore, is of the nonprogrammed kind and depends upon the voluntary and spontaneous adjustments that participants are able and willing to make in relation to their work, to each other, and to the system. Such "unplanned" coordination requires adequate communication and feedback, well-developed mutual expectations and reciprocal understandings on the part of members in related jobs, and generally depends upon whether the participants function according to one another's work problems and needs rather than unilaterally. The more complex the patterns of interdependence in the system, moreover, the less amenable coordination is to planning, and the more the solution of coordination problems depends on social-psychological variables such as these. In hospital organization research this problem area has received systematic attention only this past decade (Georgopoulos and Mann, 1962; Heydebrand, 1965; Wieland, 1965). The research done to date, however, represents no more than a good beginning compared to the significance and complexity of the problem.

Organizational coordination encompasses problems which pertain to the functional situation of the system, and especially its production and management subsystems. Organizational integration problems, on the other hand, involve the social-psychological situation of the system—its social and normative articulation at the collectivity and individual levels. Some of the most critical problems experienced by complex organizations and some of the great problems in contemporary society are integration problems.

One such problem concerns the "individual vs. the group" influence issue. And one central aspect of the issue is the "partial inclusion" (F. Allport, 1933), or rather dual partial inclusion, which characterizes organizations and their members. Increasingly, the individual is only partially incorporated into the system, and the organization is only partially incorporated into its individual members. The individual member is called upon to participate not as a total personality system, but formally and solely as an organizational role carrier. He is neither viewed nor treated as an integrated human being with capacities, needs, and goals that transcend the requirements and opportunities associated with his organizational role. He is viewed and treated as a task performer, or as an instrument of work, as a problem-solving creature, and as a potential source of dysfunctions and disturbances that make for uncertainty or unwanted deviation from the organizational work plan. In general, only insofar as his activities and output are directly contributing to the instrumental, i.e. production, concerns of the system does he count; his expressive needs and behaviors are either overlooked or not regarded seriously, or are seen as impediments to his functioning as an organizational member.

Typically, in short, the individual member is basically viewed in rational and economic terms and treated in a highly selective and fragmented manner. As a consequence the individual at best internalizes only a few of the goals and values of the organization, and identifies with the system partially and inadequately, with corresponding consequences for his participation, loyalty, and involvement. But in so doing he does not also rid himself of expressive needs, goals, and desires, nor does he dissociate these from his instrumental involvement in the system. The result is a continuous dialectic between organizational requirements and personal interests, at least for those who remain in the system. Members behave in ways which tend to protect their own identity and integrity, and the system attempts to function with maximum unity and coherence as an integrated sociotechnical system. Because of the partial inclusion with which both are confronted, however, neither can be completely successful in this respect.

Such familiar phenomena as lack of member commitment, poor morale, psychological disinterest and alienation from the system, problems of withdrawal behavior (turnover, tardiness, absenteeism), problems of deviance and compliance, and nonadaptive or maladaptive behavior, more generally, often have their origins in inadequate integration. Partial inclusion cannot be eliminated entirely either for the organization or for the members. But it could be minimized and reduced well below prevailing levels in the majority of large-scale organizations. This could be done in such ways as: more systematic and more adequate organizational socialization of members after they enter the system; better matching of people and jobs at the point of recruitment; personnel policies and reward and incentive structures that are based upon both extrinsic and intrinsic motivation and reinforcement; role redefinitions which accommodate expressive as well as instrumental needs and behavior; and more opportunities for genuine member participation and involvement in decision-making. To the extent of their implementation, these factors would help raise the social efficiency level of the system.

Integration is also affected by the openness of the system. Organizations are becoming more open, increasingly concerned with what happens in the environment, that is, more sensitive about adaptation. As the trend toward greater openness continues, the problem of organizational adaptation becomes more complex. At the same time, internal integration requirements such as the consistency and complementarity of norms (Georgopoulos, 1965) become more exacting. This is true both because the system's inputs reflect external difficulties to a higher extent than previously, and because successful adaptation depends more upon the behavior and contributions of all the members rather than just those in leadership positions, as in the past. Paradoxically, however, as organizations become more concerned for society, the social values that traditionally supported and enabled them to maintain their authority arrangements are either changing rapidly or breaking down. In the past organizations enjoyed an important advantage in this area, since society itself was successful in socializing prospective members on the basis of widely accepted values which were compatible, if not identical, with those of most organizations (Katz and Georgopoulos, 1971). Now this advantage has virtually disappeared, and while organizations may continue to emphasize rationality, members insist upon greater personal choice and more influence over the work situation.

In hospitals identification with the organization, which is an indicator of integration, varies with position in the power structure. Administrators, doctors, and trustees show generally higher commitment to the hospital as an institution than most other groups. Superior-subordinate relationships and good communication, which are important mechanisms of integration, are also more satisfactory at these levels. In this area hospitals are especially weak at the lower and intermediate levels. The identification of staff nurses and nonsupervisory employees with the organization, in particular, tends to be rather low according to hospital studies by the author and others (Searles, 1961; Georgopoulos and Matejko, 1967).

Many of the integration and coordination difficulties in the hospital are exacerbated by specialization. In general, underspecialization impairs the problem-solving capacity of the system because it makes for inefficiency, especially technical and economic inefficiency. But overspecialization can be equally dysfunctional, not so much because it may generate undue competition or conflict, as is often alleged, but because it makes the problems of organizational integration and coordination more difficult for the system and its members. Overspecialization makes for social inefficiency because it results in excessive organizational complexity and unncessarily high interdependence among unlike participants, who must relate to one another and to the system and whose specialized efforts must be collectively coordinated (V. Thompson, 1961; Georgopoulos, 1966). Victor Thompson (1961) has pointed out some of the key issues for organizational research and theory in this connection, including the issue of authority vs. specialized knowledge, or the problem of right balance between legitimate authority for decision-making and knowledge upon which decisions must rest.

The problem of organizational strain is also enduring and complex. No organization is ever completely free from strain. First, a certain amount of uncertainty is always present in the system. Second, there is always some noise in the communication network, and often the elaborate feedbacks in the system do not achieve their intended purposes for timely corrections and adjustments. Third, neither the organization nor the members can cope adequately at all times with the great complexity of the system. Fourth, because of extensive specialization and interdependence in the work situation, the possibilities for error and misunderstanding are numerous, while the impact of deficient performances can readily generalize throughout the organization. Fifth, the organization and its members are dynamic rather than static systems, and the values of the variables which make up the system in each case are subject to change within limits that are relatively broad, ill-defined, and only partially controlled. Finally, both at the collectivity and individual level, the relevant options that are open to the organization and the members in relation to the other major problems they encounter are not unlimited, and the problems themselves are never resolved completely. Inevitably, therefore, frustration and conflict can be expected to occur in the best of organizations. So long as these remain unmanaged, they impede coordination of effort (Wieland, 1965) and undermine the performances of members and the effectiveness of the system (Georgopoulos and Tannenbaum, 1957;

Georgopoulos and Mann, 1962). And although creative use of conflict might be possible at times, widespread strain of high intensity cannot be tolerated for long in organizations.

In general hospitals, intergroup tensions, as reported by the major groups, are quite common and extensive, covering the entire interaction structure of the organization. Apparently, however, they are only of moderate degree in most cases. But the level of tension tends to be relatively higher within the medical staff and between doctors and nurses than between either of them and administrators or other groups (Georgopoulos and Mann, 1962; Georgopoulos and Wieland, 1964; Georgopoulos and Matejko, 1967). Recent changes in the health care field may have altered this picture in the direction of greater intergroup tension, pressure, and conflict at the top levels of the organization.

The output problems at the organizational and individual levels are well known to researchers and practitioners alike. Issues and difficulties in this area include those of quantity, quality, and cost, the matter of reliability of individual and group performance, input-output ratio problems involving both the technical-economic and social-psychological efficiency of the system, and effort-reward balance and related motivation-to-work difficulties. The chapter by Neuhauser and Andersen highlights some of the output problems of hospitals as well as the research complexities which they entail. The measurement problem, in particular, continues to be basically unresolved, though substantial progress in assessing the quality of medical, nursing, and total patient care has been made in the last decade (e.g. see Donabedian, 1966, concerning medical care). The same may be said with reference to the study and measurement of other organizational outcomes upon which the level of patient care rendered and the hospital's contribution to the comminity's health care depend. Little else need be said regarding output other than to remind ourselves that, ultimately the output of the organization is determined by the overall problem-solving ability of the system in all major problem areas along the entire input-transformation-output work cycle.

Regarding the problem of system maintenance, which is intimately associated both with the output and adaptability of the organization, one is impressed by the paucity of relevant research. In the short run, of course, the maintenance of the system seldom appears to be of critical concern to the great majority of ongoing organizations, including hospitals. But under conditions of external threat or internal discontent, the picture changes sharply. Moreover, in the long run, the continuity, integrity, and identity of an organization can be ensured only to the extent that the system is able to solve its other enduring problems—those of output and adaptation, in particular, but also those of resource allocation, coordination, integration, and strain. System maintenance makes for regularity in the input-conversion-output cycle of the organization, and is necessary to organizational viability, growth, and effectiveness. In this light, it too must be viewed as a continuing major problem of the system.

In view of the critical adaptation and output problems of contemporary hospitals, many observers are seriously questioning the efficacy of the hospital's traditional organizational structure. It may well be that the viability of this system will require substantial internal restructuring and new adaptive mechanisms, perhaps along the lines suggested by the contributors to the present volume. To some extent, of course, this also applies to other complex organizations in modern society as well as to health care institutions (see Katz and Georgopoulos, 1971). In the case of hospitals some of the mechanisms proposed by Pellegrino below seem particularly worth considering. The proposed "community health authority," for example, could enable hospitals to deal more effectively with the adaptation problems they now face. And, internally, restructuring of control over the decision-making process, perhaps in relation to the various work teams Dr. Pellegrino discusses, may be essential to improving performance and resolving output problems.

Elsewhere, with regard to restructuring, I have written (Georgopoulos, 1969) that, considering the current problems of the system, it is likely that the general hospital eventually will require a self-governing structure which could give every professional and occupational group the opportunity to participate meaningfully in the decision-making processes of the organization. It might be advantageous, for example, to develop decision-making mechanisms and influence patterns built on the principle of multilevel federalism of semiautonomous units, which simultaneously are highly attractive to their members and can contribute effectively to the solution of system problems. Such an organizational structure could be built to provide for the representation of all the different professional-occupational groups in the hospital. It should take into account group size, specialized competencies, functions, and interests, and location in the system in relation to major organizational problems, and not only traditional power arrangements (e.g. the conventional administrator-doctor-trustee arrangement) or formal position in the authority hierarchy. Every new unit might consist of a small number of members who could choose a representative to the unit at the next higher level, etc. The highest level unit in the organization—a board of participants—would consist of members representing every major professional and occupational group in the hospital.

Boards of participants, representing the interests of all hospital personnel, and conventional boards of trustees, representing the community's interests, could work together and cooperate closely on matters of organizational policy, priorities and objectives, and major decisions affecting the hospital, its members, and the public. The board of trustees also would serve to link the hospital to the community, perhaps through close cooperation with a "Community Health Authority" such as suggested by Pellegrino. Hospital administration would function as the executive body, charged with the principal managerial, planning, financial, personnel, and coordinative functions of the organization, and having sufficient authority to discharge its responsibilities relatively free from undue internal or external pressures. It should have discretionary power in the areas of its professional competence but follow and implement the general policies and decisions made jointly by the board of trustees and the board of participants (on which the administration would be represented, as would doctors, nurses, and other groups) of the institution. Models other than the "board of participants—board of trustees—community health authority" model, of course, also would be possible and appropriate.

In any case it is amply evident that hospitals are currently being pressured heavily from all directions to be more willing to innovate and experiment with new patterns of internal social organization, new forms of operation in the areas of administration, staffing, organizational coordination, and community relations, and utilize more fully both new health knowledge and new social-psychological knowledge. Existing knowledge, both theoretical and practical, concerning the above problems and organizational behavior more generally is still inadequate and unsatisfactory, from the standpoint of structuring the organization so as to maximize the system's problem-solving capacity. At the same time, as the present volume shows, useful and dependable knowledge from organizational research in hospitals and other settings that could guide restructuring and experimentation is available. Moreover, relevant knowledge is accumulating in volume, quantity, and rates exceeding current utilization efforts on the part of hospitals and the total health care system.

Conclusions

Viewing the hospital as a complex organization in the context of modern open-system theory, this chapter proposed that a satisfactory understanding of organizational functioning and adequate explanation of human behavior in hospital settings can be achieved by the study of hospitals as dynamic, adaptive, work-performing, and problem-solving sociotechnical systems. The major problems and properties of the hospital as a system of this kind were presented and discussed, as were some of the more distinctive social-psychological features of hospital organization in its present form and state. Among basic system properties we included openness, patterning, interdependence, wholeness, internal continuity, constancy in relation to the external environment, and equifinality. Among major problems we included those of system maintenance and adaptation to the environment, the problem of output and goal attainment, and the internal problems of resource allocation, coordination of effort, social-psychological integration, and intraorganizational strain. The underlying model is that of an input-transformation-output cycle, because hospitals, like other complex organizations, face and handle not only input and output problems, but problems along this entire work cycle.

The model described may be employed at the total system level, to compare and contrast hospitals, or other types of organizations, as complex work-performing and problem-solving systems, and to study the same organization over time. Moreover, it may be used to study the functioning of particular subsystems within an organization, such as the adaptive subsystem, the instrumental or production subsystem, the management subsystem, and others, since it is possible to view each major subsystem as a mini-system (or mini-organization) which, at a less complex and less encompassing level that is defined by its own work cycle, is essentially characterized by the same major problems and properties which were specified for the total parent system. It was also pointed out that the system properties of an organization are interrelated, though not in a simple manner, and the same is true for its major problems. The basic properties in question are related also to the more unique characteristics of the system, and have consequences for the problem-solving behavior of the organization and its members in relation to the substantive problems which they encounter along the work cycle.

The major problems described, moreover, are recurring ones which are open-ended, complex, and multifaceted, and which defy perfect or once-and-for-all solutions. Furthermore, each of these problems manifests itself in the form of more specific difficulties, both at the collectivity level of organizational functioning and at the level of individual behavior and organization-member relations. The organizational effectiveness of a hospital depends upon both the technical-economic and the social-psychological efficiency of the system, and is determined by the problem-solving ability of the organization in relation to the problems discussed.

The task of assessing hospital effectiveness, of course, is an extremely complex one, for it amounts to determining the relative success and failure of the organization in all of the major problem areas of the system taken together and considered as a set. It is the overall solution the system is able to achieve in this respect that requires assessment, and such a solution depends upon the separate as well as joint outcomes of the problem-solving behavior of the organization in the various problem areas (not just the separate problem-by-problem successes and failures). Such seems to be the nature of organizational effectiveness at the total system level. Adequate assessment of the overall problem-solving effectiveness of the system, therefore, either for hospitals or other large-scale organizations, presupposes ability to answer a number of preceding questions, such as those raised in this chapter. Organization research has only recently begun to make significant inroads in this regard.

As yet we do not know with assurance the relationships among the major problems of the organization, either at the collectivity or the individual level, nor do we have sufficient dependable knowledge on how the different aspects of each problem relate to or affect one another. We know even less from available research about the interrelationships of the basic properties of the system, and about the consequences of these properties for the problem-solving behavior of the organization and its members in relation to the various problems of the system. Similarly, the relative efficacy of alternative problem-solving mechanisms used by organizations to handle the various problems is not known, nor is the extent to which success or failure in one problem area contributes to success or failure in anoher. At this stage of our knowledge it may be relatively clear that concentration of effort on internal problems can jeopardize the external relations of an organization, especially in rapidly changing environments, and vice versa. It is also clear that improvement in a particular problem area may have either positive or negative effects for another. Improving the adaptability of an organization, for example, may not necessarily result in reduction of strain within the system, and it may even result in increased strain. But, the specific conditions under which the successful solution of a major problem (e.g. coordination) would facilitate or hinder the solution of another (e.g. resource allocation), and to what degree, are not adequately understood, much less well known.

The methodological issues involved are also complex and very difficult to resolve without further research. For example, assuming adequate measures were available, the extent to which it might be possible to predict hospital performance in a given problem area from measures of performance in the other major areas could not be readily determined. It is not easy to estimate the relative "weights" that should be attached to the various measures that would serve as predictors. It might be possible, however, to make some progress in this direction if valid and reliable measures were available for assessing the problem-solving success of the hospital in each major problem area. Then it would be possible to tackle this issue on an empirical-statistical basis. For example, one could obtain the necessary measures, compute their intercorrelation, construct indices to represent overall success in each area, employ regression analysis, and ultimately assign weights to the predictors in proportion to the variance which they "explain" with respect to the problem area serving as the criterion variable in the equation. But the outcome of this approach would by no means be satisfactory, partly because the results would have limited generalizability. The prediction patterns obtained via a strictly empirical-statistical approach might not hold upon replication of the study, and would certainly differ depending on such things as the capability of available work technology, the developmental stage reached by the system, the magnitude and rate of internal change characterizing the system, the presence or absence of external threats, and other factors.

More important, purely empirical answers to basic theoretical questions, such as the question of how well could the overall problem-solving success of an organization be ascertained by measures of its success in the different problem areas of the system, do not constitute the most satisfactory resolution possible. Only increased theoretical sophistication and adequate conceptual elaboration, along with a sound organization research methodology and relevant empirical research, can be expected to lead to the best resolution feasible. The contributions presented in this book should stimulate the kind of work most needed to provide dependable answers to the questions raised in this chapter.

References

Allport, F. H. *Institutional behavior*. Chapel Hill, N.C.: University of North Carolina Press, 1933.

Ashby, W. R. *Design for a brain* (2nd ed. rev.). New York: Wiley, 1960.

Belknap, I., and Steinle, J. G. *The community and its hospitals: a comparative analysis*. Syracuse, N.Y.: Syracuse University Press, 1963.

Bennis, W. G., Schein, E. H., Berlew, D. E., and Steele, F. I. (Eds.) *Interpersonal dynamics: essays and readings on human interaction.* Homewood, Ill.: Dorsey, 1964.

Buckley, W. (Ed.) *Modern systems research for the behavioral scientist.* Chicago: Aldine, 1968.

Dalton, G. W. Influence and organizational change. In A. R. Negandhi and J. P. Schwitter (Eds.) *Organizational behavior models.* Kent, Ohio: Kent State University, 1970.

Donabedian, A. Evaluating the quality of medical care. *Milbank Memorial Fund Quarterly,* 1966, *44,* pt. 2, 166-206.

Emery, F. E. The next thirty years: concepts, methods, and anticipations. *Human Relations,* 1967, *20,* 199-237.

Emery, F. E., and Trist, E. L. Socio-technical systems. In *Management sciences models and techniques,* vol. 2. London: Pergamon Press, 1960.

Etzioni, A. *Modern organizations.* Englewood Cliffs, N.J.: Prentice-Hall, 1964.

Fleishman, E. A. (Ed.) *Studies in personnel and industrial psychology* (rev. ed.). Homewood, Ill.: Dorsey, 1967.

Georgopoulos, B. S. Normative structure variables and organizational behavior: a comparative study. *Human Relations,* 1965, *18,* 155-169.

Georgopoulos, B. S. The hospital system and nursing: some basic problems and issues. *Nursing Forum,* 1966, *5,* 8-35.

Georgopoulos, B. S. The general hospital as an organization: a social-psychological viewpoint. *The University of Michigan Medical Center Journal* (University Hospital Centennial Issue), 1969, *35,* 94-97.

Georgopoulos, B. S. An open-system theory model for organizational research. In A. R. Negandhi and J. P. Schwitter (Eds.) *Organizational behavior models.* Kent, Ohio: Kent State University, 1970.

Georgopoulos, B. S. Individual performance and job satisfaction differences explained with instrumentality theory and expectancy models as a function of path-goal relationships. In E. L. Abt and B. F. Riess (Eds.) *Clinical psychology in industrial organization.* New York: Grune and Stratton, 1971.

Georgopoulos, B. S. and Christman, L. The clinical nurse specialist: a role model. *American Journal of Nursing,* 1970, *70,* 1030-1039.

Georgopoulos, B. S., and Jackson, M. M. Nursing kardex behavior in an experimental study of patient units with and without clinical nurse specialists. *Nursing Research,* 1970, *9,* 196-218.

Georgopoulos, B. S., Mahoney, G. M., and Jones, N. W., Jr. A path-goal approach to productivity. *Journal of Applied Psychology,* 1957, *41,* 345-353.

Georgopoulos, B. S. and Mann, F. C. *The community general hospital.* New York: Macmillan, 1962.

Georgopoulos, B. S., and Matejko, A. The American general hospital as a complex social system. *Health Services Research,* 1967, *2,* 76-112.

Georgopoulos, B. S., and Sana, J. M. Clinical nursing specialization and intershift report behavior. *American Journal of Nursing,* 1971, *71,* 538-545.

Georgopoulos, B. S., and Tennenbaum, A. S. A study of organizational effectiveness. *American Sociological Review,* 1957, *22,* 534-540.

Georgopoulos, B. S., and Wieland, G. F. *Nationwide study of coordination and patient care in voluntary hospitals.* Ann Arbor, Mich.: Institute for Social Research, 1964.

Gross, B. M. The coming general systems models of social systems. *Human Relations,* 1967, *20,* 357-374.

Hall, A. D., and Fagen, R. E. Definition of system. *Yearbook of Society for General Systems Research,* 1956, *1,* 18-28.

Herzberg, F. *Work and the nature of man.* New York: World Publishing, 1966.

Heydebrand, W. V. Bureaucracy in hospitals: an analysis of complexity and coordination in formal organizations. Doctoral dissertation, University of Chicago, 1965.

Kahn, R. L., *et al. Organizational stress: studies in role conflict and ambiguity.* New York: Wiley, 1964.

Katz, D. The motivational basis of organizational behavior. *Behavioral Science,* 1964, *9,* 131-146.

Katz, D., and Georgopoulos, B. S. Organizations in a changing world. *Journal of Applied*

Behavioral Science, 1971, *7,* 342-370.

Katz, D., and Kahn, R. L. *The social psychology or organizations.* New York: Wiley, 1966.

Levine, S., and White, P. E. Exchange as a conceptual framework for the study of interorganizational relationships. *Administrative Science Quarterly,* 1961, *5,* 583-601.

Likert, R. *New patterns of management.* New York: McGraw-Hill, 1961.

Likert, R. *The human organization: its management and value.* New York: McGraw-Hill, 1967.

Maier, N. R. F. *Psychology in industry* (3rd ed.) Boston: Houghton Mifflin, 1965.

Miller, J. G. Living systems: basic concepts, and living systems: structure and process. *Behavioral Science,* 1965, *10,* 193-237, 337-411.

Morse, N. C. *Satisfactions in the white collar job.* Ann Arbor, Mich.: Institute for Social Research, 1953.

Mott, B. J. F. Coordination and inter-organizational relations in health. Paper presented at Conference on Interorganizational Relationships, The Johns Hopkins University and National Center for Health Services Research and Development, New York, January 23-24, 1970.

Mott, P. E. Sources of adaptation and flexibility in large organizations. Doctoral dissertation, University of Michigan, 1961.

Parsons, T. *Structure and process in modern societies.* New York: Free Press, 1960.

Parsons, T. *Societies.* Englewood Cliffs, N. J.: Prentice-Hall, 1966.

Perrow, C. Hospitals: technology, structure, and goals. In J. G. March (Ed.) *Handbook of organizations.* Chicago: Rand McNally, 1965.

Porter, L. W., and Lawler, E. E., Ill. *Managerial attitudes and performance.* Homewood, Ill.: Irwin-Dorsey, 1968.

Pugh, D. S. Modern organization theory: a psychological and sociological study. *Psychological Bulletin,* 1966, *66,* 235-251.

Reid, W. J. Interorganizational cooperation: a review and critique of current theory. Paper presented at Conference on Interorganizational Relationships, The Johns Hopkins University and National Center for Health Services Research and Development, New York, January 23-24, 1970.

Schein, E. H. *Organizational psychology.* Englewood Cliffs, N. J.: Prentice-Hall, 1965.

Searles, R. E. The relation between communication and social integration in the community hospital. Doctoral dissertation, University of Michigan, 1961.

Stagner, R. New designs for industrial psychology. *Contemporary Psychology,* 1966, *11,* 145-150.

Starkweather, D. B. Health facility merger and integration: a typology and some hypotheses. Paper presented at Conference on Interorganizational Relationships, The Johns Hopkins University and National Center for Health Services Research and Development, New York, January 23-24, 1970.

Thompson, J. D. *Organizations in action.* New York: McGraw-Hill, 1967.

Thompson, V., *Modern Organization.* New York: Knopf, 1961.

von Bertalanffy, L. General systems theory. *Yearbook of Society for General Systems Research,* 1956, *1,* 1-10.

von Bertalanffy, L. *General system theory: foundations, development, applications.* New York: Braziller, 1969.

Warren, R. L. Alternative strategies of inter-agency planning. Paper presented at Conference on Interorganizational Relationships, The Johns Hopkins University and National Center for Health Services Research and Development, New York, January 23-24, 1970.

Weiss, P. Animal behavior as system reaction. *Yearbook of Society for General Systems Research,* 1959, *4,* 1-44.

Wieland, G. F. Complexity and coordination in organizations. Doctoral dissertation, University of Michigan, 1965.

Woodward, J. Technology, material control, and organizational behavior. In A. R. Negandhi and J. P. Schwitter (Eds.) *Organizational behavior models.* Kent, Ohio: Kent State University, 1970.

Part Two

3

THE SOCIAL CONTROL OF GENERAL HOSPITALS*

Mayer N. Zald and Feather Davis Hair

Conformity, deviant behavior, folkways and mores, and internalization of norms and values are some of the concepts social scientists have used to explain the social control of individuals. Less clearly related to broad societal norms, exchange and reciprocity notions have focused upon interpersonal control. Yet in modern society individuals live in the shadow of large-scale organizations, as clients, members, and employees, and their behavior is often largely proscribed or prescribed by the organizations of which they are part. Consequently, our understanding of social control in modern society will remain incomplete as long as we do not explain the prescriptions and proscriptions of organizations and institutional groupings.

How does an ongoing social system control the range of performance of organizations in an institutional sector, such as the health care institutions sector? How are standards set and changed? How is "bad" performance sanctioned and eliminated, or at least contained, while "good" performance is rewarded and stimulated? These questions take on greater meaning if we give them specific institutional content. How do modern societies get rid of bad hospitals? Or do they? How is the range of hospital performance regulated? Or is it?

In some cases "society" tightly regulates performance, so that in effect almost all institutional elements adhere to relatively rigid standards. For instance, American states tightly regulate and inspect pressure boilers in commercial and group residential establishments, and to do so states have developed relatively uniform codes taking into account the amount of pressure per square inch generated and the energy source. A statistical portrait of all users would resemble a "J" curve of conforming behavior (Allport, 1934), with very few users of pressure vessels below the minimum legal standards in any one state, most users at or just above the minimum requirements, and a few far above the standards.

On the other hand, where key values related to health and safety are not

*Revised version of a paper presented at the Conference on Hospital Organization Research, May 22-23, 1970. Institute for Social Research, The University of Michigan, Ann Arbor, Michigan. Mayer N. Zald, Ph.D., is Professor of Sociology at Vanderbilt University, and Dr. Hair is now with the National Center for Health Services Research and Development. The senior author holds a career development research award from the National Institute of Mental Health, USPHS (K34, 919). The research here reported has been supported by several sources, including a grant from the Russell Sage Foundation and a grant (1-R03-MH 16391) from NIMH, USPHS. (Some modifications of the original paper have been made by the Editor.)

threatened, the range of performance of institutional elements may vary greatly, essentially providing an institutional output that matches the preference demand distribution for "products" of various size, style, and quality. Furthermore, different mechanisms of control may be brought into play at different points on a performance curve.

In this paper, using a developing research framework for the study of the social control of institutions, we will examine certain major problems concerning the control of hospitals. Unlike the excellent recent work of Somers (1969), which views problems of hospital regulation from a policy perspective, we shall look at the social control of hospitals largely as a setting for sociological and social-psychological analysis. In many respects, however, the underlying description of the facts is remarkably similar. First, we will state the basic elements of the framework (these are generally relevant to the analysis of the social control of organizations, including but not limited to hospitals). Second, we will illustrate the framework drawing on the history of hospitals in America and statistics on hospital accreditation. Finally, we will discuss how the social control matrix conditions the structure and functioning of hospitals, and especially the *decision* context of key groups and individuals within hospitals.

Basic Elements of the Research Framework

Although there is no theory of the social control of institutions presently available, much theoretical and empirical work in economics, law, political science, and sociology has relevance to such a theory. Our framework is intended to permit a synthesis of this work.

The conception of institutional control that we are developing has several distinctive features that partially set it apart from recent approaches to the environment of organizations (cf. J. Thompson, 1967). First, our focus on the social control of institutions leads us to conceive of organizations as parts of institutional arenas. We are interested in how various groups, individuals, and agencies attempt to set standards for, evaluate, and control all members of the particular institution. By institution we mean something akin to "industry," if that term is broadened to include more than profit-making industries. That is, an institutional arena or sector is any group of interlocked complex organizations providing relatively similar outputs (products, services, manifest functions) within a society.

Second, we are concerned with how different kinds of institutions are subject to different kinds of control matrices. For example, while prisons and hospitals both provide important services to society their social control matrices vary enormously. Furthermore, hospitals differ substantially in their control matrix depending upon their "ownership."

A third distinctive feature is that our emphasis upon values and normative control leads us to a broadened conception of the manner in which society sets constraints upon organizations and registers preferences. Some research, and theory, has shown how even nonmonetary exchanges, such as interorganizational exchanges of clients and cases, are related to preferences and perceived adequacy of performance (Levine and White, 1961). But we are concerned with how environmental control and exchanges are related to variations in the intensity of preferences, and with the ways in which society organizes aggregated preferences into political and professional policies to control organizations. To this date our research has focused upon the macroprocesses of the transformation of social control, but these processes work themselves out into microprocesses of organizational and professional interaction.

Although we focus upon institutional control environments, we do not assume that all institutional elements in a society face similar environments. Variations in immediately surrounding environments condition the control environments for each element. Partial social systems within the larger society present a social control matrix intersecting with and interdependent with the social control matrix of the larger society.

Social system differentiation, norms, sanctions, agents of control, structural context, and compliance characteristics of the target objects are the major components of our analysis framework. Social system differentiation is intended as a rubric for the overall level of societal "development" and provides an important part of the societal context in which the social control of institutions takes place. It is important for viewing the overall forms of social control in societies, but is less important for understanding the specific forms of institutional control in modern society. The other concepts are more integral to our approach and will be described briefly.

Norms and Performance Curves

Various groups in a society define and enforce norms of performance upon institutional elements. Norms are preferred states of behavior or behavior output, not statistical norms, i.e. modal or "average" performance. A norm is related to "Expected" *and* "sanctioned" behavior (Morris, 1956). If the output or related behavior is below the "expected," attempts will be made to sanction (reward or punish) "better" performance.

Norms range from those in which there is strong consensus, absolute clarity, and easy observability of the related behavior, to the opposite. They also vary in the level of intensity with which they are held by various groups in society. Norms can be classified as output norms, procedural norms, and facilities or custodial norms. Output norms, qualitative and quantitative, refer to products delivered to the "clients" of the institution. Procedural norms are those regulating institutional means—safety and health laws applied to a specific technology, technological design, and efficiency norms applied by professional groups. Custodial norms involve the facilities in which technology is applied (in many cases they may be the same as the technological norms).

By examining the intensity of normative preferences, the clarity of the standards, the degree of consensus among control agents, and the sanctions, one ought to be able to predict the range of institutional performance. For example, "society" will not tolerate many hospital fires, so strong sanctions are given to boiler inspectors and the codes are clearly and completely detailed. On the other hand, given the difficulty of curing some physical disorder, how much hospitals must "cure" is open to wide variation in definition and output.

The tolerance limits of norms permit variation in the range of performance of institutional elements and the emergence of normative exemplars and normative laggards. Where norms are loosely defined or subject to varying definitions, the range of performance is likely to be greater. Similarly, unless an outside agent has strong sanctions, as the costs of implementing the norms increase, the range of institutional performance is likely to increase.

Structural Context

Norms are implemented, or enforced, by control agents who operate in a structural context. Although all modern societies have highly differentiated institutions, both within and between institutions, they vary considerably in the structural context that they provide for institutional control. Structural context is defined as the *organization* of those parts of the social environment having direct control or ability to sanction institutional components (cf. Dahl and Lindblom, 1955; and Solo, 1968).

Variations in structural context between societies and between institutional arenas within societies affect the range of variation of institutional performance and the pattern and rates of change in performance. That is, the type of structural context, in conjunction with the characteristics of norms and sanctions, influences the range of performance and the amassing of demand for change. It is possible to distinguish three ideal-typical structural contexts: market, polyarchic, and hierarchic. All three are arranged along the single dimension of the relative dispersal of resources in the environment required by institutional elements. In competitive markets there are continual pressures to adaptation and change. Hierarchic contexts are (ideal-typically) characterized by relatively uniform performance. Polyarchic contexts are characterized by a large number of competing and identifiable groups attempting to influence performance.

Control Agents

In our society there are a host of different control agents comprising the structural context of any institution and its elements. These include governmental agencies that "own" the institutional elements; professional standard-setting associations; legal institutions including courts of law; organizations affecting the legitimacy of institutional performance, such as newspapers and licensing boards; labor unions; "umbrella" organizations made up of representatives of the institutional elements' *major users* or resource providers; boards of directors; and executive elites. Boards of directors are part of the institutional element but in many cases "represent" external sources of control (Zald, 1969). Executive elites are part of the organization but are held "responsible" for its performance.

Each institution and its elements are surrounded by a partially unique constellation of control agents with an interest in ensuring organizational performance. Some control agents have an interest in a specific aspect of organizational performance across nearly all institutions whereas others are specific to an institutional arena. For instance, the Tennessee Division of Boiler Inspection is interested in all pressure boilers, whether they are found in dry cleaning plants, schools, or factories, whereas the National Education Association is interested in the overall performance of primary and secondary educational institutions.

Typically, control agents are involved in a three-step process: (1) defining norms, (2) evaluating performance in relation to the norm, and (3) enforcing normative conformance where deviation is found. Depending upon several factors, including the degree of tolerance of deviation, the technical means of inspecting institutional performance, and the strength of sanctions at their command, control agents vary in their strength and effectiveness. A given agent may have strong sanctions at its command but have an internal structure which vitiates their use. For instance, state licensing laws have given hospital licensing boards and officials the power to close hospitals, yet the state boards have been understaffed and rarely carried out inspection. Or, the agent may be able to easily ascertain normative violations but unable, because of legal and other restrictions, to apply sanctions.

At this point of our work, the classification and analysis of control agents is largely tied to three dimensions: (1) the sanctions they control; (2) the extent to which they are tied to particular institutional elements (e.g. a board of directors), the total institution arena (e.g. the Interstate Commerce Commission), or cross-cut many institutions (e.g. civil courts); and (3) whether they are more effective at lower or upper ends of the performance curve.

Sanctions

Each impinging control agent may command a different kind of sanction. Sanctions are classified in several ways. They range from physical coercion, to the withholding of economic resources, to the giving or withdrawing of respect, to acclaim, and the like. At the most fundamental level sanctions can be analytically ordered in terms of the extent to which application of a sanction threatens institutional viability. Injunctive powers of a court, when backed up by police coercion, are in this sense among the most powerful sanctions. Similarly, monopolistic control of vital inputs or of output markets also represents a near coercive sanction. On the other hand, professional associations usually control only symbolic sanctions that are often quite weak. When these symbolic sanctions, such as certification, are universally used as decision cues by those who control inputs or use outputs, however, they can be extremely powerful.

It is important to remember that sanctions are used in a social context; they are symbolically and socially defined. Moreover, their application to an institutional element may have cueing effects, leading others to investigate the organization's performance and either support or negate the first agent's control attempt. When a hospital is threatened with withdrawal of accreditation, for example, other control agents may begin to survey the institutional element and either support the Joint Commission on Accreditation of Hospitals or the hospital.

A sanction can be thought of as having two values: a primary value for the target of the sanction and a secondary value for other similar organizations viewing the target. Thus sanctions have two purposes: the control of the target element and the reinforcement of norms and consequences of violating norms in the remainder of institutional elements. Analytically, this two-sidedness in the application of sanctions means that the costs of applying sanctions have to be weighed from two perspectives: the immediate cost as well as the relative deterrent benefits.

The application of sanctions involves a calculus for control agents. If a control agent fails to sanction known norm violators, he loses credibility. On the other hand, in many cases the control agent is limited in his ability to deliver sanctions. First, if surveillance is inexpensive but sanction costly, his limited resources may lead him to ignore many known violations. Second, application of sanctions to some target object may vitiate the original control purpose. For instance, disaccrediting a hospital may lead to lower medical care for a population if the hospital then loses its intern program. Accrediting associations are in the business of trying to improve medical care. We suspect, therefore, that where a hospital is the major or only supplier of service to a large population, it is less likely to be disaccredited than if it is one of many hospitals. Moreover, application of sanctions to target elements may trigger ressponses from umbrella associations and other institutional elements to change the control agency's structure, policies, and procedures.

Compliance Characteristics of Target Objects

Part of the problem of the economy of sanctions comes from deviation in the compliance *readiness* of institutional elements (for a review of the limits of judicial sanctions, see Becker, 1969). If a norm is well known, inexpensive to meet, and accepted by the elements of the institution being controlled, the control agent may rarely, if ever, have to employ sanctions. Indeed, in such a situation the control apparatus should be relatively small and institutionalized. On the other hand, norms may be ambiguous, costly to implement, or even opposed by the target organization's elite and other control agents.

Compliance characteristics of target objects may also lead to easy compliance. Thus low economic penalties for violating laws, and low surveillance rates might make it economically sound to violate laws. Yet hospitals fearing for their reputation, or having a "habit" of conformity, may comply even when sanctions are rarely applied (Lane, 1966).

CHART 1.

ANALYTIC COMPONENTS OF FRAMEWORK FOR STUDY OF SOCIAL CONTROL OF HOSPITALS.

1 Sources of Norms and Definitions of Hospitals	2 Norm Defining Agents	3 Sanctioning Organizations (Legitimate Controllers)	4 External Vectors of Placement	5 Organizational Factors	6 Normative Performance
Technology: Natural & Social Science Applied Science	Professional Associations	Governmental Agencies	Labor Market of Professionals Doctors Hospital Administrators Nurses, etc.	Effective Compliance Potential	1) Staff-Patient Ratios
	Individual Professionals	State Licensing		Leadership	2) Hospital Organization Structure
Changing Social Structure Expectations of Service	Schools: Professional Socialization	Courts: a. Liability Law b. Interpretation of corporation status and laws referring to medical practice	Market of Clientele 1) Class basis 2) Ethnic 3) Competition 4) Population Density	Community Support	3) Medical Care Criteria
	Mass Media	Medical Accrediting Agencies		Location	4) Facilities Maintenance
	Legislatures	Fund Controllers a. Medical Insurance Agencies b. Union Medical Programs c. Philanthropists d. Government & Funding Agencies e. Patients		Resources	5) Professional Qualifications

General Hospitals in America: Changes and Control Trends

The changing technology and science base of medicine has permitted both a changing function for hospitals and changing expectations of hospital performance. In very gross terms, hospitals, which were once adjuncts to a doctor's private practice or were charitable custodial institutions, have become centers for the integration of medical specialities and expensive facilities. This change in function has led to enormous changes in the capital needs of hospitals, in the nature of their funding, their control, and their internal structure.

It is impossible, short of a series of massive volumes, to seriously explicate the social control of hospitals. Such a series of studies might well be organized around the factors, processes, and groups shown in Chart 1. By and large, the general factors in the larger society and culture (listed in column 1) begin to affect specific norm definers (column 2) and control agents (column 3). External vectors of placement (column 4) are social system constraints on specific hospitals operating somewhat independently of the conscious intent of organizational decision-makers and of organizational resources (column 5). Regardless of the clarity of compliance norms or the intent of hospital decision-makers, the environment in which they exist may prohibit their acquisiton of resources with which to comply.

The preceding factors combine to affect specific hospital performance indices (column 6). Such indices (individual and aggregated), in turn, shap expectations and provide impetus for progress in technology and general standards. Here we shall concentrate on three major aspects of the transformation of social control factors in the case of hospitals: technological requirements, legal changes, and accreditation standards.

Technology

It is well known that two of the major events leading to the hospital revolution were the growth of the ability to control surgical infections through antisepsis and the diagnostic developments surrounding radiology. There are, however, little available data on the actual spread of new technologies and related facilities during the early years of this century. Recently, Wolf Heydebrand (1969) presented data on the distribution of selected facilities in hospitals for the period 1946-1961.

Table 1 shows the differential distribution of technical facilities for 1946 and 1961. In 1946, 88 percent of short-term nonfederal hospitals had diagnostic facilities, and the figure is even higher for 1961. The greatest percentage changes are found for radioactive isotope facilities (based upon research done during World War II), blood banks (related to both technological advances and growing size of hospitals), electrocardiography, and the development of clinical laboratories. These technological facilities have obvious

TABLE 1. PERCENT OF NON-FEDERAL SHORT-TERM GENER-
AL AND SPECIAL HOSPITALS WITH SELECTED TECHNI-
CAL FACILITIES, 1946 (N = 4444) and 1961 (N = 5309)

Technical Facility	Percent 1946	Percent 1961
Radioactive Isotope Facility	0.0	24.6
Electroencephalography	6.2	15.8
Dental Clinic	17.0	28.7
Blood Bank	24.7	56.2
Physical Therapy	32.3	42.8
X-Ray, Therapeutic	35.7	36.7
Pharmacy	38.2	50.7
Electrocardiography	56.3	93.8
Clinical Laboratory	79.4	96.3
X-Ray, Diagnostic	88.0	97.4

Source: Wolf Heydebrand, *Hospital Brueaucracy: A Comparative Analysis*. Unpublished Manuscript, 1969 (Table 11).

consequences for the division of labor, professional identification, and the administrative order of hospitals.

Facilities are often expensive, and sheer captial needs help account for the transformation of ownership of general hospitals during the 1935-1966 period (Table 2).

TABLE 2. DISTRIBUTION OF OWNERSHIP AND AVERAGE
NUMBER OF BEDS IN "GENERAL AND SPECIAL COMMUN-
ITY HOSPTIALS,"* 1935 and 1966

Ownership	1935			1966		
	N	Percent	Average Number of Beds	N	Percent	Average Number of Beds
State & Local Government	569	12.4	181	1,234	22.0	124
Voluntary & Non-Profit	2,469	53.9	101	3,428	61.2	155
Proprietary	1,542	33.7	30	935	16.7	56
	4,580			5,597		

*Excludes TB and psychiatric hospitals, and all federal hospitals.

Source: 1935 data from Heydebrand, *op cit,* Table 27. 1966 data from *Hospitals*, Guide Issue, Part 2, 1967, p. 446.

Table 2 clearly indicates the decline of proprietary hospitals as a significant proportion of the general and special hospitals in the country. And even if these data are somewhat biased by the underreporting of small proprietary hospitals in 1966, there is no question but that there has been a large rise in proportion of total beds in the United States in the nonproprietary hospitals. (In the late 1960s there may have been a reversal of trends for proprietary hospitals as some proprietary chains have expanded.) It is also interesting that although the number of state and local government hospitals has more than doubled, the average size has declined slightly. As management, financial, and succession problems created pressures, we suspect that local communities often have taken over small proprietary hospitals. On the other hand, Hill-Burton funds have encouraged construction of small community hospitals.

What are some of the implications of these technological, ownership, and size trends? Not all general hospitals *need* have all of the facilities listed in Table 1, nor, for that matter, many more esoteric ones (e.g. special surgical suites). Nor is there a necessary and sufficient relation between size and "quality" of performance. While a hospital must be above a certain size to be listed (Zald, 1969), licensed (Somers, 1969), and accredited (Zald, 1969), an enormous variation above that limit is possible.

But it should be apparent that from the point of view of professional personnel, professional associations, and laymen, hospitals without modern and up-to-date facilities are seen as "out-dated," "backward," "out of step," "unable to provide adequate facilities." Facilities are a necessary though not sufficient condition for meeting high standards. And both patient and professional decisions to "participate" in organizations, where they have choices, are clearly related to the quality and level of technical facilities. Thus everything else being equal, "good" facilities beget good personnel. [1]

At the same time that technological requirements change the economic requirements of hospitals, technological changes affect expected standards of care, including those standards imposed by law.

Legal Changes

Hospitals and medical practitioners are partially controlled by a legal system that employs generalized concepts, or theories, and interprets their relevance to the specific case of hospitals. Thus hospitals are affected by the changing application of legal doctrines as well as by specific changes in the condition of medical practice. Here, we shall examine briefly two important legal trends, the transformation of tort liability and the use of extralocal standards in evaluating care (a good review of other related legal trends is found in Somers, 1969, chapters 2-6).

Tort liability. Two particular aspects of hospital status partially exempted them from *liability* suits, thus lowering legal responsibility for the patient's

---

1. It should be noted that "everything else" in this case is not equal. Rushing (1970) has recently shown that between 1950 and 1967 an increase in the ratio of doctors to population in a county was positively correlated with the ratio of doctors to population in 1950. On the other hand, there was no correlation between an increase in the ratio of doctors and an increase in hospital facilities and beds.

treatment on their premises—the doctrine of charitable immunity, and the restriction of corporations from the practice of medicine.

The doctrine of charitable immunity, stemming from an English court case (*Holliday v. Leonard*, 1861), was first applied in a Massachusetts case in 1876 (*McDonald v. Massachusetts General Hospital*). Briefly, it held that a charitable institution was immune from liability to a charitable patient for the negligent act of its servants. The court ruled on the basis of the theory that the funds of a charity constituted a trust fund which could not be used to pay damage claims. Such diversion of funds would hamper the usefulness of charity and discourage future gifts. There were a variety of other interpretations, including the idea that hospital charities were like governmental units and thus immune from tort action (see Southwick, A.F., and *Bell v. Presbytery of Boise, 1966*).

Ironically, the charitable trust idea had been specifically overturned in an English case five years preceding the Massachusetts case (*Foreman v. Mayor of Canterbury*, 1871). Thus, we suspect, generally held ideas about hospitals and their role, rather than *stare decisis* and strict construction, dominated the spread of the charitable immunity doctrine. Further evidence of this predominant "world view" of hospitals is the fact that two U.S. state legislatures overruled state courts which refused to grant charitable immunity by passing legislation granting immunity or at least limiting liability (see Rhode Island, New Jersey statutes, R.I. Gen Laws. S7-1-22 and N.J. Stat. Ann 2A: 53A-7&8). A parallel "world view" interpretation of judicial decision-making is given by Friedman (1965).

In 1942 most states had, in one form or another, limited the liability of hospitals (see *President and Directors of Georgetown College v. Hughes*, 1942). However, the next two decades began to whittle away the immunity of hospitals (see *American Law Reports*, 2nd series, vol. 25; and Table 3 below). Table 3 documents the transformation in hospital immunity between 1942 and 1967.

What is important here is that tort actions against hospitals per se, not just doctors, have become increasingly feasible. Of course the mere fact that a state has or has not changed its ruling on charitable immunity is not a ready guide to the fears and practices of hospital administrators and doctors. Knowledge of the possibility of tort action crosses state boundaries. Moreover, there is almost always a discrepancy between the actual law and people's perception of the law.

At the same time that hospitals were losing their charitable immunity, another related legal process was breaching the separate responsibilities of the hospital as a corporation and the doctor as a professional practitioner.

Through World War II hospitals were responsible only for providing "adequate" facilities and for checking on the licensed status of their personnel (see e.g. Bachmeyer, 1935; and *American Jurisprudence*, 1938). Legally, hospitals had a highly limited duty:

> The extent of the duty of a hospital with respect to actual medical care of a professional nature such as is furnished by a physician is

TABLE 3. COMPARISON OF CHARITABLE IMMUNITY RUL-
INGS CONCERNING HOSPITALS IN UNITED STATES
JURISDICTIONS: 1942, 1952, 1958, 1967

Nature of Ruling	Number of States with Ruling Indicated for the Different Years Shown [a]			
	1942	1952	1958	1967
No Decision on Subject	5	2	3	3
Full Immunity	11	12[b]	10	7
Qualified Immunity	20[c]	17	13[c]	8
Trend Toward Unqualified Liability	9[d]	18	24[d]	32

a. Five states not included in the distribution for 1942, and Alaska is not
   included in the distribution for 1952; all fifty states are included
   in the distributions for 1958 and 1967.

b. Includes three states "liable if insurance carried."

c. 1942 includes seven states for which "charity not liable to beneficiaries—no decision involving strangers," twelve states for which
   "strangers may recover—beneficiaries denied relief," and one
   state in which "strangers and paying beneficiaries may recover."
   For 1958, the corresponding numbers of states are two, ten, and
   one, respectively.

d. 1942 includes seven states in which "strangers and paying beneficiaries may recover," and two states which "limit liability to
   insurance and nontrust property." For 1958, the corresponding
   numbers of states with these two forms of liability are seven and
   four, respectively.

Sources: 1942, *President and Directors of Georgetwon College v.
            Hughes*, 130 F. 2d 810, 818-821. 1952, 24 ALR 2d 29, 1942.
            1958, Emanuel Hayt, Lillian R. Hayt, August H. Groeschel, and
            Dorothy McMillan, *Law of Hospital and Nurse* (New York:
            Hospital Textbook Co., 1958), pp. 67-68. 1967, *Rabon v.
            Rowan Memorial Hospital Incorporated*. 152 S.E. 2d 485 (N.C.
            1967), 498.

to use reasonable care in selecting medical doctors. When such
care in the selection of the staff is accomplished, and nothing
indicates that a physician so selected is incompetent or that such
incompetence should have been discovered, more cannot be
expected from the hospital administration [*Darling v. Charleston
Community Memorial Hospital*, 1965].

Over the last twenty years courts have begun to reject the sharp distinction
between administrative negligence and medical negligence. In *Bing v.*

Thunig (1957), for instance, Justice Fuld, speaking for the New York Court of Appeals, said:

> While the failure of the nurses in the present case to inspect and remove the contaminated linen might, perhaps, be denominated an administrative default, we do not consider it either wise or necessary again to become embroiled in an overnice disputation as to whether it should be labeled administrative or medical. The conception that the hospital does not undertake to treat the patient, does not undertake to act through its doctors and nurses, but undertakes instead simply to procure them to act upon their own responsibility, no longer reflects the fact. Present-day hospitals, as their manner of operation plainly demonstrates, do far more than furnish facilities for treatment. They regularly employ on a salary basis a large staff of physicians, nurses and internes, as well as administrative and manual workers, and they charge patients for medical care and treatment, collecting for such services, if necessary, by legal action. Certainly the person who avails himself of "hospital facilities" expects that the hospital will attempt to cure him, not that its nurses or other employees will act on their own responsibility.

Local and professional standards. Not only have the courts begun to breach the distinction between provision of facilities and care, but they have begun to insist that hospitals have a duty to enforce *proper* medical standards, not just local community practices.

The most significant case which indicates that the hospital does have a duty regarding the quality of medical care is *Darling v. Charleston Community Memorial Hospital* (1965). This action against the hospital to recover damages for allegedly negligent medical and hospital treatment, necessitating the amputation of the plantiff's right leg, was based upon both a theory of corporate liability and the theory of *respondeat superior*. Under the corporate theory of liability the plaintiff alleged that the hospital violated the community standard of care by not requiring adequate supervision and consultation. Under the *respondeat superior* theory he alleged that the nurses were derelict in failing to report the deteriorated condition of the plaintiff to the physician and, if the doctor failed to act, to the hospital administrator (Julavits, 1967).

The hospital defended on the general basis that it could not practice medicine under the law and, therefore, was powerless to forbid or command any act of a doctor. The court ruled that a hospital may be held liable for the adverse effects of treatment approved by the doctor in charge, though not an employee of the hospital, because of what was found to be its negligent failure to review the doctor's treatment of the patient. It also held that, even though there may have been no deviation from the local standard of care, the hospital was negligent for failing to adhere to its own regulations which require that it provide qualified physicians (Boyd, 1965). As evidence of feasible standards of care, the court allowed the jury to apply the private standards of hospital accreditation, the public standards of the licensing agency, and the hospital's bylaws.

In response to the hospital's appeal to the Illinois Supreme Court (see Hallenbeck, 1966), Justice Schaefer, writing the opinion, stated that the basic dispute revolved around the duty that rested upon the defendant hospital. He noted that, strictly speaking, the duty is always the same—conformity to the legal standard of "reasonable conduct in the light of the apparent risk." Hence the question is rather one of the standard of conduct required to satisfy the duty. Although community custom "is generally admissible as bearing on what is proper conduct under the circumstances," it is not conclusive. Rather, "custom is relevant in determining the standard of care because it illustrates what is feasible, it suggests a body of knowledge of which the defendant should be aware, and warns of the possibility of far-reaching consequences if a higher standard is required."

Schaefer stated that the standards which were introduced as evidence—regulation of the Illinois Department of Public Health under the Hospital Licensing Act, the standards for hospital accreditation of the Joint Commission, and the bylaws of the defendant hospital—were poorly admitted as evidence. These standards "performed much the same function as did evidence of custom, since it aided the jury in deciding what was feasible and what the defendant knew or should have known. It did not conclusively determine the standard of care and the jury was not instructed that it did" (Schaefer, 1965).

Within the past twenty years there has been a reduction in the use of locality as a qualification of the standard of care required of physicians (see McCoid, 1959). The same trend was developing prior to *Darling* concerning the use of local standards for hospital care as a defense against liability (see e.g. *South Highlands Infirmary v. Galloway,* 1936; Leonard v. Watsonville *Community hospital,* 1956; and Boyd, 1964 and 1965). This recognition of the admissibility of standards of a nationwide organization such as the Joint Commission on Accreditation of Hospitals as evidence of what is "feasible" and of what the hospital should "know" broadens the concept of "community" considerably. It presents the possibility of using experts from any part of the country to establish specific requirements of the accrediting standards, as well as avoiding the "conspiracy of silence" frequently encountered from "a community expert testimony which may prove unfavorable to the local hospital."

Prior to the *Darling* decision some courts had held that when a standard was not imposed by the state but was adopted by the hospital itself, the private rule was admissible as evidence of the hospital's standard of care.[2]

---

2. *Moeller v. Hauser,* 237 Minn. 368, 54 N.W. 2d 639 (1952); *Judd vs. Park Ave. Hospital,* 37 Misc. 2d 614, 235, N.Y.S. 2d 843 (Sup. Ct.) Aff'd, 235 N.Y.S. 2d 1023 (1962); *Corwin v. University of Rochester,* 147 N.Y.S. 2d 571 (Sup. Ct., 1955). In *Stone v. Proctor,* 259 N.C. 633, 131 S.E. 2d 297 (1963) the court held that an adopted rule promulgated by the American Psychiatric Association could be introduced as evidence of the standard of care to which a psychiatrist should adhere. This case was cited in *Wilson v. Lowe's Asheboro Hardware,* 259 N.C. 660, 131 S.E. 2d 501 (1963), which held that an advisory safety code voluntarily adopted by the defendant was admissible to establish negligence.

However, these decisions have said that a private rule would probably not be admitted as evidence unless all of the hospitals in the community had adopted the same regulation. Here the *Darling* decision differs in that the court did not say specifically that all hospitals in the locality had to have accepted and approved a private rule before it could be used as evidence. Thus the *Darling* case indicates that a hospital may be held to a standard of care higher than the geographic area's standard.

One interpretation of the admissibility of private rules as evidence on behalf of a plaintiff could be that it would tend to discourage voluntary adoption of such rules by a hospital. Violation of such rules would not necessarily result in liability, but rather such rules would only be evidence to be considered by a jury. The hospital would be free to introduce evidence to show that a violation of the rules was not negligence, but that the rule called for more than that which is reasonable under the circumstances, and should be excluded by the court as application, therefore, The standards introduced in *Darling* were not held to be absolute, but were used as evidence of what is "feasible" (Boyd, 1965; Julavits, 1967, p. 108).

Although the use of private standards, licensing standards, and bylaws may or may not be easier for juries to use than is the "community custom" standard, the *Darling* decision did disrupt the established definition of the hospital-patient relationship, thus creating a certain amount of ambiguity on the part of both hospital and court. *Darling* introduced the concept of shared responsibilities, with the ultimate discretion in the hospital. This raises questions as to when the hospital must act, what is the extent of the hospital's liability to the patient, the hospital physician's liability, and that of the patient's private physician (Julavits, 1967, p. 109.) [3]

It does not appear that *Darling* is having much effect specifically upon the tort cases involving hospitals being presented to the courts. However, the *Darling* decision is attracting considerable attention and concern from the hospital, medical, and legal professions. Lawyers are being advised to.

. . . investigate the possibility of holding the hospital as well as the attending physician liable, even though the injury appears to

---

3. The question of the relationship between the hospital and the patient's physician was raised in *Fiorentino v. Wenger* (26 App. Div. 2d 693, 272 N.Y.S. 2d 557 1966), where the attending physician, a private practitioner and not an employee of the hospital, failed to disclose the novelty of the procedure and the risks involved to the parents of the patient. The appellate court affirmed the trial court judgment against both the attending surgeon and the hospital, holding that the hospital as an institution had a duty to ascertain whether or not the physician had made full disclosure and obtained from the patient or his authorized representative an informed consent before permitting the operation to take place. A dissent to the majority decision argued that it rendered the institution a guarantor of the conduct of all staff doctors, whether employees or not. On appeal to the New York Court of Appeals, the judgment against the hospital was reversed, but the court acknowledged that "a hospital may be liable in tort for permitting its facilities to be used by an unlicensed person or by a licensed person committing an act of malpractice with the knowledge of the hospital or under circumstances putting it on notice of such wrongful act." (*Law Week*, vol. 35, 1967, p. 2632.) Thus a hospital will not be held liable for an act of malpractice performed by a physician independently retained by the patient himself, unless the hospital management had reason to know that an act of malpractice would take place. (*American Law Reports*, vol. 14, 3rd series, p. 880; ALR 3rd 1968 Later Case Service, par. 3.)

have been the result of purely medical negligence . . . [for] even in the absence of an employer-employee or principal-agent relationship, between the negligent doctor and hospital, there now appears to be some chance, in view of the decision in *Darling v. Charleston*, to impose liability on the hospital on the theory of independent negligence in failing to review, supervise, or consult about, the treatment given by the physician directly in charge, if the situation indicates that the hospital had the opportunity for such review but failed to exercise it, or that its servants were negligent in failing to call the attention of the proper hospital authorities to the impropriety or inadequacy of the treatment being given [14 ALR 3d 873, 879].

The benefits the plaintiff receives from suing the hospital as well as, or in addition to, the attending doctor include: (1) a means of avoiding the obstacles imposed by the widely noted "conspiracy of silence" by using proof of the requirement of the professional standard other than by the use of expert testimony of a member of the same profession; (2) witnesses may be less reluctant to testify against, and jurors to find against, the impersonal institution than the individual doctor, whose career may well be wrecked by a finding of negligence; and (3) adding the hospital as a defendant will increase the resources available to the plaintiff from which to receive the damages to which he is entitled. If hospitals do, in fact, "effectively guide and control the actions of the doctors using their facilities, it is almost inevitable that, sooner or later, responsibility will follow this power" (14 ALR 3d 873, 879).

Whereas lawsuits were once found to be ineffective and unreliable methods of enforcing standards, the litigative process has slowly but surely changed the body of law concerning hospital and medical standards and hospital liability. The area of standards is being brought squarely within the scope of the courts. This legal transformation is directly and indirectly affecting the incentives and sanctions available to governmental and private standard-setting bodies such as the Joint Commission to induce compliance with standards on the part of hospitals.

If hospitals are to be responsible for these professional actions of their staff, they need a set of standards and control mechanisms which will show them to be in conformance with good practice. Aside from conformity with state licensing laws and Medicare standards, the Accreditation Agency provides the other major summary source of good practice standards. Outside of local custom, they represent a quasi-universalistic approach to the setting of standards that increasingly impinges on hospital decisions.

Some Aspects of Accreditation

As social control devices, licensing and accreditation are both mechanisms for establishing that individuals and organizations meet certain prerequisites for continuing to operate (see Gottlieb and Spaulding, 1962). The difference between licensing and accreditation is that the licensor is backed up by the police power of the state, whereas formally the accreditor only can use sanctions emanating from his prestige and consensus on the "rightness" of accreditation standards. We say "formally" because in fact accreditation gains much of its force from other agencies and individuals—including courts, funding agents, newspapers, and the like—which use accreditation as a basis for their own grants or withholding of resources.[4]

In the case of medicine, hospital accreditation developed in close relation to the perceived needs of medical education. Medical licensing preceded hospital licensing and accreditation, and the close nexus between the hospital, medical education, and postgraduate practice is a phenomenon of the last half century. Indeed, only in 1914 did Pennsylvania become the first state to require hospital internship as part of the prerequisites for a license to practice medicine (see V. Johnson, "The Council of Medical Education and Hospitals," in Fishbein's *A History of the A.M.A.*, p. 899).

As hospitals became a central site for the treating of patients and the training of students, two developments led to the establishment of hospital accredication. First, a list of approved hospitals was needed so that interns could be recommended to good practice hospitals (Johnson, *ibid*). The second development related to the growth of the College of Surgeons, which was incorporated by the State of Illinois on December 25, 1912 (Davis

---

4. In correspondence from Kenneth B. Babcock, April 9, 1969, discussing his article, "Five Years of Accreditation," *Hospitals*, 32 (Jan. 1958), p. 39, Dr. Babcock stated that while director of the Joint Commission he had letters from the United Mine Workers, the National Foundation for Infantile Paralysis and Crippled Children's Society, and the American Cancer Society about their desire to provide funds to accredited hospitals. He stated that while Hill-Burton agencies will state that they have no rulings in their grants to the effect that accredited status would receive preferential treatment, "In a letter to me, they stated that so specifically but then slyly said, 'Of course, it was possible if the local state organization responsible for distribution of their funds used it as one of their criteria.' " Dr. Babcock suggested that accreditation might be a Hill-Burton requirement in "allocating funds to the rehabilitation and renovation in already existing hospitals."

Babcock went on to state that "In Detroit, in 1965, in the allocation of funds for capital improvements by United Foundation, one of the criteria used was the existing hospital had to be accredited to be considered."

Blue Cross: Correspondence from Jane R. O'Brian, manager, Information Services, Professional Relations, Blue Cross Association (June 23, 1969) revealed that from a Blue Cross survey, 27 of the 68 responding Plans indicated that they have standards for participation for hospitals. Of those 27, 17 responded to our request for their standards. Of these 17, 3 required JCAH or AOA accreditation; 6 phrased the requirement that a hospital "should" be accredited; and the others were general requirements. Miss O'Brian observed that "Because JCAH required 25 beds for accreditation until approximately a year ago when the number was reduced to 6, many Plans could not require JCAH accreditation for participating hospitals since there were many small hospitals under this size fulfilling a real community need. On the other hand, in progressive areas of the country, such as California, Plans do not require JCAH accreditation because of the necessity of utilizing new facilities before waiting a year for the hospital to be accredited."

Responses from Blue Cross Plans to our inquiries showed that 61 Plans did not require accreditation for hospital participation in Blue Cross programs. The 12 Plans which responded affirmatively included: Arizona, Connecticut, Delaware, Chicago, Ill., Michigan, St. Louis, Mo., Northeastern Pennsylvania, Greater Philadelphia, Pa., Rhode Island, Richmond, Va., Buffalo, N.Y., and the Washington-Alaska Plan.

Fellowship of Surgeons, 1960, p. 477).

The College of Surgeons, developed in the first two decades of this century, was at first opposed by general practitioners who believed, rightly so, that College members wanted ultimately to restrict their rights to practice surgery. Aside from developing training procedures for surgery, the College also needed to develop criteria for admission based upon competence. Direct viewing of a number of operations was rejected because of costs; instead, a submission of detailed records of operations performed was requested.[5] The College found, however, that hospital records were too inadequate to be used as a base. Thus, in the first instance, the College of Surgeons accredited hospitals whose *records* systems were adequate. It should be noted that accreditation moves were bitterly resented. On the one hand, doctors resented the expenditure of time and effort required to fill out records, and, on the other, they resented anybody attempting to tell them professionally what they had to do (Davis, 1960, pp. 205-206). (Analytically, these are "compliance readiness" characteristics.)

Elsewhere we have treated the emergence of the Joint Commission on the Accreditation of Hospitals as a major private source of hospital standards. Here, since there are published statistical records indicating which hospitals are or are not accredited, it is possible to examine some of the external (environmental) and internal (organizational) correlates of accreditation.

In Table 4 we present the distribution of accredited hospitals by state. In general, in 1946 the more urbanized states had higher rates of accreditation. Furthermore, over the two decade period the states having the largest absolute percentage increases in accreditation, such as California, Florida, and Michigan, are either states with rapid growth in population or older urban states. A central part of the analysis that follows focuses on explaining how urbanization affects accreditation. Let us note, first, however, that "type of ownership" is strongly related to accreditation status. Table 5, below, relates accreditation to hospital size (number of beds) for various ownership types. As shown, both size and ownership status are related to accreditation. Larger hospitals and voluntary-nonprofit hospitals are those most likely to be accredited, while proprietary hospitals are least likely to be accredited.

TABLE 4. RANK ORDER OF STATES BY PERCENT HOSPITAL
ACCREDITATION 1946-1966

State	1946[a]	1966	Percent Change
Pennsylvania	62.7	78.0	15.3
Massachusetts	61.7	83.6	21.9
Rhode Island	60.0	84.0	24.0
New Jersey	57.7	76.6	19.9

5. In 1914, when Franklin Martin questioned A. D. Ballou about the possibility of using moving pictures for the Clinical Congress Programs, Ballou responded that it would be a long time before moving picture cameras would be used in operating rooms (Davis, 1960, pp. 147-148).

West Virginia	56.3	59.3	3.0
New York	55.0	87.0	32.3
New Hampshire	53.7	83.3	29.6
Missouri	51.7	66.9	15.2
Ohio	51.3	74.5	23.2
Connecticut	51.2	79.4	28.2
Delaware	50.0	81.3	31.3
Vermont	48.3	67.7	19.4
Illinois	47.9	84.0	36.1
North Dakota	47.8	41.5	−6.3
Virginia	47.6	78.7	31.1
North Carolina	47.4	72.9	25.5
Maryland	42.4	70.9	28.5
Washington	41.9	67.4	25.5
Michigan	41.2	80.4	39.2
Iowa	40.3	55.8	15.5
Montana	38.2	45.3	7.1
Minnesota	37.8	57.6	19.8
South Dakota	37.0	37.7	.7
Indiana	36.4	62.6	26.2
Kansas	36.2	41.5	5.3
Maine	35.9	79.7	43.8
Wisconsin	35.6	65.2	29.6
Colorado	34.3	57.8	23.5
Oregon	33.7	74.7	41.0
Louisiana	32.6	45.8	13.2
South Carolina	31.0	60.8	29.8
Kentucky	30.3	55.3	25.0
Arkansas	29.2	57.6	28.4
Arizona	29.9	52.5	22.6
Georgia	28.8	60.0	31.2
Nevada	28.6	45.5	16.9
Wyoming	28.5	55.9	27.4
California	28.4	71.3	42.9
Tennessee	27.5	51.3	23.8
Oklahoma	27.4	44.7	17.3
Idaho	26.7	45.3	18.6
Nebraska	26.2	41.5	15.3
Florida	25.4	64.8	39.4
Alabama	24.8	48.6	23.8
Utah	23.1	48.8	25.7
Texas	20.0	40.0	20.0
New Mexico	20.0	63.8	43.8
Mississippi	17.3	38.7	21.4
Alaska	--	42.3	
Hawaii	--	57.6	

a. The 1946 data report only civilian hospitals, whereas the 1966 include all hospitals listed by the American Hospital Association.

Sources: 1946: "Geographical Distribution of Approved Hospitals 1946—Civilian Hospitals," *Bulletin* of the American College of Surgeons, vo. 31 (Dec. 1946), pp. 307-308. 1966: "Table—Hospital Approvals and Affiliations, 1966; by State or U.S.-Associated Area," *Hospitals*, vol 41 (August 1, 1967), part 2, p. 475.

It is our general assumption that both size and ownership are associated with accreditation status because they set up conditions for hospital decision-makers in which seeking accreditation becomes desirable and organizational resources are sufficient to receive accreditation. On the one hand, small governmental and proprietary hospitals do not have sufficient funds and specialties to achieve accreditation; on the other, they have little pressure to become accredited.

We noted above that the more urbanized states have higher proportions of accredited hospitals. And it makes a good deal of sense to expect many aspects of hospitals to be associated with community characteristics. Thus we have analyzed a wide range of variables that might be associated with accreditation.[6]

---

6. The data for this study were collected from: American Hospital Association, *American Hospital Directory, 1947* (Chicago: American Hospital Assn., 1947); American Hospital Association, *Hospitals,* Guide Issue, vol. 35 (August 1, 1961), part 2; U.S. Bureau of the Census, *County and City Data Book, 1952* (A *Statistical Abstract* supplement), U.S. Government Printing Office, Washington, D.C., 1953; U.S. Bureau of the Census, *County and City Data Book, 1962.* (A *Statistical Abstract* supplement), U.S. Government Printing Office, 1962; U.S. Bureau of the Census, *U.S. Census of Population: 1950*, vol. II, Characteristics of the Population, part 1, U.S. Summary (U.S. Government Printing Office, 1953); U.S. Bureau of the Census, *U.S. Census of Population;* 1960, vol. 1, Characteristics of the Population, part A, Number of Inhabitants (U.S. Government Printing Office, 1961); U.S. Department of Health, Education, and Welfare, Public Health Service, Division of Public Health Methods, *Health Manpower Source Book*, section 4, County Data, Prepared by Maryland Y. Pennell and Marion E. Altenderfer (U.S. Government Printing Office, 1954); and U.S. Department of Health, Education, and Welfare, Public Health Service, Division of Public Health Methods and National Center for Health Statistics, *Health Manpower Source Book.* Section 19, Location of Manpower in 8 Occupations, prepared by Maryland Y. Pennell and Kathryn I. Baker (U.S. Government Printing Office, 1965).

A sample of 980 hospitals was randomly drawn from the 1961 *Hospitals* Guide Issue. For each hospital the following data were recorded: hospital control (ownership), service, length of stay, approvals and memberships, total number of facilities and services, number of beds, number of admissions, average daily census, total expenses, and payroll expenses. The following information was collected for the county in which the hospital is located: total population, population per square mile, percent population change 1950-1960, percent urban, percent rural farm, percent nonwhite, percent families with infomes under $3000, median family income, median school years completed by adult population, county SMSA grouping, effective buying income, number of general hospital beds, number of dentists, number of nurses, number of pharmacists, and number of M.D.s. The city population and percent increase 1950-1960 were recorded. The same information was collected for the 1950 period for all hospitals in the sample in existence in 1947 (N=688).

The variables initially used were *community factors*: percent urban, percent rural farm, population per square mile, county population change, median family income, effective buying income, percent poor, median years of school completed, and city population change; *labor pool variables:* dentists, nurses, pharmacists, and M.D.s per thousand county population; *organizational resources per patient variables:* admissions per bed, census per bed, admissions per personnel, census per personnel, and payroll expenditures per personnel; *hospital associations and approvals:* state hospital association and Blue Cross membership, cancer clinic, residency, internship approvals, maintenance of a professional nursing school, and medical school affiliation; *structural quality:* total number of facilities and services, and size (number of beds). beds).

For efficiency a number of these variables were dropped for the analysis. Data are presented for a subset of the total sample, those pertaining to general hospitals.

TABLE 5. PERCENT SHORT-TERM GENERAL HOSPITALS ACCREDITED BY SIZE (BEDS) AND OWNERSHIP, 1959

	All	Under 25	25-49	50-99	100-199	200-299	300-499	500+
Voluntary Non-Profit	54.6	00.4	27.6	68.5	95.6	98.7	100.0	100.0
Proprietary	16.3	00.0	09.5	44.2	67.3	a	a	a
State & Local	40.0	00.6	17.1	42.7	72.3	88.6	95.1	100.0

a. Under ten cases

Source: "Table 7: Accreditation, All listed hospitals, U.S.," *Hospitals*, vol. 34 (August 1, 1960), part 2, p. 400.

The data are discussed in terms of our earlier paradigm of factors affecting performance output. These are roughly grouped as: community factors; labor market potential; organizational resources per patient; structural variables; and quality-professional requirement variables. Community variables include level of urbanization and socioeconomic characteristics of the population. Labor pool variables are the ratios of doctors, nurses, and dentists to 1000 population. Organizational resources per patient variables are the ratio of beds to personnel and payroll per personnel. Finally, the quality and professional variables include two types, structural and associational. Membership in hospital associations and approval for internships are associational measures of quality, dependent upon other groups' support. Structural measures are those associated with adequate care, here size and facilities.

First let us show the overwhelming impact of urban status on accreditation and on specific variables from each variable domain. Table 6 presents these data. Note first that over time there are significant trends toward "equality" on some variables but not on others. Thus by 1960 urbanization makes no difference on the availability of Blue Cross participation, membership in the state hospital association, or admission rates per bed. On the other hand, variables such as accreditation, ratios of doctors to population, size of hospital, and number of facilities are massively affected by urban status.

Urbanization status massively, though indirectly, affects the quality of hospital performance through its effects upon the willingness of professionals to practice in rural areas; the income levels of the population affects their ability to pay for hospital service; the sparsity of population affects the size of medical facilities; and so on. Since urbanization does have this overall effect, to disentangle other variables related to accreditation we have computed correlations for 1950 and 1960 *within the urban status categories* (Table 7).

There are many interesting aspects shown by Table 7. Note, for instance, the strong relation to accreditation of M.D.s/1000 population for counties adjacent to cities, while this variable has little correlation with accreditation in independent cities or metropolitan centers. Our explanation is that both of

TABLE 6. SUMMARY MEASURES OF VARIABLES BY COUNTY GROUP, FOR 1950 and 1960 GENERAL HOSPITALS

Variable	Year	County Group [a]				
		Greater Metro-politan	Lesser Metro-politan	Adjacent to SMSA	Isolated Semi-Rural	Isolated Rural
Socio-Economic Charact.						
Median Family	1950	$3687.9	$3284.4	2764.1	$2444.9	$2156.0
Income	1960	6523.9	5740.2	4657.2	4301.8	3670.5
Median School	1950	10.4	10.2	9.3	9.0	8.7
Years Completed	1960	11.2	10.8	9.7	9.9	9.2
General Hospital	1950	5.92	6.56	3.65	4.91	4.56
Beds/1,000 Pop.	1960	4.84	4.46	3.93	4.85	4.79
Labor Pool Potential						
Dentists/1,000	1950	.730	.737	.381	.648	.263
Population	1960	.810	.570	.416	.425	.334
Nurses/1,000	1950	3.92	5.09	2.56	2.43	1.58
Population	1960	5.36	5.59	4.16	3.66	2.34
Doctors (M.D.)/	1950	2.16	2.41	0.92	0.93	0.62
1,000 Pop.	1960	2.46	1.57	0.92	1.02	0.57
Organizational Input						
Daily Census/Full	1950	.822	1.827	1.332	1.041	1.140
time Personnel	1960	.456	.497	.495	.570	.870
Admissions/Beds	1950	34.2	34.1	37.1	35.7	32.9
	1960	35.8	37.1	38.9	37.0	33.2
Organizational Structure						
Beds	1950	260.5	190.9	108.0	84.9	86.1
	1960	254.8	212.0	90.2	80.0	43.3
Number of Facil-	1950	11.0	09.2	06.9	06.3	06.3
ties	1960	16.1	15.1	11.8	11.4	09.9
Organizational Associations						
Accreditation	1950	86.2%	71.9%	48.9%	53.8%	36.0%
	1960	85.5	81.0	61.8	50.9	17.5
Membership in	1950	75.9%	75.0%	77.2%	77.8%	56.0%
State Hospital	1960	92.5	93.5	92.8	90.2	92.5
Association						
Blue Cross	1950	84.5%	72.7%	78.3%	70.8%	56.0%
Participant	1960	93.1	89.1	94.7	86.8	92.5

Approved for Internship Program	1950	51.7%	37.5%	03.3%	04.1%	04.0%
	1960	40.8	35.3	04.6	04.7	00.0
N	1950	116	128	92	171	25
N	1960	174	184	152	234	40

a. Five types of counties have been delineated, the first two being determined by the standard metropolitan statistical areas established by the Bureau of the Budget. The counties that constitute the SMSAs with populations of 1 million or more inhabitants have been called *greater metropolitan;* the counties that constitute the SMSAs with populations between 50,000 and 1 million are *lesser metropolitan.* Counties contiguous to the SMSA counties are called *adjacent:* although they may be sparsely populated, they are nevertheless relatively close the metropolitan areas and the health facilities ordinarily available in such centers. All other counties have been called isolated—*isolated semirural* if they contain at least one incorporated place of 2500 or more persons; otherwise, *isolated rural.*

the latter have a more heterogeneous social structure. Thus, although rates of M.D.s may vary by greater metropolitan and lesser metropolitan area, there are enough doctors and they are specialized enough to provide an adequate pool. However, adjacent suburbs tend to be more homogeneous and the working class suburbs have trouble recruiting staff and demand less quality.

The correlation pattern across the five county groupings clearly shows the influence of demographically related socioeconomic variables. In the less urbanized counties, where the income and education of the population are low and consequently so is the supply of medical personnel and facilities, the socioeconomic variables are significantly related to accreditation. However, when the level of these socioeconomic and personnel variables is above a certain point, as in the metropolitan areas, the variation of these factors has less effect upon accreditation.

TABLE 7. PRODUCT-MOMENT CORRELATION OF VARIABLES WITH ACCREDITATION, BY COUNTY GROUPS, FOR 1950 AND 1960 GENERAL HOSPITALS

Variables	Year	Greater Metropolitan	Lesser Metropolitan	Adjacent to SMSA	Isolated Semi-Rural	Isolated Rural
Socioeconomic Charact.						
County Data Median Fam. Income	1950	.013	.073	.353*	.192*	-.163
	1960	.138	.006	.374*	.255*	-.209
Median School Years Completed	1950	-.104	-.026	.287*	.226*	-.014
	1960	.072	.014	.286*	.175*	-.271
General Hospital Beds/1,000 Pop.	1950	-.209*	.086	.194	.224*	-.039
	1960	.064	.089	.062	.167*	-.332*

Labor Pool Potential						
Dentists/1,000	1950	-.078	.074	.316*	.140	.022
Population	1960	.095	.098	.184*	.274*	-.291
Nurses/1,000	1950	-.203*	.079	.506*	.292*	.246
Population	1960	.110	.097	.274*	.276*	-.153
M.D.s/1,000	1950	-.165	.077	.451*	.273*	.460*
Population	1960	.090	.144	.214*	.181*	.106
Organizational Input						
Daily Census/Full	1950	-.310*	-.141	-.117	-.138	-.124
time Personnel	1960	.276*	-.254*	-.206	.111	-.046
	1950	.054	.100	-.173	-.078	-.149
Admissions/bed	1960	-.079	-.135	.046	-.059	.071
Organizational Structure						
Number of	1950	.471*	.554*	.532*	.409*	.073
Facilities	1960	.464*	.596*	.504*	.511*	.451*
Beds	1950	.128	.168	.232*	.132	-.059
	1960	.299*	.397*	.389*	.455*	.615*
Organizational Association						
Approval for In-	1950	.364*	.485*	.188	.191*	.272
ternship Program	1960	.348*	.358*	.173*	.178*	.000
Membership in	1950	.300*	.482*	.273*	.379*	.161
Hosptial Associa-	1960	.304*	.152	.146	.049	.131
tions						
Blue Cross	1950	.243*	.357*	.199	.384*	.161
Participation	1960	.204*	.009	-.124	-.006	-.119

*Significant at least at .05 level. Richard G. Lathrop, *Introduction to Psychological Research: Logic, Design, Analysis* (New York: Harper & Row, Publishers, 1969). "Appendix E: Values of r significant at .05 and .01 levels," p. 287.

Within the metropolitan areas the variables more likely to differentiate between accredited and nonaccredited hospitals are internal organization and organizational input factors. Daily census per full-time personnel, a measure of staff workload, is significantly related to accreditation in the metropolitan and adjacent counties, but not in the rural county hospitals.

The single most uniformly significant variable is the number of facilities maintained by the hospital. Note that in the correlation analysis "approval of internship program" relates less strongly to accreditation than does "number of facilities." Partly, of course, this is related to sheer distributional features; fewer hospitals have internship programs than are accredited. This suggests that the motives for seeking accreditation are less clearly related to the specific possibility of gaining interns than we had originally thought. Instead, the history of hospitals, in general, is for them to strive for quality, within the limits imposed by budget, labor pool, etc. Except for the large public general hospitals—e.g. Cook County Hospital—we suggest that interns are sought both for their labor value *and* for their reflection on the teaching-quality standards of the hospital.

Before drawing any conclusions it must be remembered that a few of the facilities listed and included in the total number are facilities that are "essential" for accreditation. These include dietary services, medical records, a pharmacy or drug room, a clinical laboratory and pathological services, radiology equipment for diagnosis, and a medical library. Four of these "essentials" were included in the 27 facilities and services listed in the 1961 *Hospitals* Guide Issue. While this might contaminate the measure, it must be remembered that when a hospital maintains a service or facility not "essential" for accreditation, the standards for that facility then apply. Hence, the more comprehensive the facilities and services maintained by a hospital, the more standards with which the hospital must comply.

Through the years, the American College of Surgeons and the Joint Commission have emphasized the fact that size and physical facilities and services are not the determining factors in accreditation. They have stressed the educational and organizational aspects of the "minimum standard."

Although not possible with the available data, it would be necessary to investigate the relationship between internal organizational variables and accreditation. While it is true that hospitals with comprehensive services and facilities attract interns, residents, and other personnel, the coordination necessary to keep these facilities, services, and personnel operating smoothly and efficiently, rather than just the availability of the personnel, may be a key to the relationship of facilities to accreditation. The study of ten general hospitals, all accredited, by Basil S. Georgopoulos and Floyd C. Mann, *The Community General Hospital* (New York: The Macmillan Company, 1962) found strong positive relations between coordination and the quality of nursing care and overall patient care, but not the quality of medical care. The same study found strong negative relations between intraorganizational strain and the quality of care in these accredited hospitals (Table 48, p. 390; Table 49, p. 393; and Table 50, p. 398).

Finally, another interesting result of the correlation table (Table 7) is the seeming lack of influence of state hospital associations and Blue Cross plans on accreditation. As noted earlier (see footnote 4, p. 67), Blue Cross plans generally do not exert much effort to set or enforce quality standards for their participating hospitals. Those plans which do require that hospitals comply with standards for participation are located in those areas where the rate of accreditation is already high. Rural plans would like to be able to require compliance with standards, but are realistic about the economic and manpower factors affecting the many small hospitals in their area.

The shift from a significant relationship between state hospital association membership and accreditation in 1950 to an insignificant relationship in

1960 is perhaps more a function of the type of members than of its exertion of influence upon members to become accredited. Hospital associations originated primarily with the large urban hospitals. It would seem that as the membership has become more inclusive (90-92 percent), the relationship with accreditation would disappear. With few exceptions, the state hospital associations have not taken firm measures to ensure that their members meet accrediation standards.

Summary

In this section we have spelled out some of the massive changes in law and in technology affecting hospitals, and have attemtped to show a set of community and organizational factors associated with hospital accreditation. Both the courts and the professions have articulated complex performance norms and sanctions to match the increasing precision and complexity of hospital technology. In the process, the environment of hospitals has become populated with a wealth of control agents consciously seeking to measure and evaluate performance. Recent federal aid formulas will only further this trend, for some specifically propose to build in rewards for efficiency rather than treat all hospitals alike. Acknowledging these environmental changes and their impact on hospitals, an important question still to be answered is: What shapes a particular hospital's reaction to the environment? The final section focuses on this matter.

Decision-Making, Organizational Structure, and Control Environment

What if the doctrine of charitable immunity is changing? What if we can show the correlates of accreditation status? What differences do changes such as these make *now* to boards of directors, hospital administrators, and chiefs of service? How does the "outside" get "inside"? And what determines how much of the outside gets inside?

The basic thrust of our analysis is that the tasks of hospitals are shaped by all of the following: (1) elite, lay, and professional concepts of means and ends which are filtered through; (2) past and present education; and (3) constraints and opportunities presented to the organization by the environment and by its internal resources. Both organizational and material technologies are diffused through the larger social system.

In one sense our analysis points to the overwhelming constraints of technological change and community settings on the possibility of a hospital being completely "up-to-date." A modern hospital that had not added four or five new "facilities" by 1960 would be behind the times (see Table 6). Moreover, "keeping up-to-date" creates a more or less constant strain on the financial resources of hospitals. In Table 8 below, drawn from Heydebrand (1969), note the positive association between number of medical specialties

TABLE 8. CORRELATIONS BETWEEN ORGANIZATIONAL SIZE, DIVISION OF LABOR, AND NUMBER OF MEDICAL SPECIALTIES, BASED ON 1277 TEACHING HOSPITALS (1960)

SIZE OF TASK	Internal Division of Labor Specialiation		No. of Medical Specialties
	Functional	Departmental	
Number of Beds	.04	-.06	.03
Average Daily Census	.20	-.05	.01
SIZE OF RESOURCES			
Total Payroll, 1960	.26	.20	.45
Total Expenses, 1960	.33	.20	.49
Total Personnel, 1960	.32	.11	.52
Functional Specialization	--	.42	.33
Departmental Specialization	--	--	.35

Source: Heydebrand, 1969, Table 21.

and three measures of resources. Note also that these measures correlate with structural measures.

But we can go beyond these more or less obvious statements. The labor pool problems and the technical differentiation of hospitals has led to a massive shift in the labor composition of hospitals (Table 9). Thus the personnel mix becomes a function of forces somewhat external to hospital decision-making.

Not only are labor composition and departmental structures a result of external forces, but committees and governance structures are in part determined by legal and accreditation requirements. An adequate tissue committee and good surgical notes are required to protect staff from liability suits as well as for "teaching purposes." It might be that surgical notes of board-certified surgeons would revert to the cryptic were it not for the threat

TABLE 9. THE CHANGE IN THE STRUCTURE OF PERSONNEL BETWEEN 1935 AND 1959 BY TYPE OF SERVICE AND SIZE OF HOSPITAL

Service Type and Size (Number of beds)	Number of Hospitals		Personnel/ 100 Beds		Percent Physicians		Percent Technicians	
	1935	1959	1935	1959	1935	1959	1935	1959
General & Special	4,733	5,777	77	127	4.8	2.2	5.4	9.4
Under 25 beds	1,282	423	56	98	3.5	2.3	3.8	19.2
25-49 beds	1,150	1,391	58	99	3.4	1.2	4.4	10.9
50-149 beds	1,540	2,246	72	127	4.3	1.4	5.1	9.0
150 beds and over	761	1,717	85	156	5.3	4.0	5.8	7.8

Source: Heydebrand, *op. cit.*, Table 13.

of liability suits. A similar point could be made with regard to the "honoring" of surgical and other specialty divisions.

In some sense, of course, what we have said applies to all organizations to greater or lesser degree. Hospitals, however, are more restricted than many other organizations because their facilities are locked into hospital usages and their "ownership"-auspices status would not easily allow them to be shifted from one community to another. Moreover, their provision of a service that is critical to life and death leads society to expect higher performance standards. Whoever heard of a school teacher being sued for failing to teach! The growth of Medicare with its standards for hospital operation represents a beginning development of national performance standards.

It is clear, however, that even with this highly determined context, hospital boards and executive cadres still have considerable discretion. First, they can affect the speed of adoption of "technological (organizational and material) leading edge" developments. The "ethos" of the executive cadre interacts with their perceptions of the potential sources for resources and the costs and benefits of specific developments.

Second, again depending upon values and perception, various facilities and programs can be given different emphases, and varying images of quality may be projected for different units. The optimization of standards is not uniform across all hospital departments.

Third, introduction of new technology and facilities creates opportunities for new relations to the environment, to funding agencies, and to other hospitals. The small merger movement which has taken place in the last few years seems to be a function of the economic-technology specialization "crunch" (Starkweather, 1970). Hospitals vary in their response to this "crunch," depending upon the "foreign relations" stance of their cadre and governing bodies as well as their overlap and interaction with the relevant bodies in other organizations (Morris, 1961).

Fourth, it is important to note that all of the efficiency-oriented changes, morale-promoting factors, and new role differentiations can be influenced by the structure and characteristics of cadres and governing agents.

Finally, as long as hospitals exist in a control matrix that is organized around market and polyarchic principles, there will be wide variation in performance, and differences in performance will be related to the ability of lay and professional leadership to mobilize and coordinate resources (Belknap and Steinle, 1963).

It may be more interesting to close by speculating upon the possibility that there will be massive changes in the moral exemplars and normative bases of medicine in the next few years. A change in the norms and moral exemplars would have profound effects upon the social control of hospitals and the definition of hospital adequacy.

Boldly speaking, the norms of hospitals have been dominated by a medical concept rooted in: (1) curing diseases and repairing disorders, not preventing them; (2) the individual doctor-patient relationship, not the organization-client relationship; and (3) the fee-for-service system. As a consequence, moral examplars have been the doctors who diagnosed, cured, and developed new techniques for handling esoteric disorders. Preventive medicine and outpatient clinics have been basements of the hospital and of the medical schools. In the former case these have served as supply sources for career slots reserved for the less adequate doctors; in the latter case, they have been maintained as necessary services and used for the training of students.

From a comparative view of health systems, however, this need not be the only mode of nomative development. Furthermore, federal funds are being channeled away from the frontier research areas toward the delivery of service areas. Concerned students and doctors are pressing for a redefinition of mission. Although it is still too early to tell, it may be that there is a change in the choice of specialties and types of practice. The slow spread of group and comprehensive practice also changes the normative conception of medical ideals. The patterns of enacted law are changing the direction of rewards to hospitals, and new norms of orgnaization-client relations are coming into existence. Surely a differentiated enterprise like the hospital will not develop a single-standard exemplar; yet the definition of the leading edge will change just as it has been changing with the older concepts of practice.

Conclusion

This paper has barely begun to outline the kinds of research needed to understand the social control of hospitals. Although there are a few studies which touch on hospitals in their community context and deal with the impact of environment on boards of trustees, few have traced the processes whereby performance norms are enforced. Everyone knows that a threat of loss of malpractice insurance shakes up a hospital board, but we do not know how many have been so threatened. We have no adequate studies of the effect of liability law on performance; of the way in which boards of directors and hosptial administrators react to prospects of accreditation or disaccreditation; of the manner in which professionals conduct individual or collective battles to change the definition of good practice; or of the process by which insurance companies and other third-party agents establish standards which affect decision-making. It is clear from the contributions in the present volume that the boards of hospitals and hospital executives no longer confront mainly a local environment. What specifically shapes their reactions to this new environment, and how, remains to the studied.

References

Allport, F. H. The J-curve hypothesis of conforming behavior. *Journal of Social Psychology,* 1934, *5,* 141-183.
American Jurisprudence. Corporations. *American Jurisprudence,* 1938, *38,* 838.
American Law Reports, 2nd series, *24, 29,* 1942.
American Law Reports, 2nd series, *25, 29* at 142.

American Law Reports, Annotated, 3rd series, *14,* 873 at 878.

American Law Reports, 3rd series, *14,* 873, 879.

Babcock, K. F. Five years of accreditation. *Hospitals,* part 2, 1958, *32,* 39.

Bachmeyer, A. C. The hospital and the medical profession. *American Hospital Association Bulletin,* 1935, *9,* 35.

Becker, P. L. (Ed.) *The impact of Supreme Court decisions: empirical studies.* New York: Oxford University Press, 1969.

Belknap, I., and Steinle, J. G. *The community and its hospitals: a comparative analysis.* Syracuse, New York: Syracuse University Press, 1963.

Bing v. Thunig, 2 N.Y. 2d 656, 666; 143 N.E. 2d 3, 8, 1957.

Boyd, W. G. Notes on *Darling v. Charlestown* [sic] *Community Memorial Hospital,* 200 N. E. 2d 149 (Ill. Ct. App. 1964). *North Carolina Law Review,* 1965, *43,* 469.

Bulletin of the American College of Surgeons. Geographical distribution of approved hospitals 1946—Civilian hospitals. *Bulletin of the American College of Surgeons,* 1946, *31,* 307-308.

Corwin v. University of Rochester. 147 N.Y.S. 2d 571 (Sup. Ct., 1955).

Dahl, R. A., and Lindblom, C. E. *Politics, economics, and welfare: political economics policies resolved into their basic social processes.* New York: Harper & Row, 1965.

Darling v. Charleston Community Memorial Hospital, 33 Ill. 2d 326; 211 N.E. 2d 253, 254, 1965.

Davis, L. E. *Fellowship of Surgeons.* Springfield, Ill: Charles Thomas, 1960.

Fiorentino v. Wenger, 26 App. Div. 2d 693, 272 N.Y.S. 2d 557, 1966.

Foreman v. Mayor of Canterbury, 1871, L.R. 6Q. B. 214.

Friedman, L. J. Freedom of contract and occupational licensing, 1885-1910: a legal and social study. *California Law Review,* 1965, *52,* 487-535.

Georgopoulos, B. S., and Mann, F. C. *The community general hospital.* New York: Macmillan, 1962.

Gottlieb, S. R., and Spaulding, P. W. Controls within and upon the voluntary health system. In W. J. McNerney *et al., Hospital and medical economics,* vol. 2. Chicago: Hospital Research and Educational Trust, 1962. Pp. 1205-1459.

Hallenback, S. M. Note. *Illinois Bar Journal,* 1966, *54,* 743, 744.

Hayt, E., Hayt, L. R., Groeschel, A. H., and McMillan, D. *Law of hospital and nurse.* New York: Hospital Textbook Co., 1958.

Heydebrand, W. Hospital bureaucracy: a comparative analysis. Doctoral dissertation, Washington University, St. Louis, 1969.

Holliday v. St. Leonard, 1961, 11 c.b., N.S. 192.

Hospitals, part 2, Accreditation. *Hospitals,* 1960, *34,* 400.

Hospitals, part 2, Guide Issue, 1967.

Hospitals, part 2, 1967, *41,* 475.

Johnson, V. The council of medical education and hospitals. In M. Fishbein, *A History of the A.M.A.,* 1947, p. 899.

Judd v. Park Avenue Hospital, 37 Misc. 2d 614, 235, N.Y.S. 2d 843 (Sup. Ct.) Aff'd, 235 N.Y.S. 2d 1023, 1962.

Julavits, W. F. Hospital liability—a new duty of care. *Maine Law Review,* 1967, *15,* 102.

Lane, R. E. *The regulation of businessmen: social conditions of government economic control.* Hamden, Conn.: Shoe String Press, 1966.

Lathrop, R. G. *Introduction to psychological research: logic, design, analysis.* New York: Harper & Row, 1969.

Law Week, 1967, *35,* 2632.

Leonard v. Watsonville Community Hospital, 47 Cal. 2d 509, 306 P. 2d 36, 1956.

Levine, S. and White, P. E. Exchange as a conceptual framework for the study of interorganizational relationships. *Administrative Science Quarterly,* 1961, *5,* 583-601.

McCoid, A. H. The care required of medical practitioners. *Vanderbilt Law Review,* 1959, *12,* 549, 571.

McDonald v. Massachusetts General Hospital, 120 Mass. 432, 1876.

Moeller v. Hauser. 237 Minn. 368, 54 N.W. 2d 639, 1952.

Morris, R. T. A typology of norms. *American Sociological Review,* 1956, *21* 610-613.

Morris, R. T. New concepts in community organizations. In *The Social Welfare Forum.* New York: Columbia University Press, 1961. Pp. 128-145.

President and Directors of Georgetown College v. Hughes, 130 F 2d 810, D.C.C. 1942.

Rabon v. Rowan Memorial Hospital, Inc., 152 S.E. 2d 485 at 498 N.C. 1967.

Rushing, W. A. The distributional problem and medical care: Tennessee and Tennessee mid-south. Unpublished paper, Department of Sociology, Vanderbilt University, Nashville, Tenn., 1970.

Schaefer, J., in *Darling v. Chalreston Community Memorial Hospital,* 211 N.E. 2d 254, 257, 1965.

Solo, R. *Economic organizations and social systems.* Indianapolis: Bobbs-Merrill, 1968.

Somers, A. R. *Hospital regulation: the dilemma of public policy.* Princeton, N.J.: Industrial Relations Section, Department of Economic Research, Princeton University, Report Series #112, 1969.

South Highlands Infirmary v. Galloway, 233 Ala. 276, 171 So. 250, 1936.

Southwick, A. F., Jr. Current legal trends in hospital liability, in *Readings in hospital law.* Chicago: American Hospital Association, no date, p. 124.

Starkweather, D. Health facility merger and integration: a typology and some hypotheses. Unpublished paper presented at Conference on Inter-organizational Relationships, The Johns Hopkins University, 1970.

Stone v. Proctor, 259 N.C. 633, 131 S.E. 2d 297, 1963.

Thompson, J. D. *Organizations in action.* New York: McGraw-Hill, 1967.

Wilson v. Lowe's Asheboro Hardware, 259 N.C. 660, 131 S.E. 2d 502, 1963.

Zald, M. N. The power and function of Boards of Directors: a theoretical synthesis. *American Journal of Sociology, 1969, 75,* 97-111.

4

STRUCTURAL COMPARATIVE
STUDIES OF HOSPITALS*

Duncan Neuhauser and Ronald Andersen

The area of organization research and theory here reviewed does not have a commonly accepted name. However, it does appear to have a distinctive approach, which we will call the *structural-comparative* approach. The principal characteristics of this approach are:
1. Its chief area of concern is the formal organization.
2. The organization, division, or department is the unit of analysis rather than individual members of the organization.
3. The theoretical base is derived from Max Weber (1947), on the one hand, and Fayol (1967) and the classical management theorists, on the other. Its recent upsurge can be traced to the paper by Anderson and Warkov in 1961.
4. There is a definable set of researchers working in the area including, among others, Woodward (1965), Blau (1965, 1968) Blau, Heydebrand, and Stauffer (1966), Starbuck (1965), and Whisler (1964, 1967).
5. Structural-comparative researchers use a similar methodology. They usually compare a number of organizations, frequently 20 or more. Because they look at many organizations they tend to study them in less depth than other organization researchers. Some microeconomists use a similar methodology, and their work is also relevant here (e.g. M. Feldstein 1965, 1967; Melman, 1951; Stigler 1958, 1963). This methodology is distinct from laboratory studies, case studies, industrial engineering, participant observation, and most social surveys, which tend to limit themselves to observations in one or only a few organizations.
6. There is a cluster of variables which crop up over and over again in the structural-comparative literature, including size, complexity, the administrative component, technology, costs, and span of control.
7. This literature is largely data oriented, rather than relying heavily on personal experience and phenomenological observation as was true for much early organization literature. As a result, most of the structural-comparative propositions developed are based on empirical findings and are testable.

---

*Revised version of paper presented at Conference on Hospital Organization Research, May 22-23, 1970, Institute for Social Research, The University of Michigan, Ann Arbor, Michigan. Duncan Neuhauser, Ph.D., is Assistant Professor, Harvard University School of Public Health. Ronald Andersen, Ph.D., is Research Associate, Center for Health Administration Studies, and Assistant Professor of Sociology, University of Chicago.

8. There is much reliance on precollected data[1], as is the case with economics. This means that the researcher in this area must keep his eyes open for new data sources and existing natural experiments. Reliance on precollected data and the nonintensive nature of this research often make it possible for such research to be carried out at relatively low cost.

9. Structural-comparative studies go beyond traditional economics in that they include a wider range of variables which bear on the question of how to organize and coordinate people in organizations to promote efficiency.

10. A criticism is that questions of considerable interest to structural-comparative researchers are sometimes labeled as esoteric, or as having little practical application, by practitioners and other researchers.

A Structural-Comparative Research Framework

Our objective here is to consider the evidence from structural-comparative analyses of hospitals and to draw on similar analyses of other types or organizations which seem to have implications for the hospital field. In order to achieve a balanced perspective of the importance of structural variables, however, we need a framework which includes other types of variables that determine, interact with, and result from the structural variables. One such framework might be diagramed as in Chart 1.

CHART 1

OUTLINE OF THE RESEARCH FRAMEWORK

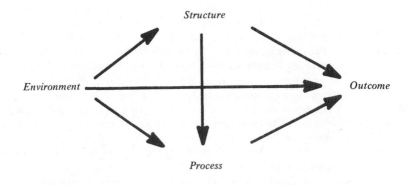

1. Frequently used sources of precollected data on hospitals include: American Hospital Association, Annual Guide Issue of *Hospitals, JAHA*, Yearly; American Hospital Association, Management Review Survey Results for All U.S.A. Hospitals Participating, Periodical; American Medical Association, Distribution of Physicians in the U.S. by State, Region, District, and County, Periodically; American Nurses Association, *Facts About Nursing*, Periodically; Hospital Administrative Services, Special Comparison, National Size Groups, Yearly; Hospital Administrative Services, Special Regional Comparison, Yearly; Ministry of Health, National Health Service, *Hospital Costing Returns* (Great Britain), Yearly.

Chart 1 indicates that the structural features of a hospital are in part determined by the external environment in which the hospital operates. Structure in turn affects the functioning of the hospital (process) and the results of hospital service (outcome). The diagram also suggests the pervasiveness of the environment in that it directly influences processes in the hospital and hospital outcome. Of course, process also has a major impact on outcome.

Variables subsumed under each of the categories in the diagram are listed in Table 1. While this list is by no means exhaustive, we feel it does give a fair indication of the variables being considered in the literature. It is beyond the scope of this paper to treat all of the variables in detail. We will focus on those which: (1) appear most frequently in structural-comparative literature; (2) have most systematically and convincingly been related to each other; and (3) provide the most fruitful leads for further research.

Specifically, we will focus on six variables which repeatedly occur in this literature and undertake to specify all the relationships between them here. These variables are: the size of the hospital (S); complexity (Cx); occupancy rate (ϕ); average length of stay (ALOS); per diem costs ($); and manhours (MH). In the future these variables and their relationships could be used as

TABLE 1. VARIABLES IN THE STRUCTURAL-COMPARATIVE FRAMEWORK FOR HOSPITAL ORGANIZATION RESEARCH

Environment	Structure	Process	Outcome
Hospital Input			*Quality of Care*
Patients	Organization size	Length of	Patient condition
Personnel	Organization	stay	Evaluation of
Supplies	complexity	Occupancy	services
Capital	Managerial com-	rate	
	ponent	Intensity of	
Community	Formal rules	care	*Efficiency*
Characteristics	Centralization	Growth	
	Number of	Employee turn-	Cost per diem
Demography	organization	over	or episode
Life style	levels	Absenteeism	Staffing ratio
Attitudes and	Relative size	Autopsy rate	
values	of departments	Manhours	*Satisfaction*
Economic			
resources			Patient
Medical care			Personnel[a]
facilities			
Health levels			
Medical tech-			
nology			

a. Whether personnel satisfaction belongs under Process or Outcome is debatable. Economists might not call it an outcome variable while social-psychologists probably would.

the basis for stimulating hospital performance.[2]

These basic variables can be generalized to a wide range of organizations. For instance, occupancy rate is comparable to the average proportion of plant capacity in use. Similarly, ALOS is a special case of the average time it takes to produce a unit of output or process one customer or client.

Our approach will be to define these key variables for each component of the framework and to consider correlations of variables *within* each component. We will then turn to interrelationships *among* the components as suggested by the arrows of Chart 1.

Unless otherwise indicated we will be referring to short-term general hospitals. Thus we are looking at a set of organizations with very much the same technology. Consequently, some care must be taken in generalizing from the following hypothesized relationships to other types of organizations, including mental hospitals and nursing homes.

The Components: Environment, Structure, Process, Outcome

Environment Variables

Table 1 suggests that the environment influences the hospital in at least two major ways. In the first place, the hospital is directly dependent upon the environment for its inputs, namely, the patients, physicians and other personnel, facilities and supplies, and capital. In addition, the hospital is shaped by characteristics and needs of the community in which it operates, including age and sex composition, occupational structure, per capita income, attitudes toward medical care, standards of living, other medical care facilities in the area, and the particular disease patterns of the population it serves (Andersen, 1965).

Some environment forces seem to have a surprisingly uniform effect on all hospitals in all industrialized countries. Those forces affecting all hospitals are best viewed as changes over time. For example, hospital costs appear to be rising faster than other goods and services for the last twenty years in the U.S.A., Canada, Sweden, and England, despite significant differences in the methods of organizing and financing medical care (Anderson and Warkov, 1961; Andersen and Hull, 1969).

However, the universal demands of the modern technology of disease treatment are not so total and pervasive as to explain all the structural characteristics of hospitals or to exclude the differential influence of other environmental forces. For example, nearly 100 percent of the births in the U.S.A. are in hospitals and attended by doctors while 70 percent of the births in the

---

2. In looking at all the relationships among these six variables, our approach has similarities to that used by Hage (1965). Hage predicts relationships between some of the same variables used here (S, Cx, ϕ, $, and MH). We will attempt to show that these relationships are known far more precisely for hospitals than Hage was able to show for organizations in general.

Netherlands are at home and 35 percent, including some hospital births, are attended by midwives. In spite of this the Netherlands has a lower infant and maternal mortality rate than the U.S.A., suggesting that the use of hospitals and doctors is sometimes poorly correlated with mortality in industrialized countries (National Center for Health Statistics, 1968).

It is precisely because the relationship between use of hospital services and human welfare is not very clear that such variations are allowed to occur and persist over time.

Structure Variables

For want of a better definition we will simply state that structure indicates the magnitude, distribution, and potential functions of the personnel and resources of the organization. In this review we will concern ourselves primarily with the structural characteristics of size, complexity, the managerial component, and formal rules.

1. *Organization size.* A key variable in the structural-comparative approach is that of organization size. Size can be measured in a number of different ways (Adelman, 1958; Rosenbluth, 1955). Several measures of hospital size are given below:

    a. Number of beds in the hospital excluding bassinets (plant capacity) (Pennel, 1939; "Hospital Administrative Services," yearly);

    b. Number of employees (Anderson and Neuhauser, 1969; Indik, 1964; Rushing 1966, 1967; Duncan, no date; Melman, 1951; Whisler, 1964; Caplow, 1957; Blau 1965, 1968);

    c. Assets of the organization (Hymer and Pashigian, 1962);

    d. Number of patient days, excluding newborn, during time period "t";

    e. Number of admissions, excluding newborn, during time period "t";

    f. Total revenue or total expense during time period "t."

For hospitals these measures appear to be very strongly correlated ($r > .90$) with each other (Heydebrand, 1965; Neuhauser, 1966; Wieland, 1965).

2. *Organization complexity.* Like size, complexity can be measured in a number of different ways. Most of the measures in the following list refer to either the range of activities undertaken by the organization of the level of skill employed to perform a certain type to task:

    a. *Environmental complexity*: the number of different types of patients seeking treatment at the hospital (but some of these patients may be turned away or referred elsewhere);

    b. *Case mix*: either the average level of difficulty of the cases being treated or the range of different cases being treated (Anderson and Neuhauser, 1969; Heydebrand, 1965; Feldstein, 1965) (case mix, of course, is not perfectly correlated with treatment);

    c. *Task complexity*: the number or average difficulty of the treatments given or tasks performed in the hospital. This is hard to measure and has been rarely used;

    d. *Division of labor*: the average educational level or the number of different types of skilled personnel working in the hospital. The assumption here is that each differently skilled person brings new activities into play (Heydebrand, 1965; Anderson, 1963, p. 51; Aiken and Hage, 1966, Hage, 1965);

e. *Technological complexity:* the number of different types of equipment in use;

f. *Departmentalization or scope of services:* the number of different departments in the hospital (Starkweather, 1970; Berry, 1965).

These measures of complexity are not as strongly positively correlated with one another as are the different size measures.

3. *Managerial component.* There is an extensive literature on the managerial component, indicating that this is a major variable in this area: Anderson and Neuhauser (1969); Baker and Davis (1954); Bell (1967); Blau (1965, 1968); Blau, Heydebrand, and Stauffer (1966); Carroll (1969); Delbecq (1968); Duncan (no date); Haire (1959); Heydebrand (1965, no date); "Hospital Administrative Services" (yearly); Indik (1964); Lindenfeld (1961); Melman (1951); Meyer (1968); Peloquin (1967); Pennel (1939); Pondy (1969); Rushing (1966, 1967); Starbuck (1965); Terrien and Mills (1955); Whisler (1964); Whilser *et al.,* (1967); Woodward (1965).

Many of the conclusions in these studies appear to contradict one another. We believe that the discrepancies in this literature can be resolved for both hospitals and organizations in general by using a model based on the following definitions:

a. First, it is necessary to distinguish between managers and clerical personnel in the following manner:

$$\frac{\text{managerial}}{\text{personnel}} + \frac{\text{clerical}}{\text{personnel}} + \frac{\text{other supporting}}{\text{personnel}} \overset{*}{=} \frac{\text{administrative}}{\text{personnel}} \quad (1)$$

As Rushing (1966) points out, this distinction is important because the managerial component declines with size while the clerical component increases with size.

$$\frac{\text{managerial personnel}}{\text{total hospital employees } (S_E)} = \frac{\text{the managerial}}{\text{component (M)}} \quad (2)$$

From now on we will be referring to the managerial component (M). A manager is defined as a person who spends most of his time supervising and directing employees directly below him in the hierarchy. Thus no one can be a manager by this definition without subordinates.

b. Secondly, it is necessary to distinguish between measures of the managerial component which include only top management and those which include managers down to first line supervisors[3] (Haire, 1959; Duncan, no

---

*A triple equal sign indicates that the equation is true by definition.

3. In the context of the model developed later in this paper, to include only top management is like assuming the span of control (α) can be infinitely large, as in Graph 1; to include all managers is like assuming a finite span of control (α), as in Graph 2

date).

4. *Formal rules.* These rules include budgets, procedure manuals, written reports, position control systems, etc. Their importance in the literature seems to stem from Weber's rational model which assumes that "decisions are made on the basis of a rational survey of the situation, utilizing certified knowledge with a deliberate orientation to an expressly codified legal apparatus" (Gouldner, 1959).

Correlations among Structural Variables

Complexity and size are positively and strongly related to each other ($r \cong .70$). They are, however, distinctly different concepts. The Anderson and Warkov study and the economics-of-scale literature are incomprehensible without this distinction. An example of the positive reslationship between hospital size and structural complexity is shown in Table 2 for Australian general hospitals (Dewdney and Thorne, 1969).

Complexity increases with size because: (1) specialized personnel and equipment must have a large case load over which to spread their costs; and (2) it is *not essential* for all hospitals to have many types of specialized services (see Table 2). Typically, only the larger hospitals will have these specialized services. Moreover, the larger hospitals can have more specialists because they can keep them busy. Elaborate referrals can modify this relationship. The tendency for general hospitals to provide a full range of services minimizes this referral effect.

In Table 2 it looks as if complexity increases exponentially with size. This is due to the unequal size intervals used in the table. It appears to be the case that complexity actually grows at a declining rate as size increases.

The positive relationship between size and complexity in the U.S.A., Canada, England, Sweden, and Australia is another example of constant technological forces at work across a variety of cultures.

The positive relationship between size and complexity may not be found for mental hospitals. This is because the larger among these hospitals tend to be custodial institutions while some of the smaller ones are intensive treatment institutions possibly offering a wider range of treatment techniques (Carroll, 1969).

Size and the managerial component can be related with the aid of the following assumptions: (1) *essentiality:* all organizations report having at least one manager; and (2) *indivisibility:* all managers are reported to be full-time employees. These assumptions can be empirically tested, and such tests show they generally hold true for hospitals.[4]

---

4. In certain special types of organizations these assumptions do not hold. For example, "essentiality" does not hold for small law firms and small physician group practices. These organizations tend to report having no manager at all. Coordination and control are probably performed on a part-time basis by the partners, who do not call themselves managers. For these organizations one would predict a positive relationship between the managerial component and size.

Although most managers appear to perform nonmanagerial tasks, they are customarily

TABLE 2. FACILITIES ON THE PREMISES OF SHORT STAY PUBLIC GENERAL HOSPITALS, AUSTRALIA [a] 1966-67

Facility	Bed complement range							
	Less than 12	12-24	25-49	50-74	75-99	100-199	200-399	400+
Labor Ward	x	x	x	x	x	x	x	x
Mobile X-Ray Unit	x	x	x	x	x	x	x	x
Mortuary	x	x	x	x	x	x	x	x
Operating Theatre	x	x	x	x	x	x	x	x
Out-patients' Dept.	x	x	x	x	x	x	x	x
Laundry		x	x	x	x	x	x	x
E.C.G.			x	x	x	x	x	x
Linen Room			x	x	x	x	x	x
Casualty Dept.				x	x	x	x	x
Catering Dept.				x	x	x	x	x
Obstet. Delivery Room				x	x	x	x	x
Premature Baby Unit				x	x	x	x	x
X-Ray (Diagnostic) Dept.				x	x	x	x	x
Pathology Dept.					x	x	x	x
Blood Bank						x	x	x
Central Sterilising Dept.						x	x	x
Haematology						x	x	x
Pharmacy						x	x	x
Physiotherapy						x	x	x
Bacteriology							x	x
Biochemistry							x	x
Medical Social Work Dept.							x	x
Postoperative Recovery Room							x	x
Chapel								x
Clinical Research Unit								x
Dental Dept.								x
E.E.G.								x
Intensive Care Unit								x
Medical Photography Dept.								x
Medical Physics Dept.								x
Occupational Therapy								x
Radiotherapy								x
Speech Therapy								x
Surgical Applicances Dept.								x
Traumatic Unit								x

a. SSPG hospitals in Queensland excluded.

Note: x indicates that the facility was available on the premises of more than half the hospitals in a particular bed complement range.

---

reported to be full-time managers (i.e. indivisible units). Hospitals occasionally employ part-time nursing supervisors, but these exceptions are too few to make a difference. Needless to say, the more exceptions to the assumptions of essentiality and indivisibility, the more inaccurate this model will be.

Note that essentiality and indivisibility can be applied to any group of workers or type of equipment in the hospital. Depending on whether these assumptions hold or not, one can predict their relationship with size. For example, clerical workers are not usually essential in small organizations and are not indivisible in that they are often part-time employees. Because of this, one

Assume one full-time manager; as the organization grows, his span of control increases apace. Thus the hyperbolic relationship [5] shown in the following graph, where $M = 1/S_E$:

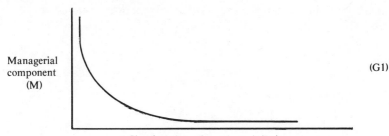

(G1)

Assume some finite upper limit on the span of control (α), and above some size ($S_E = (\alpha+1)$) the organization must hire a second full-time manager. If the organization wishes to have the largest possible span of control but never exceed α, then the relationship between the managerial component and size is as follows: [6]

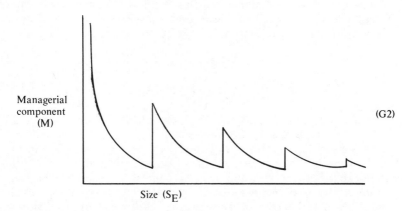

(G2)

might expect to see the clerical component increase with organization size as Rushing (1966, 1967) found. The same logic can be used to explain the relationship between complexity and size.

The introduction of these assumptions may resolve the issue of the managerial component and size, but they open up a host of other questions. which are beyond the scope of this paper.

5. One tends to observe this relationship when the managerial component is defined to include only top managers and exclude middle and lower managers (Haire, 1959; Duncan, no date).

6. To obtain this relationship it is necessary to look at individual organizations rather than clusters of organizations of different sizes which have been grouped together. It should be noted here that the managerial component is the reciprocal of the mean span of control.

This curve is discontinuous at $(\alpha +1)$, $(2\alpha +1)$, $(3\alpha +1)$, . . . , and as size increases, this curve is asymptotic to $1/\alpha$.

However, in the real world some organizations add new managers before they reach α while others lag behind, exceeding α before they add a new manager. Thus the following relationship between managerial component and size obtains:

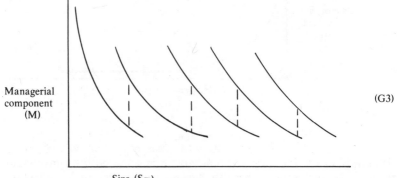

Managerial
component
(M)

(G3)

Size (S_E)

Note that for large organizations this relationship tends to disappear and the curve levels out. For this reason over a large range of organization sizes the relationship can be approximated by either of two equations:

$$M = a + b/S_E \tag{3}$$

or

$$M = a - b \log S_E \tag{4}$$

where a and b are constants and S_E is organization size as measured by the number of employees in the organization. This explains Indik's (1964) findings where log size fits his data better than linear size.[7] Perhaps because this relationship is nonlinear for small organizations Bell (1967) found no relationship between size and span of control in hospital departments.[8]

Complexity and the managerial component are positively related, as Anderson and Warkov (1961) indicate. Controlling for size shows more complexity, more departments, more managers, and smaller average span of control. It appears, however, that size has a stronger effect on the managerial component than does complexity.

---

7. From this model (G3) it can be predicted that the use of either equation (3) or (4) in regression analysis will result in heteroscedasticity with the variance in the residuals declining with organization size. From this model it can further be predicted that for very small organizations there will be an excess of managers and that they will spend more of their time in nonmanagerial tasks. This is supported by Saathoff and Kurtz (1962). Perhaps because he used rank order correlations, Rushing (1967) does not make it clear that the relationship between the managerial component and size is nonlinear for the organizations he studied.

Formal rules and the other structural variables show complex relationships. The evidence is overwhelming that the use of formal rules increases with organization size. Yet Starkweather (1970) presents evidence to the effect that the use of formal rules is more strongly related to complexity than to size and that, controlling for complexity, the effect of size washes out.

That the use of formal rules increases with size and complexity is not inconsistent with the managerial component declining with size. This is because the use of formal rules is an absolute figure while the managerial component is a ratio with size (S_E) in the denominator.[9]

The correlation between use of formal rules and size implies that management style differs systematically from one type of hospital to another (Starkweather, 1970; Neuhauser, 1966; Saathoff and Kurtz, 1962; St. Louis University, 1967; Yates, 1964; Andrews, 1968; Fearon, 1969; Hanson, 1961).

Process Variables

While the structural variables give us a somewhat static picture of hospital organization, the concept of process provides a means to consider its functioning. The variables listed under "Process" in Table 1 are selected from the many possible because they tell us something about hospital activity which has been related in the literature both to structure and outcome. Of particular interest to us, because of their bearing on hospital efficiency, are length of stay, occupancy rate, and intensity of care.

---

8. The data presented by Bell (1967) on span of control in the 30 departments of a general hospital are amenable to reanalysis using the model shown in Graph (G2), above. Assuming $\alpha = 7$, and unity of command we can estimate the mean span of control for each organization size using the following equation: $Y = (S_E\text{-}1)/m$. Thus:

S_E (employees in the department)	4	5	6	7	8	9	10	11	12	13	14	15	16	17
m (number of managers)	1	1	1	1	1	2	2	2	2	2	2	2	3	3
Y (expected span of control)	3	4	5	6	7	4	4.5	5	5.5	6	6.5	7	5	5.3

We have translated Bell's data according to the following scheme: High = 3, Medium = 2, Low = 1, and used multiple regression to predict his observed span of control (Y'). The independent variables are our expected span of control (Y). Bell's measures of supervisor's job complexity (Z_1), the subordinates' job complexity (Z_2), and closeness of supervision (Z_3). The results of the stepwise regression are:

$$Y' = +2.42 + .367\ Y - .386\ Z_1 - .345\ Z_2 - .243\ Z_3$$
$$(3.81)\quad(4.07)\quad\ (2.85)\quad\ \ (2.99)\quad\ \ (1.80)$$

$r = .79$, $r^2 = .63$, t values in parentheses, n = 30.

The first variable to enter is our expected span of control (Y), which has a first order correlation of +.52 with observed span of control (Y'). Sixty-three percent of the variance in Bell's data was explained.

9. If the measure of rules (R) is relative to size (i.e. R/S_E), then this is reciprocally related to size as in equation (3), above. As far as we know, no one has shown a strong relationship between the managerial component and the use of rules in the organization.

Assuming:

S_b = the number of beds in the hospital, excluding bassinets
P_d = the number of patient days, excluding new borns, during time period "t"
Adm. = the number of admissions, excluding newborns, during time period "t"

then, the following relationships are true by definition (American Hospital Association, 1965; Colley, 1969):

$$P_d / \text{Adm.} \equiv \text{ALOS average length of stay} \tag{5}$$
$$P_d / t \equiv C \text{ census (usually per day)} \tag{6}$$
$$C / S_b \equiv \phi \text{ occupancy rate} \tag{7}$$

Intensity of care refers to the idea that the same amount of care (as measured by lab tests, operations, therapy, etc.) can be given to the patient over a shorter or a longer period of time. This concept has important implications for average length of stay, staffing ratios, and measures of use of services per patient day. It will be discussed below.

Correlations among Process Variables

Occupancy and average length of stay vary in the following manner (Benjamin and Perkins, 1961):

Assume T is the turnover interval; that is, average time a bed remains vacant between one patient's departure and the next patient's arrival. It can be defined as bed days $(S_b \times t)$ less patient days (P_d) divided by admissions. Thus $T \equiv (S_b \times t - P_d)/\text{Adm}$. For one bed and one patient in a 10-day interval (t = 10), assume the patient stays 7 days (ALOS = 7) and the bed is vacant 3 days (T = 3). Then the occupancy is 70 percent (ϕ = .70). In the general case:

$$(\text{ALOS} + T) \text{ Adm} \equiv S_b \times t. \tag{8}$$

This is to say all the patient stays plus all the turnover intervals account for all the bed days in the hospital in time period t. Dividing through by (ALOS + T) and multiplying by ALOS gives:

$$\text{Adm} \times \text{ALOS} \equiv \frac{S_b \times t \times \text{ALOS}}{\text{ALOS} + T} \tag{9}$$

dividing through by $S_b \times t$ gives:

$$\text{Adm} \times \text{ALOS}/S_b \times t \equiv \text{ALOS}/(\text{ALOS} + T) \tag{10}$$

We know that

$$\text{Adm} \times \text{ALOS} \equiv P_d \tag{5}$$

and

$$P_d / t \equiv C \tag{6}$$

Substituting into equation (10) gives:

$$P_d/S_b \times t = C/S_b = \text{ALOS}/(\text{ALOS} + T) \tag{11}$$

since

$$C/S_b \equiv \phi \qquad (7)$$

then

$$\phi = ALOS/ (ALOS + T) \qquad (12)$$

By invoking ceteris paribus, this is to say that T is a constant. Then, for T equal to any constant greater than zero, the relationship between ALOS and ϕ is curvilinear and asymptotic to $\phi = 1.00$ as is shown below.

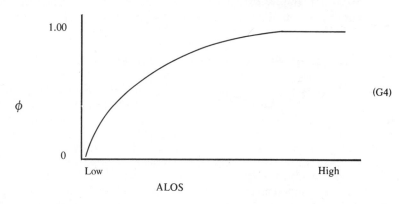

(G4)

It has been argued that T varies with ϕ in that, as ϕ rises, pressure for beds becomes greater and ALOS falls (Roemer, Moustafa, and Hopkins, 1968). On the other hand, M. Feldstein (1967) found that differences in bed availability did not lead to a shorter ALOS in the English hospital districts he examined.

Intensity and average length of stay are inversely related. The "intensity effect" says that exactly the same amount of treatment can be given over a shorter or a longer period of time (Revans, 1964a, 1964b; Deeble, 1965; Hirshleifer, 1962; Neuhauser, 1969). As we shall see, this distinction is vital in explaining the effect of ALOS on costs and man-hours. (The "intensity effect" should be differentiated from the "complexity effect" on ALOS, discussed below.)

Outcome Variables

This category is, of course, of considerable importance because it indicates measurements of the hospital's success in performing the life- and health-saving roles delegated to it by society. Unfortunately we probably know less about outcome and its correlates than is true for any of the other major categories. As Table 1 indicated, we have defined three major types of outcomes including quality of care, hospital efficiency, and satisfaction of patient and hospital personnel.

The literature on the measurement of quality of care is rather extensive: Altman, Anderson, and Barker, 1970; Bynder, 1968; Carroll, 1969; De

Geyndt and Ross, 1968; Denton, 1967; Graham and Paloveck, 1963; Kerr and Trantow, no date; Lipworth, Lee, and Morse, 1963; McNerney, 1962; Maloney, Trussell, and Elinson, 1960; Querido, no date; Roemer 1959, 1968; Roemer, Moustafa, and Hopkins, 1968; Shapiro, 1967; Thompson and Fetter, 1963. Too little work, however, has been done to check the reliability of different measures of quality of care.

Efficiency refers to some ratio of input to output. Efficiency variables include per unit costs, employees per patient day, and man-hours per unit of output (Eldor, 1969). With respect to the latter, staffing ratio is defined as the total number of employees in full time equivalents divided by the daily census, C.

Correlations among Outcome Variables

Because salary costs account for about 60 percent of total hospital costs (American Hospital Association, yearly), it comes as no surprise that per diem costs are positively related to the staffing ratio. This relationship is not perfect, however, because wage rates differ regionally and because employee skill levels change from one hospital to another (Eldor, 1969).

This concludes our discussion of the separate components of the framework shown in Chart 1. We now turn to consider some interrelationships among those components. An examination of the interrelationships of the environment and structure and process variables, and especially of the effects of all these components on outcome, may suggest important implications concerning improved hospital functioning.

Interrelationships of the Components: Findings

Environment and Structure

Large hospitals appear in urban, high per capita income communities; small hospitals appear both in urban and rural areas in the U.S.A. (Los Angeles, especially, has a large number of small hospitals). The existence of both large and small hospitals in urban areas suggests that economic forces do not require that hospitals be of any single ideal size (Shalit, 1968). The absence of large hospitals in rural areas indicates that transportation costs may limit growth (Long and Feldstein, 1967).

Over time, hospitals have been increasing in size and complexity. There remain regional differences, however (Cowan, 1963). In spite of Canada's more diffuse population, resulting in higher travel costs, on the average its hospitals appear to be larger than those in the U.S.a. (American Hospital Association, yearly; Andersen and Hull, 1969).

Environmental characteristics, such as per capita income and urban-rural differences, also define the availability of physicians and the proportion of physicians who are specialists. The availability of physicians in turn influences, and is influenced by, the size and scope of services provided in the local hospitals (Neuhauser, 1970).

The managerial component and formal rules do not appear to be strongly related to environmental characteristics.

Environment and Process

It is widely known that ALOS varies by illness, type of operation performed, complications, sex, and age of the patient (Commission on Professional and Hospital Activities, 1966, 1967, 1969). Once again, the technological requirements for treatment are flexible enough to allow for considerable additional variation (London, 1963; Slee, 1968). Controlling for illness, ALOS varies: (1) by the day of the week the patient was admitted (Lew, 1966; Altman, Anderson and Barker, 1970; London and Sigmond, 1961; London *et al.*, 1961); (2) by the physician treating the patient; (3) by the hospital (Revans, 1964a; Fisher, 1969; Heasman, 1964); (4) by the region in the United States (*Hospital Forum*, 1960); and (5) across countries (Simpson, 1968). For an example of these cross-country differences see Table 3 which compares differences between the U.S.A. and Canada (Andersen and Hull, 1969).

Some have drawn the implication from these differences, based on medical custom, that ALOS could be shortened without being disadvantageous to the patient and that this would save money. Once again the technological requirements may well allow considerable flexibility for medical and social custom.

Another interesting question is why ALOS is consistently longer for all illnesses in Canada than in the U.S.A. (Table 3). If it were purely due to local custom, then one might expect more random differences. This same pattern occurs between the U.S.A. and England (Peterson, 1967; Simpson, 1968), with English ALOS usually being longer.

There is a large body of research in the random arrival theory to explain the demand for services faced by the hospital and, consequently, occupancy rate. The underlying assumption is that requests for admission, and especially requests for maternity and emergency care, fluctuate randomly around a given mean. This will be discussed in more detail in the section "Structure and Process," below.

Occupancy also: (1) varies by day of the week—Saturday and Sunday have the lowest occupancy (London and Sigmond, 1961); (2) is lower on holidays, such as Christmas in the U.S.A.; and (3) varies by the month of the year—in the summer it is low (Hospital Administrative Services, yearly). This picture provides another example of cultural influences on the hospital. A further test would be to see if occupancy differs systematically in other cultures with different religious traditions, such as in Israel and Egypt, with different work weeks, such as in Russia when they had a 6-day work week, and with different climates, such as in southern hemisphere countries.

Environment and Outcome

Costs vary directly with the per capita income of the community the

TABLE 3. AVERAGE LENGTH OF STAY BY DIAGNOSIS IN U.S.A. AND CANADA FOR 1963

Diagnosis	ISC Code	Length of stay (days) U.S.	Canada	Canada as percent of U.S.
ACUTE CONDITION				
Hemorrhoids	461	7.2	9.5	132
Acute resp. infections	470-75	5.2	6.0	115
Pneumonia	490-93	9.3	12.2	131
Bronchitis	500-02	7.1	10.4	146
Tonsils and Adenoids	510	1.7	2.2	129
Ulcer of stomach, duodenum, and jejunum	540-42	10.7	14.5	136
Appendicitis	550-53	6.8	7.9	116
Hernia of abdom. cavity	560-61	7.1	9.4	132
Dis. of gallbladder and pancreas	584-87	11.4	13.9	122
Disorders of menstruation	634	4.0	4.9	123
Complications of pregnancy	640-49	3.1	4.5	145
Abortion	650-52	2.7	4.0	148
Delivery, uncomplicated	660	4.3	5.9	137
Delivery, specified complications	670-78	5.2	8.9	171
Head injury incl. skull fracture	800-04 and 850-56	6.1	7.5	123
Fracture, upper extremity	812-17	6.2	6.2	100
CHRONIC CONDITIONS				
Malignant neoplasm, stomach	151	17.8	27.6	155
Malignant neoplasm, rectum	154	22.0	37.7	171
Malignant neoplasm, breast	170	13.9	28.0	201
Malignant neoplasm, cervix	171	9.1	15.9	175
Malignant neplasm, prostrate	177	13.8	33.4	242
Malignant neoplasm, urinary organs	180-81	12.2	23.5	193
Diabetes mellitus	260	11.3	21.6	191
Cerebrovascular lesions and strokes	330-34	17.1	52.7	308
Inflammatory and other dis. of central nervous system	340-45 and 350-57	10.5	52.7	502
Arteriosclerotic and degenerative heart dis. and other dis. of heart	420-34	15.1	25.4	168
Hypertensive dis.	440-17	10.4	20.3	195
Dis. of arteries	450-56	15.6	48.5	311
Arthritis and rheumatism	720-27	11.2	24.0	214
Symptoms, senility, and ill-defined conditions	780-95	6.1	8.8	144

Source: Andersen and Hull (1969).

hospital is located in (Hayes, 1954, ch. 6; Robinson and MacLeod, 1965 ch. 42; Andersen and Hull, 1969). Further, M. Feldstein found that part of the cost variation in medium-sized acute nonteaching hospitals in Great Britain could be accounted for by case-mix composition.[10] These studies point to the impact that environmental factors can have on outcome measures, apart from differences in management and treatment techniques.

Structure and Process

Using first order correlations, size is positively related to average length of stay and to occupancy (McNerney, 1962; Hayes, 1954; American Hospital Association, yearly). As we shall show, however, these relationships are complicated by other factors.

Differences in ALOS are in part due to differences in *complexity*. This implies that more seriously ill patients requiring more treatment stay longer. This would explain why ALOS increases with the size of general hospitals (American Hospital Association, yearly; Dewdney and Thorne, 1969). (The Netherlands appears to be an exception here.) More seriously ill patients needing more elaborate treatment go to larger hospitals. This is the complexity effect on ALOS.

Occupancy is also positively related to hospital size, but again the relationship is not linear. A good deal of research has been done on the theory of random arrival of patients, coming out of queuing theory and industrial engineering (Blumberg, 1965; Citizens Hospital Study Committee: Northeast Ohio, 1960; Commission on Hospital Care, 1957; Drosness, 1967; Flagle and Young, 1966; London and Sigmond, 1961; London *et al.*, 1961; Long, 1964; Long and Feldstein, 1967; Thompson and Fetter, 1963; Thompson *et al.*, 1968; Young, 1965).

In its simplest form[11] this theory assumes that: (1) admissions to care are random and independent events around a given mean with a Poisson distribution (other distributions have been suggested); (2) hospitals will not wish to turn away too many patients; and (3) because arrivals are random, the census will also be Poisson-distributed. For example, say a hospital wishes to turn away patients no more than 1.4 percent of the time. Since the standard deviation of the Poisson distribution is the square root of the mean, the mean census plus three standard deviations will ensure that 98.6 percent of arriving patients will find an available bed. This results in the following equation, where the constant $K = 3$:

$$S_b = C + K C \qquad (13)$$

---

10. His case-mix measure explained 28 percent of the variance in costs per case but almost none of the variance in costs per day. Since the difference between cost per day and per case reflects ALOS, then perhaps his case-mix measure is explaining ALOS, not costs.

11. Some people will find this description superficial for their purposes, glossing over much theoretical and mathematical detail. However, our concern is to set forth the relationship between ϕ and size as observed across a large number of general hospitals. Given what we are trying to examine, we believe that this description will suffice.

Unlike the previous equations, this is not true by definition but only an approximation. Solving equation (13) for ϕ gives:

$$\phi = C/(C + K\ C) \tag{14}$$

Using $K = 3$, then a 9-bed hospital would have 50 percent occupancy, and a 100-bed hospital would have 77 percent occupancy. Plotting the relationship between ϕ and S_b shows a curve asymptotic to $\phi = 1.00$. Thus:

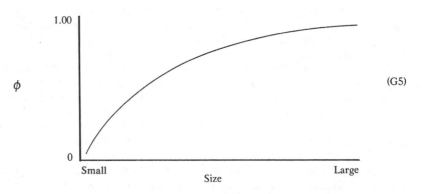

(G5)

The actual relationship between ϕ and S_b for U.S.A. and Australian general hospitals is shown in Chart 2 (American Hospital Association, yearly; Dewdney and Thorne, 1969; Commission on Hospital Care, 1957).[12]

The relationship shown is clearly curvilinear and roughly approximated by Graph (G5). There are a number of reasons why this fit is only approximate. First, the mean level of arrivals and admissions varies by day of the week, month of the year, etc. Second, many patients can queue up and wait in line, which can increase the occupancy rate. This is less true for emergencies and maternity care. For this reason these types of admissions are most frequently analyzed using this technique (Thompson and Fetter, 1963). Even for maternity care the assumptions are not precisely met. In some obstetrics cases, for example, labor may be induced and delivery performed by Caesarian section.

Third, arrivals or admissions are not always independent events; disasters and epidemics do not produce independent arrivals. Fourth, hospitals vary in their willingness to turn away patients, thus varying the value of K in the above equations. Fifth, at least in theory, average length of stay can be shortened to make room for new arrivals. Finally, patients can go to other hospitals if one is full. This is influenced by the availability of other hospitals in the area (travel costs) and by the extent of multiple hospital staff appointments for the admitting physicians. In Australia the isolated nature of many of the hospitals makes this less possible, hence the lower Australian curve in Chart 2.

---

12. To what extent ALOS explains the curve shown in Chart 2 is not known.

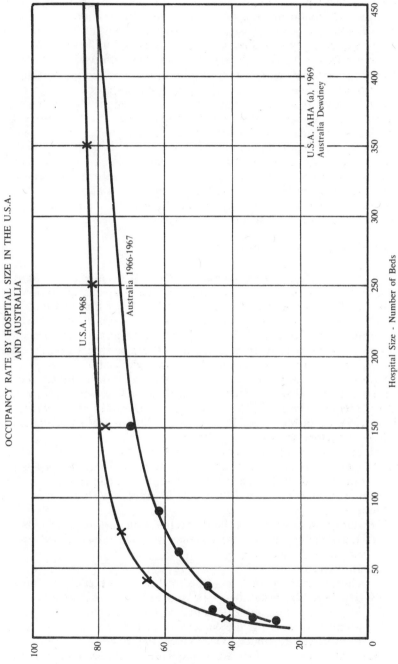

CHART 2

OCCUPANCY RATE BY HOSPITAL SIZE IN THE U.S.A. AND AUSTRALIA

U.S.A. 1968

Australia 1966-1967

U.S.A. AHA (a), 1969
Australia Dewdney

Hospital Size - Number of Beds

Percent Occupancy

In spite of these qualifications, the relationship between occupancy and size is positive and nonlinear, suggesting an important random component to arrivals, admissions, and census. Some part of the results shown in Chart 2 may be explained by ALOS increasing with size and influencing ϕ. Further research needs to be done to separate out these effects.

To the extent that complexity results in the separation of patient units into specialty areas such as medicine, surgery, and obstetrics, a large complex hospital resembles a group of small hospitals. Using the logic of the random arrival theory, we would expect lower occupancy rates in the complex hospital. The use of "swing beds," which are available to more than one service, is an attempt to mitigate this influence. An example is putting gynecological cases in the maternity service. In the same manner, extensive division of labor and departmentalization within the hospital, such as specialized laboratories which face demands for their service that are at least partially random, will lower the proportion of productive time by proportionally magnifying the random fluctuations in demand for services.

Structure and Outcome

Costs and staffing ratios increase with task complexity because it is cheaper not to employ a social worker or provide x-ray therapy than to do so. Note that this is different from Adam Smith's belief that division of labor leads to greater efficiency, because Smith was assuming the task would be performed with or without division of labor. In hospitals many tasks will be performed *only* where there are skilled workers or specialized equipment. Consequently, case costs will increase with complexity.

Without controlling for complexity, costs and staffing ratios appear to decline with size to about fifty beds and then increase with size above fifty beds (American Hospital Association, yearly; Dewdney and Thorne, 1969; Hayes 1954, ch. 6; McNerney 1962, ch. 42). What happens when complexity and other factors are controlled for will be dealt with later.

Unit costs decline up to a point in size and after that they increase with size (diseconomies of scale). The question of economies of scale is: for a constant unit of output, what is the relationship between size and per unit costs? Textbook microeconomic theory (Stigler, 1958) says that this relationship is curvilinear.

The usual reasons why costs should decline with size are (Starbuck, 1965):
1. Individisility—certain inputs come in whole units and are less costly per unit if used to capacity;
2. Bulk transactions—the purchase and sale of products in bulk is cheaper than in small lots (this may have little effect on hospitals);
3. The law of large numbers—in large numbers the demand for service is relatively more stable, thus diminishing the relative random fluctuations and lowering idle capacity which in turn is costly. (This has been discussed under "Occupancy and Size.")

The usual reason given for costs rising with size (diseconomies of scale) is that large organizations become too costly to manage. To quote Stigler: "Decreasing returns to scale arises out of the difficulties in managing a large enterprise. The larger the enterprise, the more extensive and formal its administrative organization must be in order to provide the information necessary for central decisions and the sanctions necessary to enforce these decisions" (Stigler, 1963, p. 155). About the only empirical evidence to support Stigler's belief is the extensive literature on the managerial component. The evidence for hospitals shows that the managerial component declines with size. Thus on theoretical grounds the existence of diseconomies of scale for hospitals is in doubt.

As a matter of fact, Caleb Smith (1955) and Starbuck (1965) in their reviews of this literature say the existence of diseconomies of scale is in doubt for all organizations studied. The extensive literature on economies of scale in hospitals more or less tends to bear this out (Berry, 1965; Carr and Feldstein, 1967; Cohen, 1967; Feldstein, 1961, 1967; Ingbar and Taylor, 1968; Lave, 1966; Long and Feldstein, 1967; Ro, 1966; Shalit, 1968; Wirick, 1963; Yett and Mann, 1968). The results of these studies, however, vary as much as the methodologies employed (Hefty, 1969). In general there appears to be evidence for modest economies of scale up to 200-300 beds and perhaps somewhat beyond 300. Beyond this point size appears to make little difference in costs. Graphically:

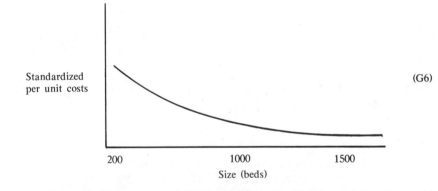

(G6)

What sets the limit on hospital size is probably not overbureaucratization but rather travel costs, i.e. the availability of patients (Long and Feldstein, 1967), the availability of doctors, or a desire on the part of existing staff members to maintain a closed shop. The cost curve shown previously (G6) suggests that one would observe hospitals of different sizes in the same market area remaining competitive with each other over time (Stigler, 1958). This, in fact, appears to be the case (Shalit, 1968).

However, a major problem here is how to standardize the unit of output. A wide variety of techniques have been used. None of these studies, however, has used particularly good controls for the quality of medical care.

Another technique for estimating optimal size is to look at changing market share over time (Eldor, 1969; Stigler, 1958). This approach makes the

Darwinian assumption of survival of the fittest. It assumes that, over time, the optimal size firms will take over a larger and larger share of the market. Data for Chicago from 1945 to 1965 on share of the market for hospital size groups are shown in Table 4. In Chicago small hospitals are declining while the size range 651-1500 beds is growing most rapidly. There is only one hospital in the 1500+ bed category, Cook County Hospital, which has declined in size. To what extent this decline in size is due to diseconomies of scale and to what extent is is due to other factors is debatable. The data seemingly would imply that the optimal size for Chicago hospitals is within the 651-1500 bed range.

TABLE 4. CHANGING SHARE OF THE MARKET FOR CHICAGO HOSPITALS BY SIZE OF THE HOSPITAL 1945 - 1965

Number of Beds	Percent Share of the Chicago Market by Size (Beds)		Absolute Difference	Percent Change
	1945	1965		
0 - 50	.5	.1	-.4	-80
51 - 100	6.7	1.8	-4.9	-73
101 - 150	9.6	7.8	-1.8	-19
151 - 200	14.2	10.4	-3.8	-27
201 - 300	22.4	20.0	-2.4	-11
301 - 650	23.4	27.7	+4.3	+18
651 - 1499	--	17.3	+17.3	--
1500 +	23.2	14.9	-8.3	-36
	100.0	100.0		

Source: American Hospital Association. Annual Guide Issues of *Hospitals*, yearly.

Unfortunately, the literature provides little information on the effects of the managerial component and formal rules on hospital efficiency. This important question is worthy of investigation (Hickson, 1966-67; Peloquin, 1967; Duncan and Neuhauser, 1969).

The evidence is fairly consistent that quality of care is positively related to size and/or complexity. It is generally believed that quality of care is better in the larger teaching hospitals which provide a wide range of services. One interesting finding here is the very high consensus among expert raters of quality of care (Georgopoulos and Mann, 1962; Denton, 1967). This indicates a strong social consensus among physicians as to which hospitals provide a better quality of care.

Relationships between structural variables and outcome measures of attitudes and behavior are generally not well defined (Porter and Lawler, 1969). Except for Revans (1964a, 1964b), who shows a difference in case adjusted ALOS (intensity) and student nurse wastage, there is strikingly little to link the structural-comparative studies with the social-psychological literature on hospitals. According to personal communication with George Wieland, an elaboration of the Revans study was unsuccessful. This casts some doubt on Revans' very unique findings.

Process and Outcome

Day-to-day fluctuations in occupancy, for a given hospital with a given number of beds, are equivalent to moving along the hospital's short-run average cost curve (Stigler, 1963). As is consistent with microeconomic theory, there are ϕ fixed and ϕ variable costs. ϕ variable costs are those which increase with the census, such as meals served and x-rays taken; ϕ fixed costs are those which are incurred regardless of changes in the census, such as personnel and overhead costs. It is widely believed that fixed costs are a large proportion of total costs in hospitals. If this is the case, short-run fluctuations in ϕ will have a marked effect on per patient costs.

As ϕ falls, ϕ fixed costs do not change, but revenue declines. Thus the difference between per diem revenue and per diem costs (called excess revenue or profits) falls.

Using the twelve monthly mean values for all HAS hospitals in 1966 within each of the eight HAS size groups one can plot ϕ against excess revenue. The relationship between ϕ and excess revenue (x) appears to be reciprocal rather than linear. There is no indication from the data that profit falls for very high ϕ as would be suggested by economic theory. The number of beds in the hospital, combined with the hospital's inability totally to control random census fluctuations, appears to set the upper limit on ϕ rather than rising costs. In other words, excess revenue (x) declines as ϕ falls within the observable range.

These correlations between excess revenue (x) and ϕ are shown in Table 5. The 50-74 bed category is excluded because of the poor correlation. These equations can be used to calculate the ϕ break-even point. Note that the break-even ϕ rises with hospital size. Very small hospitals can rarely meet or exceed their break-even ϕ (see Chart 2), and, as a result, they tend to lose money (Neuhauser, 1966) and die out (see Table 4).

As has already been stated, ALOS is influenced by complexity and intensity of care. As complexity increases ALOS increases, per diem costs increase, and per case costs increase even faster.

Intensity of care has a very different effect. For the rest of this section, we will assume constant complexity and constant ϕ. There are intensity-fixed and intensity-variable costs, and these are quite different from ϕ fixed and ϕ variable costs (Neuhauser, 1969; Deeble, 1965). [13]

Increasing ALOS does not increase the number of meals served per patient day nor the depreciation on the building. These are intensity-fixed costs.

---

13. For example, the number of meals served to patients varies directly with ϕ, but the number of meals served to patients does not vary with intensity. Thus meal costs are ϕ variable and ALOS fixed.

TABLE 5. EXCESS REVENUE (x) AND OCCUPANCY (ϕ) FOR HOSPITAL SIZE GROUPS

Number of Beds	Equation	r	p	Break-even point (x=0) (Pct. Occu.)
0 - 49	$x = 25 - \dfrac{18}{\phi}$	-.787	$\angle\ .0005$	70.6
50 - 74		-.412	NS	
75 - 99	$x = 23 - \dfrac{17}{\phi}$	-.708	$\angle\ .005$	75.5
100 - 149	$x = 31 - \dfrac{24}{\phi}$	-.837	$\angle\ .0005$	77.3
150 - 199	$x = 24 - \dfrac{19}{\phi}$	-.737	$\angle\ .005$	79.7
200 - 299	$x = 26 - \dfrac{21}{\phi}$	-.720	$\angle\ .005$	80.9
300 - 399	$x = 44 - \dfrac{37}{\phi}$	-.962	$\angle\ .0005$	82.5
400+	$x = 29 - \dfrac{25}{\phi}$	-.665	$\angle\ .005$	84.9

Source: HAS monthly averages for 1966 for all reporting HAS hospitals. n = 12. The weights in the equations are rounded to the nearest whole number and ϕ is a ratio ranging from 0 to 1.00.

Increasing intensity by shortening ALOS will increase operating room, laboratory, and x-ray use per day. These are intensity variable costs. Changing intensity produces the following results:

High intensity	Low intensity
Short ALOS	Long ALOS
High per diem costs	Low per diem costs
Low per case costs	High per case costs
High staffing ratio	Low staffing ratio.

Accordingly, lowering per diem costs may not be an efficient practice because it results in higher per case costs, and per case costs are what the patient wishes to minimize (Feldstein 1965, 1967). It appears likely that, in the U.S.A., East Coast hospitals are relatively low intensity hospitals and West Coast hospitals are relatively high intensity hospitals (American Hospital Association, yearly).

Future Research

There are other topics of interest and other unanswered problems which we have not been able to cover here. Promising areas for future research include:

1. *Turnover rates across a large number of hospitals.* It appears that there are considerable differences between hospitals and between different types of personnel. It also appears that turnover rates are negatively related to the per capita income of the community.

2. *Striking and unexplained differences in nursing staffing patterns across hospitals.* One Chicago community hospital has 65 RNs and 128 LPNs. A few miles away another similar hospital has 118 RNs and no LPNs. Once again it appears that the demands of medical technology are loose enough to allow considerable leeway here.

3. *Differences between proprietary and nonproprietary hospitals.* The health care field provides a good natural experiment where for-profit and not-for-profit firms compete in the same market (Friedman and Weiner, 1966; Holden, 1966; Johnson, no date; Niskanen, 1968; Bonnett, 1969).

4. *Organizational growth, innovation, and adaptation* (Rosner 1965, 1968; Hymer and Pashigian, 1962; Mayer and Goldenstein, 1961; Mott, 1961; Rosengren, 1968; Seldon, 1968; Boulding, 1953). With respect to growth, there are important differences when growth is measured proprotionately or absolutely. For example, small hospitals probably grow faster proportionally but large hospitals probably grow faster absolutely.

5. *Quality of care.* As discussed above, quality concerns the question: once a patient is admitted to a hospital what type of hospital will provide better care? Another question concerns the effect of the volume of hospital use by a population on the welfare of that population as measured by such things as infant and maternal mortality rates and life expectancy. A good case can be made for saying that, at a given point in time, in industrialized countries, at the margin, say plus or minus 20 percent, the use of hospital care makes no difference on mortality rates and life expectancy once per capita income and educational levels are controlled for. In other words if one were to close down 20 percent of the beds in an area, or increase the number of beds by 20 percent, one would see no noticeable differences in mortality. The lower hospital utilization rates of the prepaid group practice plans support this contention (Anderson and Andersen, to be published).[14] The findings that the use of hospital services is primarily a function of the supply of beds (Feldstein, 1967) rather than a function of morbidity or mortality characteristics of the population is not inconsistent with this hypothesis. Increasing hospital

---

14. It is argued that these plans have lower hospital use because of the provision of extensive preventive care. But a good preventive care program should increase hospital use in the short run through possibly decreasing it in the long run. To show that preventive care makes a difference one would like to see such a phenomenon. A reasonable test of our hypothesis might be to compare a matched group of Christian Scientists with another group whose religion does not discourage the use of hospital services to see which group has the longer life expectancy.

utilization may well increase type two errors (errors of commission) and decrease type one errors (errors of omission). This hypothesis is certainly subject to empirical test and is worthy of study because of its implications for public policy.

6. *There is frequently an enormous leap in the structural-comparative school between theoretical concepts and operational measures.* We have little hope for improving our knowledge if occupancy rate is used as a proxy measure for such widely varying concepts as "organizational slack," "coordination," and "efficiency."

The structural-comparative approach will stand or fall on its ability to explain such socially important issues as hospital costs and quality of care. If some other theoretical or empirical approach can explain a greater percent of the variance in these variables, it would be grounds for rejecting this approach. As of now, the structural-comparative approach is still in the running.

References

This bibliography is not exhaustive, but it covers most of the major works in our area of interest. Many of these works relate to hospitals but some do not. References are annotated using the following symbols or abbreviations, which appear after the reference in parentheses.

Symbol	Meaning
*	empirical data presented
H	about hospitals
T	compares different types of hospitals (ownership, type of patient)
S	about organization size
Cx	about complexity (division of labor, care mix)
a/e	about managerial of administrative ratio (span of control)
alos	about average length of stay
O	about occupancy
emp.	about staffing, staffing ratios
Q	about quality of care
$	about costs, efficiency
R	about rules, controls, specified procedures
env.	about environment
bibl.	includes a bibliography
morale	about morale (turnover, absenteeism, attitudes)
structure	general structural characteristics
growth	about growth, innovation
data	source of raw data on hospitals
census	about average daily census

Adelman, M. A. Measurement of industrial concentration. *Review of Economics and Statistics,* 1951, 169. Reprinted in H. J. Levin, (Ed.) *Business organization and public policy.* New York: Rinehart, 1959 (S)

Aiken, M., and Hage, J. Organizational alienation: a comparative analysis. *American Sociological Review,* 1966, *31,* 497-507 (*, R, morale)

Altman, I., Anderson, A. J., and Barker, K. Methodology in evaluating the quality of medical care: an annotated bibliography 1955-1968. University of Pittsburgh Press, 1970. (H, Q, bibl.)

American Hospital Association. Annual Guide Issues of *Hospitals, JAHA*. Chicago: American Hospital Association, Yearly. (H, data)

American Hospital Association. Management review survey results, for all USA hospitals participating. Chicago: American Hospital Association Periodical (*, H, data)

American Hospital Association. Uniform chart of accounts and definitions for hospitals. Chicago: American Hosptial Association, 1965. (H definitions)

American Medical Association, Department of Economics, Division of Socio-Economic Activities. Distribution of physicians in the U.S. by state, region, district, and county. Chicago, Illinois: American Medical Association, Periodically. (*, data)

American Nurses Association. *Facts about nursing*. New York: American Nurses Association, Periodically. (*, data)

Andersen, R. Factors influencing hospital-use statistics. In *Applications of studies in health administration. Proceedings of the Eighth Annual Symposium on Hospital Affairs*. Chicago: Center for Health Administration Studies, University of Chicago, 1965. (H, env.)

Andersen, R., and Hull, J. T. Hospital utilization and cost trends in Canada and the United States. *Health Services Research*, 1969, *4*, 198-222. (*, H, alos, $, emp.)

Anderson, O. W. Health service systems in the United States and other countries: critical comparisons. *New England Journal of Medicine*, 1963, *269*, 896-900. (*, H, emp., alos.)

Anderson, O. W. and Andersen, R. Patterns of use of health services. In H. Freeman (Ed.) *Handbook of medical sociology* (2nd ed.). Englewood Cliffs N.J.: Prentice-Hall, 1972.

Anderson, O. W., and Neuhauser, D. Rising costs are inherent in modern health care systems. *Hospitals*, 1969, *43*, 50-52. (*, H, $)

Anderson, T., and Warkov, S. Organizational size and functional complexity. *American Sociological Review*, 1961, *26*, 23-28. (*, H, S, a/e, Cx)

Andrews, C. Financial and statistical reports for administrative decision-making in hospitals. Doctoral dissertation, Indiana University, 1968. (*, H, R.)

Baker, A. W., and Davis, R. C. Ratios of staff to line employees and stages of differentiation of staff functions. Reseach monograph 72. Industrial Management Studies, Bureau of Business Research. Columbus: Ohio State University, 1954. (*, a/e, emp., S)

Bell, G. D. Determinants of span of control. *American Journal of Sociology*, 1967, *73*, 100-109. (*, H, S, Cx, a/e, R)

Benjamin, B., and Perkins, T. A. The measurement of bed use and demand. *The Hospital*, 1961, 31-33. (H, alos, O)

Berry, R. E. Competition and efficiency in the market of hospital services: the structure of the American hospital industry. Doctoral dissertation, Harvard University, 1965. (*, H, $, S, Cx)

Blau, P. M. The comparative study of organizations. *Industrial and Labor Relations Review*, 1965, *18*, 323-338.

Blau, P. M. The hierarchy of authority in organizations. *American Journal of Sociology*, 1968, *73*, 453-467. (*, R, structure)

Blau, P. M., Heydebrand, W. V., and Stauffer, R. E. The structure of small bureaucracies. *American Sociological Review*, 1966, *31*, 179-191. (*, S, Cx, a/e, structure)

Blumberg, M. The effects of size and specialism on utilization of urban hospitals. *Hospitals*, 1965, *39*, 43-47. (H, S. O, census, Cx)

Bonnett, P. The proprietary hospital: its past, present, and speculations on its future. Paper presented at the 1969 National Forum on Hospital and Health Affairs, Duke University, May, 1969. (Mimeographed.) (*, H, T)

Boulding, K. E. Toward a general theory of growth. *Canadian Journal of Economics and Political Science*, 1953, *19*, 326-340. (S, growth)

Bynder, H. Doctors as patients: a study of the medical care of physicians and their families. *Medical Care*, 1968, *6*, 157-167. (*, H, Q)

Caplow, T. Organizational size. *Aministrative Science Quarterly*, 1957, *1*, 484-505. (S)

Carr, J. W., and Feldstein, P. J. The relationship of cost to hospital size. *Inquiry*, 1967, *4*, 45-65.

(*, H, $, S)

Carroll, J. The structure of teaching hospitals. Doctoral dissertation, Department of Sociology, University of Chicago, 1969. (*, H, a/e, O, Q, S)

Citizens Hospital Study Committee: Northeast Ohio. Questions on hospital utilization and costs: special studies. *Hospitals and their use in northeast Ohio 1960*, Part XIII, 1960. (*, H, O, S, census)

Cohen, H. A. Variations in cost among hospitals of different sizes. *The Southern Economic Journal*, 1967, *33*, 355-366. (H, S, $)

Colley, D. G. A more precise formula for 'average length of stay'. *Hospital Management*, 1969, *108*, 28 (*, H, alos)

Commission on Hospital Care. *Hospital care in the United States*. Cambridge: Harvard University Press, 1957. (*, H, O, S, T)

Commission on Professional and Hospital Activities. How much longer do patients stay in major teaching hospitals? *The Record*, 1969, *7*. (*, H, alos, S)

Commission on Professional and Hospital Activities. Length of stay: Friday and Saturday admissions to surgery. *The Record*, 1967, *5*. (*, H, alos, S)

Commission on Professional and Hospital Activities. *Length of stay in short term general hospitals*. New York: McGraw-Hill, 1966. (*, H, alos.)

Cowan, P. The size of hospitals. *Medical Care*, 1963, *1*, 1-9. (*, H, S)

Deeble, J. S. An economic analysis of hospital costs. *Medical Care*, 1965, *3*, 138-146. (*, H, alos, $)

DeGeyndt, W., and Ross, K. B. Evaluation of health programs: an annotated bibliography. Systems Development Project, Minneapolis, Minn., 1968. (mimeographed.) (H, Q, bibl.)

Delbecq, A. L. The world within the "span of control." *Business Horizons*. Bloomington: Graduate School of Business, Indiana University, 1968. (R, a/e, bibl.)

Denton, J. C., *et al.* Predicting judged quality of patient care in general hospitals. *Health Services Research*, 1967, *2*, 26-33. (*, H, S, Q)

Dewdney, J. C. H., and Thorne, J., *Australian short stay public hospitals 1966-67*. Australian Studies in Health Service Administration, No. 8, School of Hospital Administration, University of New South Wales, 1969. (*, H, S, emp, Cx, $)

Drosness, D. L., *et al.* Uses of daily census data in determining efficiency of units. *Hospitals*, 1967, *41*, 45+. (*, H, O, $, census)

Duncan, O. D. Size and structure of organizations: manufacturing establishments. Unpublished paper. (No date). (*, S, a/e)

Duncan, S. F., and Neuhauser, D. The hospital administrator with a Master's degree in hospital administration: does he do a better job? *Program Notes*, AUPHA* 1969, No. 22. (*, $, R)

Eldor, D. An empirical investigation of hospital output, input and productivity. Doctoral dissertation, Department of Economics, New York University, 1969. (*, H, emp.)

Fayol, H. *General and industrial management*. London: Pitman, 1967.

Fearon, H. Inventory management: survey and analysis of current practice in 55 hospitals. *Hospital Progress*, 1969, *50*, 84. (*, H, R, S)

Feldstein, M. S. *Economic analysis for health service efficiency*. Amsterdam: North Holland Publishing, 1967. (*, H, S, Cx, $, alos.)

Feldstein, M. S. Hospial cost variation and case mix differences. *Medical Care*, 1965, *3*, 95-103. (*, H, Cx, $)

Feldstein, P. J. An empirical investigation of the marginal cost of hospital services. Graduate Program in Hospital Administration Research Series, University of Chicago, 1961. (*, H, $, S)

Fisher, D. H. A national comparison of length of stay between federal short term general hospitals and non-federal short term general hospitals. Iowa City: University of Iowa, 1969. (University Microfilms #HE1125.) (H, alos., T)

Flagle, C. D., and Young, J. P. Application of operations research and industrial engineering to problems of health services, hospitals and public health. *Journal of Industrial Engineering*, 1966, *17*, 609. (H, bibl.)

Friedman, J. W., and Weiner, T. A small proprietary hospital closes its doors. *Hospitals*, 1966, *40*, 46-51. (H, S)

Georgopoulos, B. S., and Mann, F. C. *The community general hospital*. New York: The Macmillan Co., 1962. (*, H, Q, R)

Gouldner, A. W. Organizational analysis. In R. K. Merton, L. Broom, and L. S. Cattrell (Eds.) *Sociology today.* New York; Basic Books, 1959.

Graham, J. B. and Palovcek, F. Where should cancer of the cervix be treated: a preliminary report. *American Journal of Obstetrics and Gynecology,* 1963, *87,* 405-409. (*, H, S, Q)

Hage, J. An axiomatic theory or organizations. *Administrative Science Quarterly,* 1965, *10,* 289-320. (S, Cx, O)

Haire, M. Biological models and empirical histories of the growth of organizations. *Modern Organization Theory,* Chapter 10. New York: John Wiley & Sons, 1959. (*, S, a/e, growth)

Hanson, R. C. Administrator responsibility in large and small hospitals in a metropolitan community, *Journal of Health and Human Behavior,* 1961, *2,* 199-204. (H, R, S)

Hayes, J. H. *Financing hospital care in the U.S..* Vol. I of *Factors affecting the costs of hospital care.* 3 vols. New York: Blakiston, 1954. (*, H, $, S, O, alos.)

Heasman, M. A. How long in hospital? A study in variation in duration of stay for two common surgical conditions. *Lancet,* (Sept. 12, 1964), 539-541. (*, H, alos.)

Hefty, T. R. Returns to scale in hospitals: a critical review of recent research. *Health Services Research,* 1969, *4,* 267-280. (H, $, S, bibl.)

Heydebrand, W. Bureaucracy in hospitals. Doctoral dissertation, Department of Sociology, University of Chicago, 1965. (*, H, S, Cx, a/e, T)

Heydebrand, W. Bureaucracy in hospitals: an analysis of division of labor and coordination in organizations. Unpublished paper, University of Chicago, no date. (Mimeographed.) (*, H, S. Cx, a/e, T)

Hickson, D. J. A convergence in organization theory *Administrative Science Quarterly,* 1966-67, *11.* 224-237. (R, bibl.)

Hirshleifer, J. The firm's cost function: a successful reconstruction. *The Journal of Business,* 1962, *35,* 235-255. (S, alos., $, Volume of production, rate of output.)

Holden, H. The case for doctor-owned hospitals. *Medical Economics,* 1966, *43,* 240-245. (H)

"Hospital Administrative Services." Special comparison, national size groups. Chicago, Illinois: American Hospital Association, Yearly (Mimeographed.) (*, H, emp., $, S, data)

"Hospital Administrative Services." Special regional comparison. Chicago, Illinois: American Hospital Association, Yearly. (Mimeographed.) (*, H, emp., $, S, data)

"Hospital Administrative Services." "Spotlight" series. Chicago, Illinois: American Hospital Association, Periodical. (Mimeographed.) (*, H, $, S, emp.)

Hospital Forum. Pentagon compares hospital stays. *Hospital Forum,* 1960, *3,* 40. (*, H. alos.)

Hymer, S., and Pashigian, P. Firm size and rate of growth. *Journal of Political Economy,* 1962, *70,* 555-569. (*, S, growth)

Indik, B. P. The relationship between organization size and supervision ratio. *Administrative Science Quarterly,* 1964, *9,* 301-312. (*, S, a/e)

Ingbar, M. L., and Taylor, L. D. *Hospital costs in Massachusetts.* Massachusetts: Harvard University Press, 1968. (*, H, $, S)

Johnson, R. L. Capital financing of proprietary hospitals. Unpublished paper, no date. (Mimeographed.) (*, H, $, alos, O, S)

Kerr, M., and Trantow, D. J. Defining, measuring and assessing the quality of health services: an annotated bibliography. Minneapolis, Minnesota: Institute for Interdisciplinary Studies, American Rehabilitation Foundation, no date. (Mimeographed.) (H, Q, bibl.)

Lave, J. R. A review of the methods used to study hospital costs. *Inquiry,* 1966, *3,* 57-81. (H, $)

Lew, I. Day of the week and other variables affecting hospital admissions, discharges, and length of stay for patients in the Pittsburgh area. *Inquiry,* 1966, *3,* 3-39. (*, H, alos.)

Lindenfeld, F. Does administrative staff grow as fast as organizations? *School Life,* 1961, *43,* 20-23. (*, S, a/e)

Lipworth, L., Lee, J. A. H., and Morse, J. N. Case fatality in teaching and nonteaching hospitals. *Medical Care,* 1963, *1,* 71. (*, H, Q, S)

London M. Variations in postoperative stay among appendectomy patients. *Hospital Management,* 1963, *96,* 45-57. (*, H, alos)

London, M., and Sigmond, R. M. How weekends and holidays affect occupancy. *Modern Hospital,* 1961, *97,* 79-83. (*, H, O)

London, M., *et al.* Small specialized bed units lower occupancy. *Modern Hospital,* 1961, *96,* 95-100. (*, H, S, O, census)

Long, M. F. Efficient use of hospitals. In *The economics of health and medical care. Proceedings of the Conference of the Economics of Health and Medical Care,* University of Michigan, 1962. Michigan: Bureau of Public Health Economics and Department of Economics, University of Michigan, 1964. (H, S, O, census)

Long, M. F., and Feldstein, P. Economics of hospital systems: peak loads and regional coordination. *American Economic Review,* 1967, *57,* 119-129. (*, H, env., S, census, $)

McNerney, W., and study staff. *Hospital and medical economics.* Chicago:. Hospital Research and Educational Trust, 1962. (*, H, R. S. Q, $)

Maloney, M. C., Trussell, R. E., and Elinson, J. Physicians choose medical care: a sociometric approach to quality appraisal. *American Journal of Public Health,* 1960, *50,* 1678-1686. (*, H, Q, S)

Mayer, K. B., and Goldstein, S. *The first two years: problems of small firm growth and survival.* Small Business Research Series No. 2, Small Business Administration. Washington, D.C.: Government Printing Office, 1961. (S, growth, bibl.)

Melman, S. The rise of administrative overhead. *Oxford Economics Papers,* 1951, *3,* 69-102, (*, S, growth, a/e)

Meyer, M. W. Expertness and the span of control. *American Sociological Review,* 1968, *33,* 944-951. (*, R)

Ministry of Health, National Health Service. *Hospital costing returns.* London: Her Majesty's Stationery Office, Yearly (*, H, data, S, alos, $, O)

Mott, P. E. Sources of adaptation and flexibility in large organizations. Doctoral dissertation. University of Michigan, Department of Sociology, 1961. (*, H, Growth)

National Center for Health Statistics. *Infant Loss in the Netherlands,* Series 3, No. 11, 1968. USPHS, Department of Health, Education, and Welfare, Washington, D.C.

Neuhauser, D. Average length of stay and hospital staffing ratios. *Abstracts of hospital management studies,* 1969, *4,* 34-35. (Mimeographed.) (University Microfilm #NU1166). (*, H, emp., $, alos., Cx)

Neuhauser, D. Hospital size and structure. *Hospital size and efficiency. Proceedings of the Ninth Annual Symposium on Hospital Affairs.* Center for Health Administration Studies, University of Chicago, 1966. (*, H, env., S, growth, Cx, $, a/e, O, R)

Neuhauser, D. Evidence for change: the urban community hospital and its environment. *The Urban hospital in transition. Proceedings of the 13th Annual Symposium on Hospital Affairs.* Center for Health Administration Studies, University of Chicago, 1970. (To be published.) (*, H, Env., S, $)

Niskanen, W. A. Non market decision making: the peculiar economics of bureaucracy. *American Economic Review,* 1968, *58,* 293-305. ($, T)

Peloquin, R. J. Hospital organization: span of control. Unpublished paper, University of Chicago, 1967. (*, H, S, $, R)

Pennel, E. H., *et al. Business census of hospitals 1935.* Public Health Reports, Supplement No. 154, p. 32, Table 27. Washington, D.C.: Government Printing Office, 1939. (*, H, data, a/e, S)

Peterson, O. L., *et al.* What is value for money in medical care? *Lancet,* 1967, no. 7493, 771-776. (*, H, alos)

Pondy, L. R. Effects of size, complexity and ownership on administrative intensity. *Administrative Science Quarterly,* 1969, *14,* 47-61. (*, S, Cx, a/e, $, bibl.)

Porter, L., and Lawler, E. Properties of organization structure in relation to job attitudes and job behavior. In L. L. Cummings and W. E. Scott (Eds.) *Organization behavior and human performance.* Illinois: Richard D. Irwin, 1969. (a/e, morale, S, structure, bibl.)

Querido, A. *The efficiency of medical care.* Leiden, Holland: H. E. Stenfert Kroese N. V. (*, H, Q)

Revans, R. W. *Morale and effectiveness of general hospitals: problems and progress in medical care.* England: Oxford University Press, 1964a. (*, H, morale, alos.)

Revans, R. W. *Standards for morale: cause and effect in hospitals.* England: Oxford University press, 1964b. (*, H, morale, alos.)

Ro, K.K. A statistical study of factors affecting the unit cost of short term hospital care. Doctoral dissertation, Yale University, 1966 (Mimeographed.) (*, H, $, S)

Robinson, G. J., and MacLeod, L. An analysis of costs in thirty-five short term general hospitals in Connecticut. Connecticut: Yale University, 1965. (Mimeographed.) (*, H, $)

Roemer, M. I. Is surgery safer in larger hospitals? *Hospital Management*, 1959, *87*, 35 (H, S, Q)
Bureau of Economic Research. New Jersey: Princeton University Press, 1955. (S)
death rates adjusted for case severity. *Health Services Research*, 1968, *3*, 96-118. (*, H, Q, alos, Cx)

Roemer, M. I., Moustafa, A. T., and Hopkins, C. E. Hospital death rates as a quality index. *Hospitals*, 1968, *42*, 43. (*, H, Q, alos.)

Rosenbluth, G. Measures of concentration. *Business concentration and price policy*. National Bureau of Economic Research. New Jersey: Princeton Universeity Press, 1955. (S)

Rosner, M. M. An analysis of organizational influences on hospital adoption of new drugs. Doctoral dissertation, University of Chicago, 1965. (*, H, R, growth)

Rosener, M. M. An analysis of organizational influences on hospital adoption of new drugs. Unpublished Ph.D. dissertation, University of Chicago, 1965. (*, H, R, growth)

Rosner, M. M. Economic determinants of organizational innovation. *Administrative Science Quarterly*, 1968, *12*, 614-625. (*, H, growth)

Rushing, W. A. Organizational size and administration: the problems of causal homogeneity and a heterogeneous category. *Pacific Sociological Review*, 1966, *9*, 100-108. (*, S, a/e)

Rushing, W. A. Two patterns of industrial administration. *Human Organization*, 1967, *26*, 32-39. (*, S, a/e)

Saathoff, D. E., and Kurtz, R. A. What administrators of small hospitals do. *Modern Hospital*, 1962, *99*, 85. (*, H, R, S)

St. Louis University. Curriculum study: Graduate program in hospital administration, St. Louis University, 2nd year report. St. Louis, Mo., 1967. (Mimoegraphed.) (*, H, R, S)

Seldon, J. B. A national survey of the acceptance of progressive techniques by hospitals. Unpublished Master's thesis, University of Iowa, 1968. (University Microfilm #AB0022.) (*, H, growth, S, R.)

Shalit, S. Barriers to entry in the American hospital industry. Unpublished paper, Graduate School of Business, University of Chicago, 1968. (Mimeographed.) (*, H, S, $)

Shapiro, S. End result measurements of quality of medical care. *Milbank Memorial Fund Quarterly*, 1967, *45*, 127-150. (H, Q)

Simpson, J., *et al. Custom and practice in medical care*. England: Oxford University Press, 1968. (*, H, alos.)

Slee, V. N. Uniform methods of measuring utilization. *Utilization review*, Illinois: American Medical Association, Council on Medical Service, Committee on Medical Facilities, 1968. (*, H, alos.)

Smith, C. A. Survey of the empirical evidence on economics of scale. *Business concentration and price policy*, National Bureau of Economic Research. New Jersey: Princeton University Press, 1955. ($, S)

Starbuck, W. H. Organizational growth and development. In J. March (Ed.) *Handbook of organizations*. Chicago, Illinois: Rand McNalley & Co., 1965. (S, growth, a/e, $, bibl.)

Starkweather, D. B. Hospital size, complexity, and formalization. University of California, Berkeley, 1970 (Mimeographed.) (*, H, S, Cx, R)

Stigler, G. The economies of scale. *Journal of Law and Economics*, 1958, *1*, 54-71. (*, $, S)

Stigler, G. *The theory of price*. New York: The Macmillan Co., 1963.

Terrien, F. T., and Mills, D. C. The effects of changing size on the internal structure of the organization. *American Sociological Review*, 1955, *20*, 11-13. (*, S, a/e)

Thompson, J. D. and Fetter, R. B. The economics of the maternity service. *Yale Journal of Biology and Medicine*, 1963, *36*, 91-103. (H, O)

Thompson, J. D., *et al.* End-result measurements of the quality of obstetrical care in two U.S. Air Force hospitals. *Medical Care*, 1968, *6*, 131-143. (*, H, Q)

Weber, M. *The theory of social and economic organization*. Glencoe, Ill.: The Free Press, 1947.

Whisler, T. Measuring centralization of control in business organizations. In W. W. Cooper, H. J. Leavitt, and M. W. Shelly (Eds.) *New perspectives in organization research*. New York: John Wiley & Sons, 1964. (*, R)

Whisler, T., *et al*. Centralization of organization control. *The Journal of Business*, 1967, *40*, 10-26. (*, R)

Wieland, G. F. Complexity and coordination in organizations. Doctoral dissertation, University of Michigan, 1965. (*, H, S, Cx, R)

Wirick, G. C., Jr. An econometric analysis of the cost of hospital care in the Buffalo, New York area. Michigan Bureau of Hospital Administration, University of Michigan, Unpublished paper, 1963. (*, H, $)

Woodward J. *Industrial organization: theory and practice*. London: Oxford University Press, 1965. (*, S, Cx, a/e, structure)

Yates, W. L. An analysis of selected personnel policies and practices in North Carolina general hospitals with 100 beds. The Duke Endowment, 1964. (Mimeographed.) (*, H, R)

Yett, D. E., and Mann, J. An analysis of hospital costs: a review article. *The Journal of Business*, 1968, *41*, 191-202. (H, S, $, bibl.)

Young, J. P. Stabilization of inpatient bed occupancy through control of admissions. *Hospitals*, 1965, *39*, 41-48. (H, O)

5

ISSUES AND DISCUSSION
OF PART TWO

The Social Control of Hospitals

Presentation Highlights: M. N. Zald

What I want to do is briefly to talk about a particular framework for the study of the social control of institutions, about the major elements of this framework, and about the goals of our approach. Then, I will briefly summarize selected findings from a study that Mrs. Hair and I have been conducting within this framework for the last two and a half years or so.

The problem in this area is that we do not have, either in sociology or in the other social sciences, a comprehensive approach to how organizations are controlled. How do organizations such as hospitals get rid of bad performance? How are norms set for organizations? How do you get rid of bad school systems, or do you? How does a society establish criteria for performance, and how does it develop moral exemplars and criteria for laggards—the criteria of deviance at the institutional level? We clearly have knowledge on these matters at the individual level. To most of us who have worked in organizations of one kind or another, it is clear that a major part of the society is conducted through large-scale organizations. Yet we do not really study (sociologists have tended to ignore) how society or the community impacts on organizations to establish their norms or constrain their functioning.

Your rejoinder may be: "Well, what is economics all about?" Certainly, the theory of the competitive market is a theory of social control. However, no one would argue that the market phenomenon (at least not the clientele market) is the major determinant of constraint on hospitals. Labor markets are a much more important constraint on the performance levels of hospitals. In the case of hospitals, labor involves questions about the norms of professionals: what will the professionals support and what they will not support in establishing the input markets for hospitals, or where will they commit their labor and where they will not commit their labor?

Similar questions immediately come up if you are talking about universities. The major constraint on universities is clearly not the market of students. To some extent this is a constraint, and it is a determinant. But such things as the accrediting agencies and governmental regulating agencies are very important determinants of control. Yet in sociological theory and in social science in general, there is no comprehensive framework that encompasses all major sources of control. Everybody goes his own way. You may have an economist studying markets, a lawyer studying regulatory agencies, and a political scientist studying state legislatures, but it seems that very few people try to study and understand how all of these interact to determine the performance level of institutions. This is our goal.

At this point, we do not have a theory of social control of institutions. Yet we will be able here to develop subpropositions for specific institutional arenas, and for certain specific concepts we will be able to develop propositions—indeed, a fairly dense network of propositions. At least we will be able to, on the one hand, block in some concepts and propositions and, on the other hand, point to lines of research that have been missed because they seemed to have fallen into the interstices between feilds.

What are some of the main points in this area? First, there are five or six key conceptual domains or conceptual areas of concern. One is *sanctions*.

Any theory of social control has to look at sanctions. The important thing about sanctions, however, that seems to me to be missed in much of the literature, is that every sanction is two-headed in the sense that it has a value both for the specific object or organization being sanctioned, rewarded or punished (I use sanctioned in the sense of both negative and positive rewards), and for what everybody else is doing in that kind of organization. Whenever you sanction a hospital and somebody knows that, then other hospitals say: "We had better avoid that condition." Whenever a liability suit or tort suit is brought against a doctor, other doctors say: "We had better watch out on that score." It means that they know about it. If you are calculating the costs of sanctioning organizations such as hospitals and are talking about taking away the accreditation of a hospital, it may be that the calculus of the sanction not only involves whether you want to punish that particular hospital, but also how everybody else is going to view it. Is it going to have a positive spillover for the performance of other hospitals?

In other words, sanctioning an organization is not like a father punishing his son, in which case he is doing it just to get the son in line. This is how most of our theory of deviance looks at a sanction if you keep the individual in mind. But at the institutional level a sanction is aimed at changing both the performance of the particular organization being sanctioned and also the performance of everybody else in the arena. This becomes a key issue when dealing with highly symbolic sanctions. Accreditation, for example, is clearly and mainly a symbolic sanction.

Another line that we have been exploring is the *performance curve*, or normative curve. How do different norms vary in their tolerance? What is the society's or the community's willingness to tolerate deviance? How sloppy can an organization be, one might ask? What range of performance standards will be allowed? Perhaps a hospital might allow much greater variation in standards of nursing care in general medical wards, for example, than in the operating room. By and large the risks and cost of violation of a tolerance norm are related to how tight the performance curve and standards are.

I doubt very much that any rural 30-bed hospital is going to try open-heart surgery. They are going to rule themselves out of the game. In short, there is an interaction between the performance curve and what different people and professionals will try to do. Professionals are often quite conscious in this respect. When they say "That is not in our league, we could not attempt that," they are making a normative statement, a statement about their capabilities for performing in some areas but not in others. A small study I did of a hospital made it quite clear the urologist felt that the general surgeons in the hospital were not recognizing his specialization and were going in on cases that they should have been referring to him. This happens all the time. It happens more, I suspect, in cases where the professional controls over the hospital are lower. In any event, another key question is where and how do the norms get defined, and what is the toleration level?

A third kind of concern that we have is with the sociology of the *control agents*. One part of the study that we are presenting today is an historical analysis largely of the development of the Joint Commission on Accreditation of Hospitals, and how it grew out of the College of Surgeons. We are interested in this kind of thing because the control agent becomes the key funnel for the societal norm definition. He becomes the keeper of the sanctions. What determines how strong his sanctions are? What is the interaction process with the objects being controlled in the hospital matrix—the hospitals, the professions, and the society? Is hospital accreditation strictly a professional operation? Is there any relationship to the society? Are there no serious external (outside of the professional arena) forces impinging upon the Commission?

An example from a different arena is also instructive. In our study of the growth of the accrediting agencies for colleges it became clear that they were partly a defensive organization. At the turn of the last century educators were saying about the creation of the College Accreditation Agency, "If we do not do this, the government will move in," and "If we do not do this, we will get like the European system." In the American context of emphasis upon private enterprise, antifederalism, and antinational government (which goes back clearly to the Revolution) this was seen as a bad thing. The reasoning of those involved was, "We'll set up an organization to control ourselves to avoid federal intervention." This has always been an underlying theme in the whole social control arena. The entire independent regulatory agency structure, many political scientists who study these things say, was a massive mistake because what it essentially did was destroy the needed potential for fine-tuning adjustments to the changing political scene or the changing demands of society. Yet at the time the independent agencies were set up, this was a way of protecting them from the society, from the political executive; it was an insulating move. In order to understand it you have to go into the sociology of the accrediting agencies and control agents.

A fourth aspect that we look at has to do with the *characteristics of the objects being regulated or controlled*. If everybody wants the rule that a control agent is attempting to enforce, then there are not many problems. If the hospital is already performing at the level that the commission on accreditation wants it to perform, then there is no problem. All you have to do is to state the rule, and they say "Yes, that is a good idea." There are no costs to it. If you get into this area at all, you soon find that it is the compliance readiness characteristics of the target population or organization which become a key factor.

The last general concept in our research framework is *structural context*. This provides a way of getting us into the possibilities of total control of institutions when dealing with a strong hierarchical system rather than a pure market.

Let me now turn to some substantive findings. First, when you are interested in social control, you are obviously interested in social change at the same time. Virtually the only way that you can begin to understand social control is to see what norms are developing and how the context of the organization has changed, and why, and then try to unravel this and look at new norms developing. In the first section of our paper we talk about changing technology, just to get a feel for this as an indication of what would be expected of a hospital. There are very few studies that really cover this; there are good historical studies of changing medical technology, but we do not really know the adoption rates of hospitals. When does a hospital, for example, move into a new kind of surgical suite? When does it move into a new kind of blood bank? Wolf Heydebrand's thesis tends to move in this direction. He managed to get data for 1935 and 1960 and chart out the spread of technological change in hospitals.

Technological change places constraints on the captial budget of organizations. Accordingly, there is an interpenetration between changing medical standards, and what a good hospital has, and the ownership capital matrix of the organization. You start getting a changing distribution along with the federal tax policy, and you start getting pressures for different size hospitals because only certain size hospitals can support certain kinds of facilities. This is fairly straight forward and I will not sell it to you as a startling breakthrough.

Let me turn to where we have dug in more. Our own substantive work on the social control of hospitals has focused on three pieces: (1) the evolution of hospital law; (2) the evolution of the College of Surgeons into the Joint Commission on Accreditation of Hospitals, and the sociological history of the evolution of medical standards as they apply to hospitals; and (3) the changing rates of accreditation and the factors associated with those changing rates—the socioeconomic and organizational factors related to each hospital that account for its level of accreditation.

There are some very interesting general points in the sociology of law that I will not cover in any detail. I will summarize only a few basic findings. The first key point with regard to the evolution of hospital law is that for a variety of reasons the courts wanted to exempt hospitals from suit. I say "wanted" because the law and the basis upon which it first started exempting hospitals from suit provide no adequate explanation. The American law was based upon an English case that a few years later was found to be a bad decision. The courts in England reversed their earlier decision exempting hospital charitable trusts from liability suits for tort cases. Yet this principle spread rapidly in the United States. Therefore, it cannot be argued that it was inherent in the law that hospitals be exempted from liability suits. Instead one must ask something about the nature of hospitals in the United States. I suspect that a lot of judges were on the boards of hospitals, and the friendliness of judges may account for this phenomenon. It is much like the treatment of a licensing case where the values of the judges become a key determinant.

But from our point of view the key thing in this area is the clear trend in hospital law to eliminate the distinction between "administrative" and "medical," as in the *Darling* case. However, other things may be actually more important both in the *Darling* case and in the change since then. It may be more important that the courts, when they started looking for what kind of criterion to apply, have said that the criterion of local custom is not sufficient. For a long time, the level of care, i.e. the normative level, was based not upon what the medical profession and good hospital administrators would say ought to be, but upon what was prevalent in the local community. This is no longer the case. The law has changed as we have developed national norms. The movement to say that an expert witness could be brought in from outside the city is part of the development of a national norm system for the law and for the hospitals.

The other important point in the evolution of hospital law is the recognition of the standards of private agencies, e.g. accrediting agencies, as one potential definer of norms. Such agencies typically claim such things as: "We are a private organization"; "We are not legal"; "We do not have any standing at law"; "We are just a group of your peers in the profession attempting to establish good standards." Every profession tries the self-regulation approach when setting norms for peers. The sanctions of peers, however, take on more meaning than implied by self-regulation if they control some key resource. One such resource may be medical education and intern programs. If a hospital does not have an intern program, accreditation might mean very little in this connection. But it begins to mean something when a hospital goes into court and the judge asks: "Are you in conformance with the policies of the Joint Commission on Accreditation?" In this case, accreditation obviously has a lot of meaning, and the state law and licensing acts, along with the standards of a private agency, now get introduced as normative standards whereas earlier only the local community norms were invoked.

Some of the most interesting aspects of our study, from the point of view of an organizational analyst at least, are those on the evolution of the Joint Commission on Accreditation of Hospitals out of the College of Surgeons. The fighting within the professions about this development, the resistance to control, and the opposition to setting up such a normative agency, are all well documented. We have spared you these details in our short paper. Let me just comment, however, on the statistics related to accreditation.

The problems of data reduction here are terrible because we are working with a yes/no value on the dependent variable—accreditated or nonaccreditated. Consequently, even though we present correlation coefficients and get a systematic pattern from the data, we do not interpret the correlations in terms of percentage of variance accounted for. The statistical assumptions are a bit sloppy here. But the key points are, I think, very interesting. For example, the data show that the number of facilities in the hospital is the major correlate of accreditation. There is an interesting contradiction here. Theoretically, the hospitals which are the most easily accredited by Commission standards are those which have the fewest facilities, because the standards emphasize "how well you coordinate what you have" as the major criterion. More facilities, it is reasonable to expect, would lead to more problems in coordination. Yet it is clear that hospitals which have more and more of the advanced facilities also have higher rates of accreditation. I suspect this means that they are attracting a kind of staff which insists upon professionalism.

There is an interplay then between having up-to-date facilities, the variety and quality of staff that a hospital is able to attract and hold, and staff involvement in the management of the hospital, on the one hand, and accreditation, on the other. All of these together seem to determine accreditation. The Commission, I think, has about sixteen doctors who go to the hospitals for accreditation site visits. We have looked at their questionnaire and have interviewed individuals associated with the Commission, but we have not talked to the person who has to do the fundamental evaluation in terms of how he knows when the coordination level is adequate. The fact that our findings go the way they do suggests that if this person is not being faked out by sheer number of facilities (and this is a possibility), then professionalism (the quality of staff and commitment to professional definition) becomes a key intervening process behind our correlations.

Clearly, as all of you know, urbanization and the factors related to urbanization are fundamental aspects to consider in relation to accreditation. In any work that we do, it is quite clear that we have to control for two or more such variables. Two particular variables that should be used as major independent variables when studying accreditation would be hospital organization and hospital size, but it is no easy task to control for these variables.

Discussion

Comment: One of your tables shows something about proprietary hospitals and accreditation. Similar tables for a later year, 1966, showed practically no difference between proprietary and nonproprietary on percent of hospitals accredited when size is controlled for regarding proprietary and nonproprietary institutions.

Zald: Yes, proprietaries have move up.

Question: Are proprietary hospitals sluggish in adapting?

Zald: They were, probably because they had no real reason to be at earlier points. That is, if you did not have an intern program, and most proprietary hospitals were relatively small (you know, four or five doctors at most was sometimes a fairly large staffing pattern), there was really very little motivation to seek accreditation. Our argument would be that change in the courts stimulated the accreditation movement (sometimes this is a very difficult problem—you have to be accredited in order to be funded or to be in the good graces of third paties such as the courts or the insurance groups). Some people will say you do have to be accredited. We have surveyed every Blue Cross program in the country, however, and sometimes they do not even know themselves whether they expect that from the hospitals that they are funding.

Our general assumption is that, more and more, accreditation has become a kind of baseline. At some point it just became important to be accredited, and all hospitals moved toward it. Incidently, this is exactly what we find and, as a result, accreditation loses some of its strength. When everybody gets above the norm, then a new normative process is going on. This same kind of process, incidently, applies to colleges. If you looked at the history of colleges from 1900 to 1960, around 1920 or 1930 about 40 percent of the colleges would have been accredited, whereas in the North Central Association today roughly 90 percent would be accredited. Here too you see this movement toward accreditation. Large colleges got accredited first, and then the movement spread throughout.

Question: Do you not think that accreditation agencies really establish lower limits? After those limits are reached, other kinds of control processes take over, like prestige ratings and things of that kind.

Zald: Yes. But the interesting thing is that, historically, there was a switch. In the early phases they were often the prestige hospitals and the prestige universities that first established accreditation standards. They were the ones which were meeting the norms, and everyone else was below. In contrast, at the present time, both in the college case and the hospital case, accreditation standards define the lower base of the norm rather than the upper limits. This an interesting process. Why it had to go quite this way—why the accrediting agencies could not stay ahead of the game and always be raising their standards—is not clear.

Comment: You mentioned earlier, when you talked about the conditions of control, the two-directional component of sanctions. If you assume that sanctions are communicated to others, do you not also have to assume that the necessity of exposure to sanctions (in other words, to be involved in the sanctioning process) must be a precondition in order for the sanction to become a threatening or contagious influence? In other words, one of the consequences of sanctions may be: "Let me stay out of the condition in which I can be sanctioned." Therefore, the accreditation process is both a sanctioning process as well as a process of border defining; it may keep people from outside of the border.

Zald: Yes. Both in the hospital and the university case, attempts to insulate oneself from the normative requirements, from the norms of that particular social system, can be found. For example, a college may say: "We are not that kind of institution; therefore, your standards do not apply."

Comment: I think we need to talk about internal as well as external forms of control, like accrediting agencies. People from outside come and say: "Hey look, what are you guys doing?" This is different from internal forms of control. I think there is a fundamental reality problem (for want of a better term) in trying to assess performance of tasks, or specific role functions, such as those of the physician, the surgeon, or the nurse. Medicine is a long way yet from being an exact science. To the extent that it lacks this precision (I do not mean orthopedic surgery which is a pretty cut-and-dried subject), internal as well as external controls are required. Performance standards often can be more precise for certain surgical procedures than in internal medicine or pediatrics, or even obstetrics. The issue is one of the right methodology and technique of control—one of how to do it, rather than one of whether control of performance is necessary.

Comment: I had the priviledge about two years ago to talk to Dr. Kenneth Babcock when he was the head of the Joint Commission. He discussed some of the problems they have had over the years in devising precise measures for evaluation. He mentioned that they used to have a rating scale for hospitals, by departments and so forth, which did not last because they had to defend the scores when asked questions, such as "How come you rated that operating room five points higher than our operating room?" They could not defend this very well, and when they would say it was expedient they would get into more hot water. Consequently, they abandoned this system, but now they are going back to it. The main point is that this precision business of performance is quite different from the simpler task of "weeding out the bad apples." The latter is not a major problem. The problem is with evaluating professional standards of performance. Such evaluation implies a certain precision, but the assumption of precision may be questionable. To the extent that there is precision in performance, however, there are going to be problems in controlling performance according to standards.

Comment: I have a related comment, which is also related to the problem of the correlations mentioned earlier. The very problem of precision or a lack of it is what is interesting to the social scientist. Why are hospitals not accredited at different periods? Can you find out any trends? Is accreditation related to fads and fashions of certain sorts, such as the introduction of particular technologies or techniques? In the American system we have a very interesting special case in medicine in that only one form of medicine is accredited. It would be very interesting if one examined a system like that in India or Pakistan, where they have to worry about two systems—a native medicine system and a Western medicine system in competition. The two systems are using different standards, and the problem of control becomes very interesting because there the whole system of medicine is controlled in several ways, whereas in America we tend to forget about the cult practitioners. In the case of competing systems, one may raise the level of legitimate medicine but lose much of the clientele to those who are not licensed.

Comment: I would like to make two small comments? First, I doubt whether surgery is as exact as we are often led to believe. Surgeons may be quite exact about an organ, but also make an awful lot of mistakes of other kinds—for example, about the incidence of infections, the poor way that surgeons often manage infections, and the way they cause infections. It may well be that one small aspect of the process is exact, but surgeons make many other gross errors which may be even larger than the errors people in other fields make.

Second, concerning the proprietary hospitals, it might be interesting simply to look at the pattern of use, because there is a kind of middle-class family which uses these hospitals, as well as the middle-class physician, and there is a network of interesting relationships here. Only simple, easily managed illnesses get into proprietary hospitals. The dirty, costly, and difficult cases are referred to the medical centers or to large community hospitals, partly because the doctors are shareholders in the proprietary hospitals. The profit motive may make it easier to maintain such an arrangement, with or without accreditation.

Comment: There may be regional differences, here, however. In my own area on Long Island, for example, where half of the hospitals are proprietary (this may be surprising to those who may regard this as a sophisticated area), the movement is almost toward powerism in the kinds of service offered. The proprietary hospitals are faced with the same kinds of social functions as the so-called voluntary community hospitals. Their reasons for moving toward accreditation are just plain good business. There are enough people who want to know if the hospital, whether or not proprietary, is accredited, and part of the byline of every statement that the institution puts out is: "We are an accredited hospital."

As the only clinician here [Dr. Pellegrino speaking], I would also like to say that I am delighted with the comments made earlier about the issue of precision in medicine. What I would like to say is that the measurement of clinical performance now can become more precise. If we think in terms of "prudential decision-making" rather than merely in terms of whether "the right diagnosis has been made" on the part of the physician, we can move toward greater precision. A number of us are very concerned with this problem. What is required is to assess the output of the physician's action in terms of whether or not this is the most prudent thing situationally, here and now, phenomonally, for this patient. We can do this, now, through a true peer review approach—something that the accreditation process currently lacks.

The people who do the reviewing for hospital accreditation, with all due respect to these gentlemen, follow a checklist. They are alerted to certain very obvious gross deficiencies by the checklist. Obviously, however, the best clinicians are not going to be spending their time going to every hill and dale and hamlet in this country looking at hospitals. The reviewers are a group of individuals who have the language of medicine and can interpret whether or not the checklist is satisfied. But this does not get at the question of prudential decision-making. Yet for greater precision we have to move in this direction. This can be done now. For example, I can lay down for you the criteria for the proper prudential handling of a sore throat, having nothing to do with diagnosis. Having done that, of course, the next step should be to take it out of the hands of medicine and put it into other hands, as part of the extension of the system. We can do it, and it can be judged. I think we are moving in that direction.

Comment: From a social control point of view, the interesting thing about the evaluation of prudential decision-making is that it is a costly (expensive) process.

Answer: It need not be.

Comment: One component of social control is always how much does it cost you to establish a normative base? The present accreditation system is relatively inexpensive. There may be all kinds of ways of establishing a normative base for the evaluation of performance, but the cost function of the control process must be considered.

Answer: I do think that I can offer to you the hope, and the possibility, that we can systematize the assessment process in such a way that the cost will not be excessive. We are now developing in our continuing medical education program a mode whereby we can judge (we are going to have to do this) the performance of individual practitioners.

Comment: This is a perfect time for trying to do precisely what you say. Looking at nursing home administrators, for example, we find licensure laws just passed, with the usual grandfather clause. In their surveyors' program, external agents apparently are able to move in to regulate the lower-status occupational roles. This does not cover the higher status professional roles where there is more autonomy; professional autonomy almost by definition means freedom from control. But I think in the case of the nursing home administrators the government is moving in with the economic weapon of Medicare payments. This may be a step toward upgrading quality through governmental control. This is a perfect time to be studying this because right now I think it is the hottest thing in the health care field, and it is the biggest mess you can imagine.

Comment: As another example, one of the greatest sources of poor practice in a hospital is not covered by the Joint Commission of Accreditation at all, even though assessment standards, including mental standards, are available. This is the area of drug usage. The accreditation process does not get at how drugs are in fact used in the hospital. Yet standards that can be met can be set up, and performance can be readily evaluated, with existing techniques.

Question: You mean they do a better job with horses in the stables than with people in hospitals in the area of drug usage?

Answer: No; they do not do that very well either. They use some drugs on animals in ways which are worse than in medicine. I happen to know this since I have had some research in veterinary medicine.

Question: In a few instances, relating unfortunately to closing the barn door, in pathology conferences they are beginning to get at this kind of error. Are they not?

Answer: You are quite right, these are some of the errors. But the overall issue has to do with the institutionalization of an ongoing evaluation of the decision-making of individual clinicians against the standards of their peers rather than with more limited mechanisms such as pathology conferences.

Comment: Let me make a comment which takes us back into the problem of the sociologist. I think some of this discussion is quite relevant to our attempt at this conference. What do we synthesize? It strikes me that there is a danger here for the sociologist to be almost co-opted into studying what is visible rather than what is essential. The example of surgery, for instance, as against that of the sore throat, with respect to prudential decision-making by the clinicians, might suggest in a sense that what is more dramatic is defined as more precise by virtue of its dramatic properties, regardless of the very essence of the thing. This is what I would call a trap for the social scientist—a matter which I think has important implications for the study of control.

Question: Could I just ask for a clarification from Dr. Zald? I am concerned about the focus of social control in that it does not seem to provide a framework for interactive control. That is, it seems to place an emphasis on outsider groups and on the one-way exercise of control rather than on the tradeoffs between participants in a system. I am concerned about this, in part because it seems to favor one normative position over another. This concern is also responsive to a question raised earlier in the discussion: "Will we only look and see what participants have for goals and use those in our analyses?" Yet, I would argue, your framework does provide an opportunity to identify efforts of outsiders. For example, the Joint Commission on Accreditation of Hospitals suggests a kind of uniformity in control systems which may be extremely inappropriate if there is a great diversity in the social system. The focus that you use leads to the identification of certain control agents, but the approach does not focus upon the great diversity in the social system.

Answer: I do not find this contradictory to our framework. It is true that we have not pushed in that direction, partly because Dr. White and his group's work over the years has been directed exactly at that—at the tradeoffs going on in the interacting matrix. We come in at the boundaries of their work and take for granted the kind of exchange relationships and bargaining going on between agencies in a community. Various functions, for instance, which are forms of social control determine the referral pattern between hospitals and among agencies. In any community where there are five hospitals there is a tradeoff process which includes not only the hospitals and medical profession but other community agencies as well—the city planning body, the tax policies of that community, and so on. Similarly, in college systems we see among the accrediting agencies the beginning of real diversification in standard setting for different types of colleges. The associations have said: "We will have one set of procedures for the four-year college, another set of standards for the university, and another for the two-year colleges."

I think we have just found that this other hole was so gross in the sociological literature that, if we came ten years after the Levine and White work was started, we could still say: "There is this approach already going on, and we do not rule it out at all. Our work, however, tends to have a broader historical sweep to it, partly because you can see the norm changes easier over long sweeps of time than you can at the microlevel. And the microlevels are working out of those lower historical sweeps." Consequently, I do not see a problem. You are right, however, that in our approach to the study of the social control of institutions we do not focus on the diversity in the social system as much as might be desirable.

Structural-Comparative Studies

Presentation Highlights: D. Neuhauser

The title of the paper says we are concerned with something that might be called, for lack of a better name, the structural-comparative approach to the study of organizations. Briefly, this approach is a useful tool when you have at least 30, and usually 100 or 200, organizations to examine comparatively. If you are looking at one or two hospitals highly intensively, what we are discussing is much less appropriate.

Structural-comparative studies tend to rely heavily on precollected information. They also tend to rely on natural experiments. A good example of a natural experiment of this sort is that conducted by Mark Feldstein, which showed that demand for hospital services in England adjusted to the supply of beds over time. He could show that because the supply of hospital beds in the English hospital regions was constant for a 25-year period.

Our paper could be divided up in a number of different ways for categorizing its contents. The way we chose was to look first at the environment of hospitals; then to look at the internal processes and structural characteristics of hospitals, and how these relate to each other; and, finally, to look at organizational outcomes, primarily the quality of medical care and some measures of efficiency. Another way to put this is to say that we tried to define all of the relationships, in a theoretical way, among five major variables which occur frequently in structural comparative studies of hospitals. These are: average length of stay; occupancy rate; size; complexity, measured in various ways; and costs for the staffing ratio. We have tried to show how all of these things are related to each other.

There is still another way in which to view our paper. This involves the examination of a number of underlying concepts which seem to appear over and over again in the research reviewed. One is that of essentiality. This refers to the fact that all hospitals have to have certain types of staff and equipment. All hospitals have to have at least one manager, for example; they all have to have at least one operating room. This has certain consequences. It results in a declining proportion of these services as a total dollar volume— e.g. a declining proportion of managers as a percent of all employees in the hospital. Because certain types of services such as social work are not "essential," on the other hand, they may exist only in large hospitals where their costs can be spread over a larger number of patients. Because managers are essential, I suggest, essentiality may explain why the managerial component is negatively related to hospial size. Conversely, because the scope and complexity of services used involve many departments or things which are not essential, organizational complexity measures are positively related to size.

Another concept is that of indivisibility. In organizations some things come in whole units. For example, this is true of operating rooms; a hospital cannot have half an operating room. Because of this, a fairly large volume of service is required in order to spread the costs of such indivisible facilities and make them a paying proposition.

A third major concept is that of intensity. Hospital care can be given to an individual patient or to the average patient over a shorter or a longer period of time. In England the average obstetrical patient stays 13 days, in New England about 8 days, and in California only 6 days. This results in quite different staffing patterns. Intensity results in short average length of stay and in a high cost per patient day, but perhaps a low cost per patient case or per admission. One can also predict from this kind of intensity phenomena that certain types of services in a high intensity hospital will take up a larger share of the number of employees, the total budget, or the total costs.

Another underlying concept is that of uncertainty. The use of hospital services is to some degree unpredictable and uncontrollable. The fluctuations involved are partly random and result in idle standby capacity which, in turn, raises costs. Such fluctuations appear to be proportionately greater in small hospitals than in large hospitals.

In the paper we also talk briefly about environment. We do not have any grand or good theory about the impact of the environment on hospitals. There are some interesting things, however, which come out in our research review. For instance, in this country, states which have the most rapidly growing populations also have the greatest rise in the proportion of proprietary hospitals. And my guess for Long Island is that the county which has the greatest growth in population has the highest increase in the number of proprietary hospitals.

Another issue is, what might be called, that of technology versus medical or social custom. In a sense, technology constrains all hospitals at a given point in time in very much the same way. Hospitals have to have certain techniques, certain equipment, and certain types of personnel. But technology of this sort is not totally constraining. There is room for some variation above and beyond this. Nursing staffing patterns provide a good example. All hospitals have to have a certain number of nurses, but the ratio of registered nurses to licensed practical nurses in a number of different hospitals varies enormously. One hospital in Chicago has 130 registered nurses and no licensed practical nurses. Another hospital, a mile or two away, has one licensed practical nurse for every registered nurse on its staff. I do not see any rhyme or reason to attribute this variation to technological or to economic reasons, even though I do not know why it occurs.

Another example is shown in our paper (Table 3) with respect to average length of stay. Specifically, controlling for various classifications of illness, patients stay longer in Canadian than in American hospitals uniformly within illness categories. The same thing appears to hold when comparing the United States with Sweden or with England. Why should this occur? I do not think it can be explained by the requirements of the patients being treated. I believe it has to be explained by something like medical custom or social custom. As far as I know, for example, it appears that California has the lowest average length of stay anywhere in the world. Why should this be true, and why should it persist over time? Some people attribute this to a shortage of beds; because there is a shortage of beds, they argue, there has got to be a rapid turnover of patients to get people in and out. But Feldstein in England found that the average length of stay did not adjust to scarcity of beds there. We are left with an unexplained problem.

We also talk about the managerial component of hospitals. We tried to present a reason why it varies with hospital size and, I hope, resolve some of the morass of the empirical literature on this topic. The managerial component is important for two reasons. One is economics, and the other is a methodological reason. The major reason given is that "diseconomies of scale" (diseconomies of scale meaning that beyond a certain organization size costs will go up and efficiency will decline). Some use this argument to suggest that there is some ideal size for organizations such as hospitals. There is only one reason given for this in economics, namely that the costs of coordination (the costs of management controlled) become proportionately greater beyond a certain size. As far as I know, there is absolutely no empirical evidence in economics to show whether this is or is not true. It seems simply that this is a fondly believed view among a large number of people. I venture to propose that the literature on the managerial component is the only empirical evidence relating to this issue.

As far as I can tell, however, there is no strong evidence in managerial component studies which shows that the managerial component does begin to rise in organizations at some upper level of size. I, therefore, raise a fundamental doubt as to the concept of diseconomies of scale in economics in general. This is quite consistent with the findings in hospitals which show that there is very little evidence that there are diseconomies of scale—that very large hospitals are inefficient. Perhaps the reason why hospitals are not too large may have something to do with transportation costs; it may have something to do with the fact that there are only so many patients around who want to use the services; or it may have something to do with the fact that physicians want to keep a fairly closed shop and do not want to have a hospital open to all comers. Second, the managerial component is important because it provides a measure of control in organizations, and control is an appropriate issue.

With respect to outcome, the quality of care, there is only one major conclusion that we try to make in the paper: in most of the studies, the quality of care appears to be positively related to a cluster of variables that includes size, complexity, and teaching versus nonteaching. These are all highly correlated, and most of the studies of quality of care tend to pick up this cluster.

One of the intriguing findings in this area, I think, is shown in the study by Denton—one that I have replicated for community hospitals in Chicago. If you get a panel of experts, not connected with the hospitals, the agreement among experts as to which hospitals are well run and which hospitals are poorly run is very high. Denton found an interrater reliability of .86. I found an interrater reliability of .74. Personally, I find this to be quite a remarkable phenomenon.

With respect to efficiency, I think the major issue is that ultimately we must deal with cost measures. I think that is the most appropriate thing to use.

With respect to further research, I would like to talk about two things. First, I would like to make a proposition, which I think is empirically testable but I have yet to see the information that would disprove it. The hypothesis is this: at the present time, at the margin of, say, plus or minus 20 percent, the use of hospital services makes no difference on any measurable aspect of human welfare such as infant mortality, maternal mortality, or life expectancy rates, when such things as education and income levels are controlled for. The admission rates in the Kaiser hospitals, as you know, are lower than Blue Cross admissions. In contrast, Saskatchewan has an admission rate which, I believe, is nearly twice that of the United States. Corresponding differences in health do not seem to exist. Again, unlike the situation in the United States, where almost all children are delivered in hospitals, in the Netherlands 70 percent of all children are born outside of the hospital and 35 percent are delivered by midwives. Yet in the Netherlands the mothers and children appear to be no worse off due to this difference. I propose this as a hypothesis which is empirically testable.

Secondly, I would like to talk briefly about the relationship between structural variables, such as size and occupancy rate, and variables used in social-psychological and attitudinal studies. There is a real gap between these two kinds of research. There is very little information that links the structural-comparative studies with the social-psychological studies in the field. The only study that I know of which relates the two is Revans' study in England, in which he compared nursing wastage with average length of stay, controlling for case-mix differences. He found high nursing wastage; the nurses quit, left, and dropped out of school in a greater proportion when the average length of stay, case-mix controlled, was longer. As I understand, George Wieland undertook a replication of this study but did not come up with anything similar; he tried to change one of these variables and found no change in the other. A great deal of research remains to be done if we are to close the gap. I will stop here.

Chairman: Perhaps Dr. Andersen would like to add some comments before moving on into our discussion.

Dr. Andersen: Let me make just one point. When we started working on this paper I thought it would be very worthwhile, and perhaps also particularly appropriate in terms of social policy. If you look at the relationship between environment, structure, and process, primarily in terms of outcome, as Dr. Neuhauser points out, there are some relationships which do get over to the set of outcome variables. But these are relatively few and far between, given the vast amount of literature available (it is fairly vast if you take into account the structural literature concerning organizations as a whole). The kinds of measures we think of as related to outcome are largely economic measures, and many of the variables in this model drop out or they have not been considered by economists or by other people looking at outcome measures. It seems to me that this is one area where we can do a great deal of useful research. We do have some reasonable outcome measures now, particularly in the case of hospitals. When we look at either quality or efficiency, it seems to me that the primary requisite is that we control for the other. When we look at quality of care, we have to consider a standard product in terms of unit cost efficiency. Conversely, when we look at efficiency, we have to be sure that the hospitals are turning out the same kind of product in terms of quality. Now this is not an easy task as, I am sure, all of you are aware. But it is a task, I think, that we need to perform in order to relate the kind of work that is going on in this area to social policy.

Discussion

Comment: I have a problem with the use of professional experts in determining quality of care, although I recognize that this is probably the soundest approach to take when making judgments in this area. There have been other efforts, so far not very successful, to use some kind of a rating system which looks at the patient, the patient's chart, the patient condition, safety, medications administered, and the like. These have relied not on the professional competence of the expert, but on the uniform training of raters or observers. We used this technique (based on some of the work that the Veterans' Administration had done) in a study of 8 hospitals, all of which were fairly large, and looked only at a uniform set of data concerning medical, surgical, or medical-surgical units. But we did not find, even within that rather uniform set, that quality increased with the size of the hospital. On the contrary, some of the smaller nonteaching hospitals offered, according to this instrument, better quality of care. We might have not found that if we had used experts who were impressed with teaching competence or with the breadth and size of some of the institutions.

Some hospitals are awesome just in their titles, but in fact one of the most awesome that we looked at did have the lowest average quality of nursing care of the patient units studied. This is not directly challenging your position, because we were looking at a very narrow band at the high part of the range. But in view of our results I would no longer be thunderstruck if it were found that a 30-bed hospital in a town of 5000 provided a better quality of care than was offered at, say, a major university hospital.

Dr. Neuhauser: Let me state two things here. First, you are right about the possibility of negative relationships. Jean Carroll, in a recent dissertation looking at teaching hospitals, tended to find that there was a negative relationship within teaching hospitals between quality of care and size variables. I do not suggest that there is a perfect correlation between quality and size. Nor do I propose that mean evaluation is the final or the best measure of the quality of care. Quality of care is such a difficult thing to measure. Yet it is very interesting that the experts seem to agree. There is rather strong consensus among experts about which hospitals they consider good.

The second point I would like to make is that average patient day costs rise with the size of the hospital. Typically, this is explained on the basis of more complexity of service, more difficult diagnoses, and the like. But regardless of the explanation, costs rise with hospital size. At the same time I have some data which make me suspect that quality may drop with increased hospital size. The point is that we have at least some leads to suggest that there may be an optimum size which is exceeded in some cases and may be resulting in a diseconomy-of-scale phenomenon.

Chairman: We have some interesting data on some of these issues too. In our study of Michigan hospitals we used a group of expert raters, including some members of the Commission on Accreditation and other physicians, to evaluate the quality of medical care. The interrater agreement was significant and at about the same level as you mention in your paper. Moreover, the ratings given to the hospitals by these experts correlated significantly with the judgment of the medical staffs and of the professional nursing staffs within the hospitals. The latter finding perhaps is even more impressive than the agreement among experts. There may be general norms in the health professions that all these people are using as criteria for assessment.

With respect to economic measures, in the same study we found that the lower-cost hospitals were rated more highly by the experts and by the medical staffs. And with regard to size, we found a curvilinear relationship. The hospitals that were rated best were neither the smallest nor the largest; they were those in the middle of the size range. These results just reinforce the conclusion that we are dealing with an extremely complex task when attempting to assess the quality of care in hospitals. The point that one should control for unit costs when studying quality, and for quality when studying costs or efficiency, is very well taken.

Comment: Some ratings by so-called experts, like those used by a national magazine a year or so ago to name the 10 best hospitals in the country, may be misleading. Much depends upon the composition of the panel. In that case there was a high correlation between some prior administrative association with those particular hospitals and panel membership. This is reminiscent of the ratings of leading sociology departments—there was agreement as to leading departments because the Ph.D.s they have turned out were doing the voting. I am hoping for quantitative assessment which would take into account both social-psychological and structural variables. This may be one way of achieving progress in the assessment area, and it is feasible. But concerning the structural variables that you mentioned, Dr. Neuhauser, are you implying here that, as a result of your very good and extensive study, that these perhaps lack validity for evaluating hospital organization or certain functions of the system?

Answer: I suppose that this may be true if you take a social-psychological point of view. Then obviously the structural measures lack validity. But if you take a structural point of view the social-psychological measures lack validity. At the same time the two kinds of variables are not unrelated. If I am not mistaken, the Kaiser hospital system in California has a low admission rate, and the physicians in the Kaiser group are rewarded for keeping their patients healthy and out of the hospital by the bonus method. In other words, there is a relationship between structure and social-psychological variables in this case.

Comment: One also has to consider the fact that since one third of the beds of acute hospitals in California are still proprietary—the highest proportion in the country—it may be that there is a high percentage of unnecessary hospitalization for minor things, which is always related to short length of stay. We have had some studies in acute hospitals in a metropolitan area done by masters students who have taken patients with a length of stay under three days and compared them with those staying over ten days, the average being eight to nine days. They have run the data by diagnosis, doctor, and so on, and it is amazing how they have come out with two separate patient populations. And it is just a big can of worms; we have not been able yet, even with the computer, to determine what accounts for length of stay. This is a very ambiguous variable.

A long length of stay may be due to medical custom, but in one sense it is a social-ecological outcome as well. In British Columbia or Saskatchewan compared to New England, for example the length of stay may be high because they do not want to discharge a surgical patient back up in the boondocks, in the upper provinces, where if he has a relapse or develops an infection he cannot be reached. It takes two weeks to drive back up to the northern part of Canada to get home and to get back. Because no doctor is available and no hospital is within a close distance, they are reluctantly practicing conservative medicine. Because of the ecological-spatial factor, the normal length of stay in the northwest territories in Canada is exceedingly long. For exactly this reason, I believe, British Columbia has a very long average length of stay.

Comment: You can get some excellent comparative data closer to home in military hospitals where, for different reasons, they also have a long length of stay. If the soldier cannot march, there is no other place but the hospital. Ther are some very significant contrasts on patient census and occupancy rates between military and nonmilitary hospitals due to social-psychological factors.

Comment: It is also true that if you are admitted to a hospital on Friday you are going to stay in longer than if you are admitted on Monday. These structural variables—length of stay, admission rate, occupancy rate, etc.— are confusing. Hospitals can manipulate occupancy—they just do not count that empty wing any more to keep their occupancy figure high, as is being done by some hospitals. The measurement of structural variables, as a result, is a nonexact science.

Comment: The problem of structure when looking at hospitals is also related to function. If you look at growth and other aspects of structure in terms of what kinds of functions the hospital is carrying out, you can look at it as a system. Certainly the question of why hospitals grow, or which ones grow, is related to getting all feudal barons in the community together. We do have a kind of system wherein certain hospitals grow because of change in their functions or increased services to the community, or because of support from influential elements in the community.

There is also a problem concerning outcomes. Of the specific outcomes mentioned, those which caught my attention involve maternal and child health. This is a very dangerous area. Holland was mentioned in this connection. Denmark has a similar system. Finland, on the other hand, has 99.7 percent hospital deliveries. But there what goes into prenatal care is not a medical input; rather it is things such as nutrition. From the standpoint of quality of care outcomes, then, maternal and child care is a very dangerous kind of area. One can standardize for diagnosis, for example, and still come up with similar results in these countries.

Comment: I do not think that this is the issue, however. I think the point, which is really one of the most tantalizing points of sociological knowledge, is that when we compare things, we tend to use a "salami" technique of cutting when a "submarine sandwich" approach may be a much better model because when you cut longitudinally you cut across the processes that you are describing. This is the frustrating aspect of many of our comparative studies in the social sciences. They make assumptions about comparability when in fact the continuity of covert and overt behaviors may be the real core of the data.

Dr. Andersen: Would it be fair to say, though, that most of the questions raised about our framework concern environmental variables? I think one of the points that we have tried to make is that the environment is a prior condition which has a great deal of influence on process and outcome as well as structure.

Answer: If you include the internal environment in it, I will go along. If you go back to Zald's paper and include what might be called the normative present, which superlays almost all judgments of all pocesses and which sometimes is a prison, sometimes a blanket, and sometimes a mirror with which we see something only when we look at the things we put in, I have no problem with you framework. If you consider that part of the environment, in other words, and consider that the measures themselves are normative inputs and forms of control, then I would go along with it.

Comment: I think that what is implied here is the desirability of looking at the hospital as one part of the total health care delivery system. What you are suggesting is that the hospital can play relatively larger and smaller roles in the total health care of particular patients. When looking at the total system, the outcome measures, such as efficiency, will correlate to some of these social variables (e.g. normative and control measures) more than they will correlate to how the parts of the system are structured. For example, assuming that there is some consistency in quality, and I think you are suggesting that there is, people with higher education and higher income are apt to receive higher quality care from the total system and to be able to utilize the system more effectively. This would mean that the impact of the hospital per se is less important than these other factors.

Dr. Andersen: I think I can speak for both Duncan and myself on this point. We would say that education and income, even controlling for intervening variables, still would play a major part in determining the kinds of outcome measures we might look at to measure the health or the illness level of a population.

Comment: This is looking at the total system though. Recognizing that hospitalization in most instances does not terminate an episode of medical care, the benefit of hospitalization may still depend to a very great extent upon both the patient's ability to maximize the gains in the hospital and upon the environment, or the family and community setting to which the patient returns and their ability to complete the job, so to speak.

Comment: I agree, but none of you have mentioned the matter of quality in relationship to the end that the hospital has set for itself—its function. One of the greatest problems, I believe, is that all hospitals essentially set the same goals for themselves. This may go counter to the idea of an effective health care system. For example, if you evaluate care in terms of the proper clinical decisions and the needs of the patient when he enters the hospital, 85 percent of all illnesses can be handled better in a small than in a middle-sized hospital. Certainly, assessing this kind of thing must take into account differences in the functions of hospitals in the rural area, secondary care hospitals, and university hosptials. One of the most important questions, then, is what is the end point of the function a hospital sees itself performing in the milieu within which it exists. To me, the social function of the institution, or what the hospital is trying to achieve, is a prime determinant.

The experts are susceptible to bias. They are staying within their own cultural system and may be inclined to rate university hospitals high on the quality of care. There is no question that at Johns Hopkins a mitral valve is better taken care of than it would be somewhere else. But a very serious question in my mind is whether they take care of pneumonia or an ordinary gall bladder disease any better, or perhaps less well, than in the community hospital. The paraphernalia of medical care to which we bow are geared for tertiary care. But the assessment of quality must be made in relation to primary and secondary as well as tertiary care. If so, is there any validity, from a social scientist's point of view, for starting the process with the frame of: "What is the function of this hospital, or what is this hospital intended for in social terms?"

Comment: In my view, and others will disagree, the question is whether the social scientist assumes the goals of the hospital as held by the people there or tries to specify the functions of the institution. We, by and large, and I think you too, essentially start from the concept of goal as the people in the organization are at present defining it, and we really assume it.

Comment: But that is not the social purpose of the institution. How the people who are performing it see or define the function of the hospital is not necessarily the social function of the institution.

Comment: You say that is not the social purpose of the hospital. This means that you, in this case a health care professional, have a definition of what its social function should be. And this, then, becomes the process by which new norms get defined. Consequently, I accept your point and say that medical sociologists, as opposed to lowly organizational types like myself, ought to be concerned with helping doctors, medical professions, and nursing professions to define what the goals of the organization are.

Comment: No; they should not define the hospital's goals. That is precisely my point. This function has to come from an agency outside the professions. I realize that we are in the metaphysics of hospitals, but without it we may skirt the issue.

Question: What agency would that be? The Joint Commission? They are a part of the medical profession. The courts? Probably not.

Answer: The hospital's board of trustees, since it represents the society and the voluntary health system.

Comment: But the board is only a part of the system. The charter of the institution, the whole legislative document that makes up the hospital in an administrative sense, should be the source of definition.

Comment: But you are an organizational analyst. You know that the charter itself represents a sociological process that requires examination.

Comment: But unless you set up an initial effort to define the role and function of that facility in the community, you have no *terminus ad quem.* And that is the basic function of trustees—to be responsible for the quality of care practiced in that facility.

Comment: To the social scientist, there is no *terminus ad quem.*

Comment: If you say there is none, then I think, if I amy say so, you cannot measure the quality of care. I am not attacking sociology; I am merely saying that if you are looking at the quality of care in a hospital, you must have some operational definition (granted, this takes it out of the realm of metaphysics) of what you expect. I really think the definitional determination has to arrive from the board or some other group, who are the advocates for society for the use of this instrument for social purposes. The minute you throw this task back to professionals like myself, you are doomed to an endless measuring of things that are set before you without relationship to what it is that society wants. Because your point is very significant, I would be willing to state that the same thing can be said about medicine in total. If you remove medicine from the scene today, for example, what are the evils that will occur to society? And I do not suggest to remove it altogether.

Comment: No; I got you. But even that is an open question, for society might be willing to give up those things.

Question: Are any of you familiar with the studies that were done at Michigan State about ten or twelve years ago, in which the boards of hospitals defined the goals for the hospitals? Trustees defined the social function of the institution, but they did it for a particular segment of the population—the population they represented in society—and not for the total community. They decided for middle-class and upper-class services but not for services to the total population.

Comment: That is changing, now, however.

Comment: Yes, but it is not changing much because of the initiative of the boards.

Comment: That is true. However, the boards have been made to feel that they have a moral, legal, and social responsibility as advocates for whatever it is that the community wants in the case of community hospitals.

Comments: I doubt that there is a board of directors in America, except one that owns the organization, which takes the kind of role that you are talking about. Boards just are not the authorities in organizations. If you observe hospital boards in action, you will see that in most cases the administrator can exert decisive influence over the trustees. Of course there are a few administrators who do not do that. If you try to find a singular source of authority on goal setting, you just will not get there. You are going to find such things as an insurance company coming in and applying pressure, a commission with its own expectations, the local professional association, and other sources of influence. In effect, the goal-setting process just cannot be tied down that way.

Chairman: The issue of defining the organizational function of the hospital or the institutional function which it serves within the community is critical to many evaluative studies. We can also accept the fact that there are many defining agents in the external system whose definitions may overlap and sometimes contradict one another. It would be worthwhile to take into account, and occasionally use as a basis for analysis, the definitions provided by several of these relevant defining agents. Partly because of differences in functions and definitions of functions, moreover, it is desirable for hospital research to separate the community hospitals from teaching hospitals, the rural area from metropolitan area hospitals, the large hospitals from small hospitals, and so on, because their functions tend to vary systematically. Methodological and theoretical differentiation along these lines is important to keep in mind in our studies.

Comment: I would like to make a comment on another aspect of the Neuhauser and Andersen paper, which is an extraordinary pulling together of this area, that takes us back also to the problem of the cross-sectional versus the longitudinal slice process. In part the issue is just a data problem posed by the absence of relevant materials. If we use the comparative method for looking at anything that would give us a lever on change over time, however, there is some interesting economic theory that has not been sufficiently explored. You may know Penrose's work, **The Growth of a Firm,** in which he tries to take the individual firm and look at the factors that lead to growth or not. This may have relevance to comparative hospital research. In part the issue is reflected in the falsity of the notion of diseconomy of scale for the management component.

Under constant technology, and this means not only material technology but also social technology, there probably is a diseconomy of scale in organizations. But the economic literature has tended to ignore social technology changes and changes in administrative style, including work restructuring, divisionalization, and others. Someone has drawn attention, for example, to the phenomenon of the transformation of the hospital into, essentially, a set of subdivisions, treating the institution not as a single hospital but as, maybe, eight related hospials. Much like the divisional corporation, a hospital may have a centralized computer system for financing and for patient billing, and yet be structured or run as a group of subhospitals each being run almost like an autonomous division of a corporation. We have always had separate children's hospitals, and separate women's hospitals as components of large hospitals. Some real economies of managerial scale are probably realized in these cases, the entire hospital being run under one managerial system for cental administration and yet maximizing the benefits of decentralized operation. The economics literature is really very weak in this area because it has not yet learned G.M.'s lesson.

Chairman: I think perhaps this is a good point to stop. Thank you.

Part Three

6

PROFESSIONALS IN HOSPITALS: TECHNOLOGY AND THE ORGANIZATION OF WORK*

W. Richard Scott

Among the many developments in hospital research over the past decade or so, I would like to single out for brief attention certain trends which seem of general significance and at the same time form a context for the exploration of my more limited subject.

It is important to note that these trends are evident not just in research on hospitals, but more generally characterize research on formal organizations. This is as it should be, since the value of studies of specific types of organizations is greatly enhanced when the both profit from and contribute to our general knowledge of organizations.

Three Trends in Hospital Research

The trends to be considered are: (1) the shift from case to comparative studies; (2) the movement from closed to open system models of organizational structure; and (3) the more recent tendency to replace the entrepreneurial model of the professional with an interdependent model.

From Case Studies to Comparative Studies

In the postwar period and during the relative peace and quiet of the Eisenhower years, sociologists discovered the hospital. From the late forties and early fifties to the middle sixties the case study served as the vehicle by which sociologists traveled around, in, and through this alien and exotic environment. Smith (1949) and Wessen (1951) carried out their doctoral research in hospitals and, together with Argyris (1956) and Burling and his colleagues (1956), were among the first to provide descriptive accounts of the structure and functioning of hospitals as complex organizations. Historical perspective was provided by Perrow's case study (1961, 1963) of shifting power structures and goals in a voluntary hospital as well as by Lentz's general description (1956) of the evolution of hospital structure. Throughout this

---

*Revised version of paper presented at the Conference on Hospital Organization Research, May 22-23, 1970, Institute for Social Research, The University of Michigan, Ann Arbor, Michigan. W. Richard Scott, Ph.D., is Professor of Sociology at Stanford University.

period the case study was also utilized by investigators to pursue a wide range of more specialized topics, from "teamwork in the operating room" among physicians and nurses (Wilson, 1954) to "laughter in the ward" among patients (Coser, 1962).

The theoretically informed, carefully conducted case study performs important functions in the social sciences, not the least of which is a descriptive mapping of uncharted territories. Where little is known, much of value can be learned through this approach. It is also true, however, that as more is learned about a given subject area, case studies have a rapidly diminishing value. Weick (1969, pp. 18-21) has recently reminded us of the importance of an adequate empirical base upon which to build and test our theories, and at the same time he questions the capability of case studies to provide us with such a data base.

Among the drawbacks to case studies, Weick emphasizes the following: (1) their *situation-specific* character: "We can learn from it what to do and not to do to survive in that particular environment, but we learn much less about the environment itself and why those particular adjustments are the best ones"; (2) their *ahistorical* nature: the focus of such studies is often on special arrangements for dealing with a particular problem or crisis rather than on the regularities of behavior which precede, continue during, and survive the crisis; (3) their *tacitly prescriptive* character: the instigator tells us what worked or did not work in a particular situation without informing us sufficiently as to the conditions under which the solutions solved or the failures failed; and (4) their *one-sided* nature. As Zelditch (1962, p. 574) notes, when the observer wishes to examine a relation between *a* and *b*, it is characteristic of unplanned and unsystematic observation that " 'a' will be more frequently recorded than 'not-a' and 'a and b' more frequently than 'not-a and b' or 'a and not-b'." Such limitations, while not inherent in the case study approach, are sufficiently common as to raise questions concerning the adequacy of much of the data collected by this method.

The case study has come under criticism not only because of the low quality of the data it generates, but also because of the *type* of data it elicits. Case studies of one or a few organizations may permit the systematic collection of data on the behavior or attitudes of individual participants or work groups as these exist within the context of an organization. But they do not allow the generation and testing of propositions concerning the interrelations, determinants, and consequences of various aspects of organizational structures. As Blau and I noted ealy in the decade under review, "To arrive at the latter type of generalizations requires systematic comparison of a fair number of different organizations." (Blau and Scott, 1962, p. 13).

The decade of the sixties saw the completion of a number of comparative studies of organizational structure, and a small subset of these focused on hospitals. A few of these studies (Columbia University, 1960; Heydebrand, 1965) make use of preexisting statistics such as those regularly collected by the American Hospital Association. We also now have a handful of studies which use fragmentary existing data from such sources as the World Health

Organization to make descriptive comparisons of American and European hospitals (Glaser, 1963; Roemer, 1962). Other comparative studies are based primarily on survey methods by which data are gathered from a sizable number of participants in selected hospitals (Georgopoulos and Mann, 1962; Revans, 1964; Georgopoulos and Matejko, 1967). Still other studies rely for data on the reports of one or a few informants who are asked to report data for the organization as a whole.

Distinct problems are associated with each of these data-gathering approaches which merit brief comment. The obvious deficiency associated with the use of preexisting statistics is that the researcher has no control over either the type or the quality of the data collected. Distinctions useful for administrative purposes may be of little value for, or work at cross-purposes to, theoretical concerns. And no student of organizations should need to be reminded of the political nature of official documents or of the administrative biases which may characterize organizational records and reports.

Comparative studies which rely for data on the reports of all or most (or stratified random samples of) participants collected by survey methods are confronted with the problem of weighting. It is common in such approaches for the response of one member to be given equal weight to that of another in spite of Vidich and Bensman's (1960, p. 201) warning that "all answers to the same question on a questionnaire are not of equal weight, and cannot be treated as such." Equal weighting flys in the face of everything we know about social structure—both formal and informal—the most important characteristic of which is differentiation: differentiation of knowledge, of competence, of influence, of commitment, of power, etc. From the standpoint of its effect on the organization, for example, one physician's opinion may not be of equal importance with another's, and to treat them as equal in the analysis of responses may provide a very misleading description of the system under investigation. One of the few empirical studies which has attempted to deal with this issue is that by Aiken and Hage (1968). Their solution—to give equal weight to each social position regardless of the number of occupants— is not especially attractive, but does represent recognition of the problem.

The use of one or a few representatives of the organization as "surrogate observers" or as "expert respondents" (Scott, 1965, pp. 291-293) is increasingly being employed in organizational research. Perhaps a single questionnaire is sent to the organization to be filled out by the administrator or, more likely, his assistant. Such a practice seems justified for the collection of certain types of data but not for others. For example, one may expect to obtain reasonably valid and reliable reports on the numbers of persons occupying certain generally recognized statuses in the organization, or on the number of hospital beds and the average rate of their occupancy. Administrators are apt to keep fairly accurate records concerning such matters. The interests of social scientists commonly extend beyond such mundane matters, however, with the result that informants are sometimes asked to provide information on matters beyond their competence. One questionnaire sent to administrators to collect information relating to the problem of hospital mergers asked informants to report the number of other organizations with which the hospital had regular contract. It seems unlikely that a single, sociologically unsophisticated informant could provide valid data on such a complex matter.

Indeed, what little research we have suggests that participants' views of the organization's environment is a function of their location in the organizational structure. Informants are sometimes asked to report the number of levels of authority within their organization or to report the turnover rate for particular categories of employees. But notions as to what constitutes an "authority level" may vary, and accurate statistics may not be available on matters such as turnover. In short, in some cases informants are being asked to report information concerning their organization which they are not qualified to report. As comparative studies relying on expert respondents become increasingly popular, it is essential that we move toward the development of criteria or guidelines for determining the types of information which can appropriately be collected from such sources.

While many unsolved problems remain with respect to the collection and analysis of these types of data, the move toward systematic comparative studies of hospital structure is an important indicator of the maturation of this field of inquiry.

From Closed to Open System Models

The movement from closed to open system models now occurring in the parent discipline of organization theory has yet to make its impact on the analysis of hospital organization with full force, but there is little doubt that it will during the next decade. The full implications of the transition to open system models are only imperfectly understood—indeed, they are often misunderstood—but the following points may be briefly noted:

1. As Walter Buckley (1967, p. 50) notes: "That a system is *open* means not simply that it engages in interchanges with the environment, but that this interchange is an essential factor underlying the system's viability, its reproductive ability or continuity, and its ability to change." Organizations depend upon their environment for sources of inputs—materials, socialized personnel, etc.—and for markets for outputs (Levine and White, 1961). The environment is not only the source for and recipient of these exchanges; through various institutional mechanisms—e.g. governmental regulations, judicial decisions, the actions of the "market"—it also has a large role in setting the terms of these exchanges. Who can doubt that the number and types of clients available in close proximity to the hospital, the general economic resources of the community, and the number and types of competitors for these resources (see Elling and Halebsky, 1961), the policies and practices of licensing boards and local and state medical societies—who can doubt that such factors have profound implications for the structure and functioning of a hospital facility?

Lawrence and Lorsch (1967), for example, used cross-sectional data to show that industrial firms vary in their effectiveness by the degree to which they adopt coordinating mechanisms appropriate to the characteristics of their particular environments. It would appear to follow that the analysis of internal structure which does not take into account relevant aspects of the environmental context of the organization is likely to be not simply limited, but misleading.

2. Mechanistic models which presume a rigid and unchanging structure and organic models which presume a tendency toward equilibrium are inadequate in that they do not take account of the capacity of organizations for growth and change. Organizations as open systems can import energy from their environment. Further, in the process of adapting to environment, organizations typically become more differentiated in form, more elaborate in structure. Unlike physical and organic systems, social systems can and do fundamentally change their structures without any breach of continuity. Organic models tend to emphasize the conserving, deviation-counterbalancing processes that act to preserve or maintain a given form of the system ("morphostatic processes") at the expense of structure elaborating, deviation-promoting processes which operate to change the form of the system ("morphogenic processes") and which are central to an understanding of "higher level" systems.

Few studies of hospital structure have focused on structural change. One exception has already been mentioned: Perrow's (1961) analysis of changing power structures and goal systems in a voluntary hospital. Another is represented by the work of Strauss and his colleagues with their emphasis on "negotiated order." As Strauss and his associates (1963, p. 148) note: "Our model bears upon that most central of sociological problems, namely, how a measure of order is maintained in the face of inevitable changes (derivable from sources both external and internal to the organization). Students of formal organization tend to underplay the processes of internal change as well as overestimate the more stable features of organizations—including its rules and its hierarchical statuses." Elaborating the concept of "negotiated order," they continue (p. 164): "Since agreements are patterned and temporal, today's sum total of agreements can be visualized as different from tomorrow's—and surely as quite different from next week's. The hospital can be visualized as a place where numerous agreements are continually being terminated or forgotten, but also as continually being established, renewed, reviewed, revoked, revised. Hence at any moment those that are in effect are considerably different from those that were or will be." Unfortunately, the work of both Perrow and the Strauss group is based on non-systematic, impressionistic observation within a single hospital.

3. The open system approach emphasizes that there are various degrees or levels of "organization." At the tight end of the continuum, relations among the elements making up the system or organization are completely determined: only one set of relationships is possible and all elements are then cogs in a rigid structure. Moving up the continuum, we have systems in which there is some degree of interdependence, in which the presence of certain elements exerts certain constraints on the behavior of others. At the far end of the continuum, we have zero organization—mere aggregates of unrelated

elements.

Human organizations tend toward the loose end of the continuum. In comparison with other types of organizations, hospitals are even farther out, exhibiting a high degree of structural "looseness." In the predominant form of hospital organization—the so-called voluntary hospital—physicians are not full-time participants in the structure but episodic, powerful visitors enjoying a large degree of autonomy and freedom from responsibility for the enterprise as a whole. Also, many hospital departments function as "parallel" rather than "interdependent" structural units (Blau and Scott, 1962, pp. 183-84), in the sense that they are organized to function relatively autonomously of other segments of the organization. Models which approach hospitals as if they were tightly organized, highly integrated systems, and sharply differentiated from "external" structures are not likely to advance our understanding of this type of organization.

4. Finally, this suggests that the boundary between an organization and its environment is an entirely arbitrary line drawn only for purposes of analysis. What elements of the system we choose to label "the organization" are entirely a matter of analytical convenience. To the extent that one element is related to another, in the sense that it is exerting constraints on the behavior of the other, it is a part of the system whether we choose to label it "organization" or "environment."

Other features of the open system approach could have been included, for example the suggestion that purposive systems can be better analyzed by utilizing the notion of feedback mechanisms which allow a system to include the results of its own action in the new information by which it modifies its own subsequent behavior. Since at this point the open system approach is more promise that accomplishment, however, perhaps enough has been said to indicate some of the directions which may be taken during the next decade. (See also Georgopoulos, 1970.)

From Entrepreneurial to Interdependent Models

The traditional sociological model of the professional is that of an individual who, by virtue of extensive, theoretically based technical training and a long period of socialization during which he has internalized appropriate norms and standards governing his performance, is capable of autonomous functioning. The practitioner's sphere of autonomous functioning is protected by licensure and other legal arrangements with the claim that the profession itself, and only the profession, is competent to undertake regulatory action when warranted by the misbehavior of individual practitioners. These characteristics have been presumed to describe the professional from early times down to the present in spite of the fact that two important changes have taken place. First, it is a well-documented historical trend that members of the "free" professions, such as physicians, are in increasing numbers moving the locus of their practice from individually maintained private offices to some niche within the framework of an organization, whether private group-practice clinics or hospital-based practice. And second, the general practitioner is being rapidly supplanted by a diverse array of specialists.

Under these changed circumstances, it seems time to reconsider the model which was initially developed to describe the behavior of the professional acting as a private entrepreneur. In this connection I agree very much with Freidson's (1970, pp. 88-89) appraisal of the situation:

> Far too much attention has been paid to the personal characteristics and attitudes of individual members of occupations and far too little to the work-settings. This is particularly the case for the professions. On the whole, students of the professions in general and medicine in particular have adopted the same individualistic value position of the men they study. They have been inclined to postulate and search for personal qualities manifested in views of work, of self, and of clients which are supposed to be inculcated or at least intensified and stabilized in the course of professional education . . . . Education is a less important variable than work environment. There is some very persuasive evidence that "socialization" does not explain some important elements of professional performance half so well as does the organization of the immediate work environment.

The work environments of professionals in medicine are complex and diverse, but more and more they are situations characterized by a division of labor among professionals taking place within the context of an organization. These are changes which we propose to explore now in more detail.

Technology and Structure

Some of the most interesting and promising work of the past decade concerns the relation of technology to organizational structure. Although there are some exceptions, organizations by and large do not create their own technologies but import them from the environment in the form of machines or equipment, packaged programs or sets of instructions, or trained workers. This, then, is one of the significant ways in which the environment affects the form and activities of an organization.

This is not the place to review the general literature pertaining to technology and organizational structure. Rather, we will focus on the more limited problem of technology, the professional worker, and appropriate forms of organizational structure. We will begin by proposing some dimensions of technology having implications for structural arrangements. Then, after considering some of the difficulties associated with the assessment of technology, we shall conclude with an examination of physician tasks as they relate to some aspects of hospital structure.

Dimensions of Technology

To focus on the "technology" of an organization is to view the organization as a mechanism for transforming inputs into outputs. We mean to define technology very broadly as including the characteristics of the inputs; the characteristics of the transformation activities performed by men or machines on these inputs; and the characteristics of the outputs. Several dimensions have been proposed as useful for the analysis of technology, but we will concentrate attention on three. The first, "uniformity," is employed to characterize both organizational inputs and outputs. The second, "efficacy," is used to characterize the transformation process; and the third, "social valuation," will be applied primarily to the outputs.

Uniformity. The significance for structural arrangements of the relative uniformity of inputs has been emphasized by many analysts, including Litwak (1961) and Thompson (1967). Referring to the same dimension, I have earlier proposed that tasks be categorized in terms of the extent to which the "resistance to be encountered by a given task performance is predictable" (Scott, 1966), and Perrow (1967, pp. 195-96) emphasizes the "number of exceptional cases encountered in the work, that is, the degree to which stimuli are perceived as familiar or unfamiliar." In his discussion of organizations which socialize, Wheeler (1966, p. 78) has suggested that we differentiate between those which "aim for what might be called homogenizing settings that tend to reduce the relevance of prior experience for present adjustment" and differentiating settings in which "authorities may urge recruits to give expression to the different backgrounds and intrersts they bring into the organization." Wheeler's distinctions could be applied with equal value to describe the characteristics desired for the outputs. Is the organization's goal one of producing a collection of uniform and homogeneous products or is it one of producing a set of relatively diverse, if not unique, outputs? Finally, in his empirical study of technology and structure, Harvey (1968) appears to focus attention on uniformity of outputs, although he describes his distinction as being one of "technical diffuseness" versus "technical specificity." He characterizes this dimension as follows (p. 249): "Technical diffuseness implies a firm in which a number of technical processes yield a wide range of products. Furthermore, the actual products included in this range are more likely to vary from year to year as a result of model changes and changes in technological production processes. The more technically diffuse a firm, then, the greater the degree of 'made to orderness' in its products."

The predictions and findings across these various studies relating uniformity of both inputs and outputs to structural features of the organization are remarkably consistent. In its simplest terms the theoretical argument is that given unpredictable variations in inputs or desired customizing of outputs (nonuniformity), decisions concerning work activities should be made by individual performers. More specifically this suggests that:

1. Formalization will be relatively low. Attempts to specify in detail the work activities or roles of participants will be unsuccessful. Where coordination of activities among the various performers is required—as it usually is in complex work situations involving the contributions of many different specialists—it cannot be achieved by standardization but can be attempted by

"plan" (the establishment of schedules to govern the actions of the inter-dependent units) or by "mutual adjustment" among the performers (Thompson, 1967, p. 56).

2. Bureaucratization will be relatively low. More discretion will be given to the "production" workers—participants directly engaged in the transformation tasks—with fewer decisions remaining for those higher in the hierarchy. A smaller administrative overhead usually results since less planning, supervision, and coordination through the hierarchy are required. This implies that fewer levels of formal authority will be needed and that there will be a smaller ratio of administrative to production employees.

3. The division of labor will be relatively low. Since problems cannot be predicted in advance, arrangements for dividing labor on these tasks cannot be predetermined. Because choice of later activities is affected by the success or failure of earlier activities (feedback from the task object), a single per-former or set of performers working in concert is better able to carry out the entire sequence of required activities. If work is passed on to others, a bulky record detailing the previous history of task activities usually accompanies the transaction.

Efficacy. By efficacy we mean the extent to which there exists a rational-ized transformation process such that there is a known chain of cause-effect events which produces the desired outputs. Perrow (1965) has indicated that among the correlates of high efficacy are the presence of a system of feedback such that the consequences of acts can be assessed in an objective manner, the definition of an acceptable, reasonable, and determinant range of tolerance, and the ability to communicate the techniques to others sufficient-ly to train them to carry out the activities and achieve results within accept-able limits of tolerance. Thompson (1967, p. 85) describes a similar dimension in his discussion of the relative completeness of the "under-standing of cause-effect relations."

Closely related to, and yet somewhat distinct from, the dimension of efficacy is the "clarity" of goals—the relative specificity or diffuseness with which the desired characteristics of outputs are defined. There is an obvious and also a not-so-obvious reason for the relative close association of efficacy and goal clarity. Obviously, a clear view of the goals to be attained may en-able workers to improve their performance by helping them to focus attention on the relevant attributes of the task object and by providing a clear set of criteria for selecting among alternative activities. Less obviously, the direction of the association may be reversed: ability to produce certain effects or to measure readily changes in certain properties of the task object may cause performers to concentrate attention on these aspects of the work process and eventually define what they can do as what they want to do. ("When I'm not near the goals I love, I love the goals I'm near.") In such cases original or vague goals are displaced by specific ones, not because these are desired, but because there is an efficacious technology for producing them. (Some colleges, for example, apparently seek not so much to produce "educated" persons as to turn out persons who have achieved enough credit units to graduate.)

Other things being equal, the more efficacious (rationalized) the transformation process, the more possible it is to plan the work process in advance, prescribe performance programs for participants, and subdivide labor among workers. In short, rationalization's effects on the work structure are virtually the opposite of nonuniformity. This is not to say the formalization, bureaucratization, and the presence of specialization will not be found among organizations possessing a technology low on efficacy—only that high values on these dimensions are more likely to occur given high efficacy.

Indeed, one of the important consequences of low efficacy appears to be the absence of any clear basis for predicting organizational arrangements. As Freidson (1967, p. 498) notes: "It seems no accident that the most marked variations in organization and in staff-patient and staff relations are to be found in mental rather than general hospitals. It is not in general hospitals that conditions can so easily vary from those of a concentration camp to those of a partially self-governing community. The organization of mental hospitals can vary so markedly because there is no clearly efficacious method of 'curing' the mentally ill." There can be enormous differences in the structure of organizations possessing low efficacy since the basis for their organization appears to be ideology rather than technology, and there are few constraints on variations in ideology (see Perrow, 1965).

Finally, in situations characterized by low efficacy, Thompson (1967, p. 87) argues that "efficiency" and "instrumental" tests of adequacy of functioning are not likely to be employed. In their place organizations typically resort to "social" tests in which they compare themselves on a broad range of criteria with organizations viewed as comparable.

Social Valuation. This dimension of technology has received less attention than the previous two. As a result it is less clearly formulated and we have little empirical research bearing upon its effects. By "social valuation" we refer to the importance placed upon the inputs and/or outputs of the organization by some social group or by society at large.

First, with respect to inputs we may distinguish between organizations which process people and those which process nonhuman material. In general, because of certain cultural values which attach to individual human life, more social importance is usually attributed to human than to nonhuman material (Perrow, 1965). If we restrict attention to people-processing organizations, however, there are clearly differences in value associated with different types of clientele. In general, less value is probably attached to prisoners, social welfare clients, and inmates of mental institutions than to students, other types of trainees, and patients in general hospitals. Reasons for such differences are undoubtedly many and varied but surely include such considerations as whether the person is there because he wants to be or because he has to be, whether the person is paying for the services he receives or has them paid for by others, and whether the person himself is the object of services dispensed by the organization in contrast to other groups, such as the public at large, being the beneficiary of the organization's efforts (see the distinction between "service" and "commonweal" organizations in Blau and Scott, 1962, pp. 51-57).

Turning to outputs, let us continue to restrict attention to those organizations which process human beings. One way to view the importance attached to outputs is to utilize the economic concept of "value added." The importance of what has transpired as the object moves through the organization's transformation processes may be assessed in terms of the value of the object after, as compared with before, it entered the process. Two components of valuation may be noted: first, how much change has occurred in the object? This component is clearly related to the previous dimension, efficacy. Second, how much social value is placed on the kinds of change which have been effected? Thus considerable social value might be placed on the rehabilitation of prisoners, but because of the low efficacy of prison technology little social value is placed on the output of prisons.[1]   Conversely, little social value might be placed on the ability to cut hair even though barber's colleges may be quite effective in transmitting the requisite skills.

The consequences for organizational structures of differing values associated with their inputs and outputs may be briefly stated. The greater the social importance attached to their inputs and their outputs, the more likely they are to develop structures which allow individualized (nonuniform) production techniques. Thus, following our first set of propositions, this means that the higher the social valuation, the less the formalization, bureacratization, and division of labor of the structure.

Some Problems in Relating Technology to Structure

Before applying some of these general notions concerning dimensions of technology and work structures to the organization of work within the hospital, we should remind ourselves of some of the complexities involved in this association. First, there is not one professional group but many types of professionals involved in the work of the hospital: physicians, nurses, and social workers, among others. In one sense these groups all work within a set of arrangements which is called the hospital structure; however, if we look more closely, we see that the work arrangements for the physician are different from those for the nurse, which in turn are different from those structuring the performance of the social worker.

Second, even for a given professional group, such as physicians, there are significant differences among the various specialty groups in the activities they perform, the methodology and techniques they employ, and the nature of their relations with clients and colleagues (Bucher and Strauss, 1961). Such differences are reflected also in the organization of the various wards:

---

1. It is important here to comment that while the "objective" efficacy of an organization is important in determining the valuation of its outputs, efficacy is in part a matter of social definition. Using various kinds of objective indicators, it does not appear that colleges and universities are particularly effective organizations. Profound changes do not typically occur in individuals as they pass through our institutions of higher learning. Yet relatively high value is placed in our society on the college graduate. Some organizations apparently perform "well" because they are believed to perform well. Other organizations, such as prisons, may suffer from a self-fulfilling prophesy running in the opposite direction (see Meyer, 1970).

"There is a fair amount of evidence of significant variation in the organization of interaction and performance within the wards of the general hospital, differences apparently stemming from the presence of different specialties, which is to say different practices, different tasks, and different requirements for the performance of those tasks, (or 'technologies')." (Freidson, 1970, p. 128.)

Third, when we examine the work practices of a single professional practitioner of whatever specialty, we discover that he typically carries out not one but many types of tasks with which are associated quite diverse technologies. For some of these tasks his efficacy may be quite high, for others, low; for some tasks inputs may reflect high uniformity, for others they may be quite diverse. Of the many tasks a worker performs, which will determine the overall structure of his work arrangements? One can argue with Hughes (1958, pp. 121-122) that there exists a core set of tasks which comes to define the "symbolic work" of the particular set of practitioners. It is probably the case that structural arrangements, to the extent that they relate to task characteristics, are more likely to be affected by these core tasks than by others regarded by performers as peripheral to their central activities.

We would suggest, for example, that the differences in work structure between medical and surgical wards reported by Coser (1958) reflect differences in the core tasks performed by these medical groups. The medical wards place central importance on the task of "diagnosis," and the "oak tree" structure reported as characteristic of such wards is well suited for extensive consultation among colleagues and joint decision-making and problem-solving. On the other hand, it may be argued that patients on surgical wards have already been diagnosed, and hence the "pine tree" structure reported for these wards is a reflection of the need for centralization of control in order to coordinate the many activities necessary to carry out surgical treatment. All of this is merely to suggest that different professional groups within the hospital perform different tasks and that a fairly clear understanding of the central tasks associated with each group may be necessary before it is possible to relate their activities to structural arrangements.

Another source of difficulty in attempting to relate types of tasks to types of structural arrangements must be raised. To this point we have argued as though the various characteristics of dimensions or tasks were objective features associated with particular types of work. In fact, task dimensions are at least in part socially defined. We have already argued that degree of success or efficacy is in part socially determined. Some types of performances succeed merely because sufficient numbers of people believe that they do. Similarly, the uniformity or nonuniformity of the objects processed is partly a matter of the way in which they are defined or conceived. Given the same set of objects (e.g. students) it is possible for performers to emphasize their similarity or their diversity. Do performers focus attention on the differences that are present or direct attention to the basic similarities of the set of objects? The type of work arrangements which exist (or those which are preferred by participants) will depend then not simply on the "objective" nature of the technology but on the social definition or conception of that technology. This fact makes the study of technology of even greater interest to social scientists. In positing a relation between technology and work arrangements, it is not only the dependent but also the independent variable which requires sociological formulation.

These considerations concerning task conceptions raise one final problem to be considered here: if conceptions of task in fact do vary from group to group (and from time to time), whose conception shall we consider in attempting to relate technology to structure? We would argue that for most purposes it is appropriate to focus on the conceptions of task held by organizational managers or administrators. This is the segment of the organization most clearly involved in establishing the structure of the organization and in designing work arrangements for participants. We would begin, then, by expecting to find an association between managerial conceptions of technology and organizational work arrangements.

It is clearly the case, however, that the task conception held by rank-and-file participants may differ from those held by management. Task conceptions held by participants will undoubtedly be affected by the work arrangements present in the organization, but their conceptions may also be shaped by forces external to the organization, for example by professional training centers. To the extent that task conceptions held by participants differ from those held by managers, we would expect participants to collectively strive to change managerial conceptions to correspond more closely with their own, and, failing that, we would expect considerable dissatisfaction among workers and conflict between workers and the administrative sectors.

Some groups, for example physicians, have sufficient power to bring to bear on the organization that they are able to force administrators to take their preferences into account when work arrangements are devised. Other groups, such as nurses and social workers, have been much less successful in persuading administrators to adopt their task conceptions and establish appropriate work arrangements.

Technology and the Organization of Work

We now propose to apply some of these general notions concerning dimensions of technology and work structure to the organization of work within the hospital, in particular to the work arrangements for the physician. Emphasis will be placed on the differing conceptions of medical tasks held by physicians and by administrators. Since systematic data on physicians' and administrators' task conceptions are lacking at the present time, all our descriptions and conclusions are tentative and need to be subjected to empirical verification.

Divergent Task Conceptions

Physicians' task conceptions. Most physicians appear to place great emphasis on the nonuniformity of both the inputs (patient conditions) and outputs (what is regarded as an appropriate goal to be realized for a given patient). With respect to the second dimension, in spite of the enormous strides, in medical science and the splendid array of medical instrumentation, phsycians view their transformational procedures as only partially rationalized. As Freidson (1970, p. 164) notes: "Even when general scientific knowledge may be available, the mere fact of individual variability poses a constant problem for assessment that emphasizes the necessity for personal firsthand examination of every individual case and the difficulty of disposition on some formal, abstract scientific basis." As for the dimension of social valuation, great value is placed in this culture on health, and considerable faith is held in the ability of the medical practitioner to furnish this commodity. Further, most individual patients pay in one way or another for the services they receive and are in a position to make some demands on the medical system for personalized, quality care. Physicians tend to ally themselves with these sentiments, insisting that quality medical care is customized, individualized care under the direction of a competent practitioner.

Physicians' conceptions of technology exert pressures toward the creation of work arrangements which will allow maximum autonomy for individual practitioners. Conceptions emphasizing the nonuniformity of inputs and the customized nature of outputs, the absence of a completely rationalized set of therapeutic procedures, and the high value placed upon the "raw material" and on the services provided are inconsistent with a high degree of formalization, bureaucratization, and specialization of work functions. Practitioners holding such views will insist that rules be held to a minimum, that administrators concentrate their energies on providing necessary support services and refrain from exercising close control over medical tasks, and that physicians' tasks cannot be subdivided and parceled out among a collection of workers.

These conceptions of the nature of work are in large measure acquired during the lengthy period of professional socialization. They are consistent with an entrepreneurial model of medical practice in which geographically dispersed and independent practitioners provide services to a distinct client group. What they do not take into account is the increasing degree of specialization in the work of physicians.

Given the tremendous growth of technical knowledge and the multiplicity of skills involved in ministering to the patient, physicians are increasingly confronted with the choice of becoming incompetent generalists or competent specialists. The latter career choice is made by the overwhelming majority of physicians. It appears that increased rationalization of technology does indeed lead to increases in the division of labor.

The proliferation of specialist professionals has had important direct and indirect effects on the organization of medical work in hospitals. One direct effect is described by Heydebrand (1965): "In contrast to the specialist form of professionalization, the generalist form as found in the traditional professions may in fact provide integration and coordination of specialized work functions and thus reduce procedural communications and supervisory enforcement of operative rules. Professional specialists, on the other hand, are themselves part of a system of division of labor, especially when they are employees of an organization. Rather than contributing to coordination, they are likely to require additional coordination and administrative regulation."

In short, when tasks are divided and subdivided, integration and coordination of effort are required. Some of the necessary coordination is provided by the specialists themselves functioning as a "temporary system"—a transitory system of relations among a team of physicians and other medical personnel brought together around a particular patient and existing for the duration of that patient's illness. [2] Much of the burden of coordination, however, falls upon medical, nonmedical, and nursing administrators. An important indirect effect of specialization is the fragmentation of the professional community as numerous speciality segments emerge with differing competencies, identities, vocabularies, values, and interests (see Bucher and Strauss, 1961). The medical staff of the modern hospital finds it increasingly difficult to speak with one voice on the variety of issues confronting the hospital as an organization.

The growth of coordination problems and the increased segmentalization of the medical profession have both contributed to a shift in power from physicians to administrators (see Perrow, 1961). Administrators are concerned with coordinating the flow of work among medical, paramedical, and nonmedical participants and increasingly are called upon to coordinate work and adjudicate among the conflicting needs and demands of medical specialties. Thus while the individual physician remains a central actor on the scene, and while he has sufficient power to see to it that some of his preferences for work arrangements are taken into account, his preferences do not completely determine work arrangements. Since administrators have acquired considerable power in hospital settings, it is important to consider the conceptions which they hold of medical technology and the consequences of these conceptions for work arrangements.

Administrators' task conceptions. Most of the important differences in conceptions of medical tasks held by administrators (who may be physicians with administrative responsibilities) as contrasted with those of practicing physicians are due to differences in the level and scope of task definition. Whereas practitioners tend to view the medical task as ministering to the needs of individual patients, administrators are much more likely to view the medical task as ministering to the needs of a patient population. Also, whereas individual practitioners view the patient from the perspective of a relatively narrow set of needs which they as individual physicians are competent to service, administrators must take into account a much broader spectrum of needs—routine care, hotel services, ancillary facilities and services, communication and preservation of information, financial accounting, coordination of specialist activities—generated by the presence of a large number of patients requiring round-the-clock care.

---

2. Miles (1964) has analyzed the peculiar strengths and weaknesses of such temporary systems. His insights might well be applied to and extended by research on the functioning of medical teams in hospitals.

Reviewing our task dimensions from the administrator's point of view, then, patients, while certainly not interchangeable, present many common characteristics and make many similar demands on the organizational system. Patients can be roughly categorized according to the type of services required, and reasonably accurate predictions can be made concerning such matters as locus of primary care, type of consultation and other services which will be utilized, length of stay, etc. With respect to the dimension of efficacy, administrators readily acknowledge that all activities within the system cannot be completely rationalized, but would also insist that many can and more will be. Activities which can be routinized whenever possible are removed from physicians. For example, since the number and types of laboratory tests which will be required during a given period can be accurately estimated, specialized personnel with relatively small amounts of training can be employed and instructed to follow a given set of procedures. Automated multiphasic testing equipment is rapidly being installed in the larger medical centers, and current attempts to evaluate the effectiveness of diagnosis by computer suggest the extent to which even the core medical tasks are in the process of being rationalized.

Predictability of inputs and rationalization of techniques make possible increasing degrees of specialization and formalization. The presence of many different types of personnel whose work must be supervised and coordinated requires bureaucratization of work arrangements. Supervision and control of physicians' work tends to remain primarily in the hands of physicians, but these activities are also becoming more centralized. For example, in her study of an out-patient clinic, Goss (1961) reports that physicians in the position of assistant clinic director exercised "authority"—issued directives to which complicance was expected—with respect to such administrative matters as scheduling of patients, but were only able to proffer "advice" in the area of patient care. Nevertheless, what is important to note in this report is the extent to which surveillance duties had been concentrated in a few positions rather than distributed through the colleague group,[3] so that physicians holding these positions were granted the "right" to routinely review all case records and to make suggestions to individual practitioners. In addition, as Goss (1961, p. 44) notes, these rank-and-file physicians "considered it their duty to take supervisory suggestions about patient care into account, and in this sense they accepted supervision." Also, other types of surveillance are possible given the aggregation of sizable numbers of physicians in common settings. Thus McNerney's (1962) survey of control in hospitals reveals that 26 percent of the small hospitals, 47 percent of those with between 100 and 500 beds, and most larger hospitals have imposed restrictions on the types of work which medical staff can perform. In addition, 37 percent of the hospitals surveyed reported that medical-record committees used the records to determine whether the care given by the physician is adequate, and 61

---

3. Colleague control is, of course, the type of control emphasized by the model of the "free" professional. The effectiveness of this form of control leaves much to be desired, if the conclusions of Freidson and Rhea's (1963, 1965) study of a medical clinic are found to hold generally.

percent of the hospitals had tissue committees which functioned to detect and protect against inappropriate use of surgery.

Turning to the final dimension, the high valuation placed upon the patient, or to put it another way the seriousness with which mistakes are viewed, has given the individual physician some leverage in the system. This has been bolstered by statutes which place legal responsibility for the welfare of the patient on the individual physician. Motivated by such accountability, physicians have been able to cry "emergency" and by this device cut through standard operating procedures and institutionalized arrangements. An alliance between the needs of individual patients (for customized care) and physicians (for autonomy) has preserved some flexibility in the system. But this situation may also be changing. Faced with the rising costs of hospitalization, the public (the patient population) has strengthened the hand of the administrators who are calling for greater efficiency of operations—which means a greater division of labor, more formalization, and, as a consequence, more bureaucratization.

Recent legislation in a few states has attempted to shift responsibility for the quality of medical care from individual physicians to the hospital as an organizational unit. As the "service module" in modern medicine moves from the individual practitioner to the organizational unit, and as the locus of responsibility begins to shift to become more consistent with these service arrangements, we can expect to see increased efforts to improve and extend organizational control systems. The current interest in process and outcome evaluation as techniques to compare and assess the level of performance among various medical systems is only one indicator of this more general trend (see Donabedian, 1966, 1968; Shapiro, 1967).[4]

Task Conceptions and Conflict

The foregoing discussion attempts to sketch in the outline of two divergent conceptions of medical technology. These conceptions are held by two powerful classes of actors within the hospital organization: physicians and administrators. Physicians as a professional group whose skills are essential to the operation of this type of organization have sufficient power to insist that their conceptions of medical tasks be taken into account in devising appropriate work arrangements. And, as we have argued, administrators, who have primary responsibility for devising work arrangements in the hospital, have over time increased their power in relation to the medical staff.

Not too surprisingly, the conceptions of medical technology held by each of these groups are self-serving in the sense that each supports and justifies work arrangements preferred by each of the parties. Physicians prefer autonomy—freedom from administrative interference and supervisory control—and their conception of their work helps to justify this preference.

---

4. For a general theoretical discussion of task evaluation as a means of organizational control, see Scott *et al.*, 1967. The concepts developed in this paper are applied to health organizations in Scott, 1966.

Physicians need some freedom from administrative regulations and procedural rules if they are to provide appropriate services to individual patients presenting unusual problems. Administrators prefer order—a degree of coherence and predictability in the mass of activities which together comprise the technology of the hospital. Administrators need some tools for controlling and regulating the contributions of diverse occupational groups and medical specialists, and increased specialization and formulization are required if the economies demanded by client groups are to be effected.

Much of the conflict currently characterizing physician-administrator relations centers around the issue of what constitutes appropriate work arrangements in the hospital. And, if our analysis is correct, disagreements over work arrangements stem in part from differing conceptions of medical technology and from differences in the level from which physicians and administrators view the technology.

Conclusion

Hospitals are settings within which work is done, and it seemed to us worthwhile to attempt to examine certain aspects of this organization by focusing attention on its technology. Unfortunately, upon inspection, technology does not appear to be the sort of solid, unambiguous matter that the term connotes. Rather, its dimensions—we have rather arbitrarily chosen to focus on three of them—appear to vary depending upon the perspective of the observer. In particular, physicians appear to share certain conceptions of their technology which differ from those held by administrators. Conceptions of technology seem particularly worthy of study because they appear to underlie—provide a basis for or a justification of—work arrangements. The way in which tasks are conceived will determine in part the arrangements under which they are carried out. Because of differences in the conception of medical tasks held by these two powerful groups, one expects to find considerable tension and conflict between administrators and physicians on the question of how work is best organized.

History does seem to be on the side of the administrators. The increasing rationalization of technology serves as a foundation for increased division of labor, formalization, and bureaucratization within medical organizations. But to the extent that medical technology is not completely rationalized so that individual judgment continues to play a significant role in the performance of medical tasks, and to the extent that the customized ministration to the needs of individual patients continues to be a primary goal of health systems, there remains justification for the physician's demand for some autonomy in his practice. The issue would seem to be how much autonomy in what areas of functioning can be accorded individual physicians consistent with the requirements of coordination and efficiency in the provision of quality medical care?

References

Aiken, M., and Hage, J. Organizational interdependence and intra-organizational structure. *American Sociological Review,* 1968, *33,* 912-930.

Argyris, C. *Diagnosing human relations in organizations: a case study of a hospital.* New Haven: Yale University Press, 1956.

Blau, P. M., and Scott, W. R. *Formal organizations.* San Francisco: Chandler, 1962.

Bucker, R., and Strauss, A. Professions in process. *American Journal of Sociology,* 1961, *66,* 325-334.

Buckley, W. *Sociology and modern systems theory.* Englewood Cliffs, N.J.: Prentice-Hall, 1967.

Burling, T., Lentz, E. M., and Wilson, R. N. *The give and take in hospitals.* New York: Putnam, 1956.

Columbia University School of Public Health and Administrative Medicine. *The quantity, quality, and costs of medical and hospital care.* New York: Columbia University Press, 1960.

Coser, R. L. Authority and decision-making in a hospital. *American Sociological Review,* 1958, *23,* 56-63.

Coser, R. L. *Life in the ward.* East Lansing: Michigan State University Press, 1962.

Donabedian, A. Evaluating the quality of medical care. *Milbank Memorial Fund Quarterly,* 1966, *44,* 166-206.

Donabedian, A. Promoting quality through evaluating the process of patient care. *Medical Care,* 1968, *6.* 181-202.

Elling, R. H. and Halebsky, S. Organizational differentiation and support: a conceptual framework. *Administrative Science Quarterly,* 1961, *6,* 185-209.

Freidson, E. Review essay: health factories, the new industrial sociology. *Social Problems,* 1967, *14,* 493-500.

Freidson, E. *Profession of medicine.* New York: Dodd, Mead, 1970.

Freidson, E., and Rhea B. Processes of control in a company of equals. *Social Problems,* 1963, *11,* 119-131.

Freidson, E., and Rhea, B. Knowledge and judgment in professional evaluations. *Administrative Science Quarterly,* 1965, *10,* 107-125.

Glaser, W. A. American and foreign hospitals: some sociological comparisons. In E. Freidson (Ed.) *The hospital in modern society.* New York: Free Press, 1963.

Georgopoulos, B. S. An open-system theory model for organizational research. In A. R. Negandhi and J. P. Schwitter (Eds.) *Organizational behavior models.* Kent, Ohio: Comparative Administration Research Institute, Kent State University, 1970.

Georgopoulos, B. S., and Mann, F. C. *The community general hospital.* New York: Macmillan, 1962.

Georgopoulos, B. S., and Matejko, A. The American general hospital as a complex social system. *Health Services Research,* 1967, *2,* 76-112.

Goss, M. E. W. Influence and authority among physicians in an outpatient clinic. *American Sociological Review.* 1961, *26,* 39-50.

Harvey, E. Technology and the structure of organizations. *American Sociological Review,* 1968, *32,* 247-259.

Heydebrand, W. V. Bureacracy in hospitals: an analysis of complexity and coordination in formal organizations. Dissertation, Department of Sociology, University of Chicago, 1965.

Hughes, E. C. *Men and their work.* Glencoe, Ill.: Free Press, 1958.

Lawrence, P. R. and Lorsch, J. W. *Organization and environment.* Boston: Graduate School of Business Administration, Harvard University, 1967.

Lentz, Edith M. The American voluntary hospital as an example of institutional change. Doctoral dissertation, Cornell University, 1956.

Levine S., and White, P. E. Exchange as a conceptual framework for the study of interorganizational relationships. *Administrative Science Quarterly,* 1961, *5,* 583-601.

Litwak, E. Models of bureaucracy which permit conflict. *American Journal of Sociology,* 1961, *67,* 177-184.

158 Organization Research on Health Institutions

McNerney, W. J. *et al. Hospital and medical economics: a study of population, services, costs, methods of payment, and controls.* Chicago: Hospital Research and Educational Trust, 1962.

Meyer, J. E. The charter: conditions of diffuse socialization in shcools. In W. R. Scott (Ed.) *Social processes and social structures.* New York: Holt, Rinehart and Winston, 1970.

Miles, M. B. On temporary systems. In M. B. Miles (Ed.) *Innovations in education.* New York: Teachers College Press, 1964.

Perrow, C. The analysis of goals in complex organizations. *American Sociological Review,* 1961, *26,* 854-866.

Perrow, C. Goals and power structures—a historical case study. In E. Freidson (Ed.) *The hospital in modern society.* New York: Free Press, 1963.

Perrow, C. Hospitals: technology, structure, and goals. In J. G. March (Ed.) *Handbook of organizations.* Chicago: Rand McNally, 1965.

Perrow, C. A framework for the comparative analysis of organizations. *American Sociological Review,* 1967, *32,* 194-208.

Revans, R. W. *Standards for morale: cause and effect in hospitals.* London: Oxford University Press, 1964.

Roemer, M. I. General hospitals in Europe. In J. K. Owen (Ed.) *Modern concepts of hopsital administration.* Philadelphia: Saunders, 1962.

Scott, W. R. Field methods in the study of organizations. In J. G. March (Ed.) *Handbook of organizations.* Chicago: Rand McNally, 1965.

Scott, W. R. Some implications of organization theory for research on health services. *Milbank Memorial Fund Quarterly,* 1966, *44,* 35-59.

Scott, W. R., Dornbusch, S. M., Busching, B. C., and Laing, J. D. Organizational evaluation and authority. *Administrative Science Quarterly,* 1967, *12,* 93-117.

Shapiro, S. End result measurement of quality of medical care. *Milbank Memorial Fund Quarterly,* 1967, *45,* Part 1, 7-30.

Smith, H. L. The sociological study of hospitals. Doctoral dissertation, Department of Sociology, University of Chicago, 1949.

Strauss, A., Schatzman, L., Ehrlich, D., Bucher, R., and Sabshin, M. The hospital and its negotiated order. In E. Freidson (Ed.) *The hospital in modern society.* New York: Free Press, 1963.

Thompson, J. D. *Organizations in action.* New York: McGraw-Hill, 1967.

Vidich, A., and Bensman, J. The validity of field data. In R. N. Adams and J. J. Preiss (Eds.) Human organization research. *Homewood, Ill.: Dorsey Press, 1960.*

Weick, K. The social psychology of organizing. *Reading, Mass.:* Addison-Wesley Publishing Company, 1969.

Wessen, A. F. The social structure of a modern hospital. Doctoral dissertation, Yale University, 1951.

Wheeler, S. The structure of formally organized socialization settings. In O. G. Brim, Jr., and S. Wheeler, (Eds.) *Socialization after childhood: two essays.* New York: Wiley, 1966.

Wilson, R. N. Teamwork in the operating room. *Human Organization,* 1954, *12,* 9-14.

Zelditch, M., Jr. Some methodological problems of field studies. *American Journal of Sociology,* 1962. *67,* 566-576.

7

PATIENT CARE AS A PERSPECTIVE FOR HOSPITAL ORGANIZATION RESEARCH*

Hans O. Mauksch

The study of organizations has traditionally been motivated by the fascination inherent in the complex arrangements of human resources in institutional matrices. The utility of such research has been rooted in the concerns of management science and human engineering. Most of the well-known approaches have addressed themselves to the maintenance of the organizational system itself. This might have taken the form of concern with the nature of organizational properties (Anderson and Warkov, 1961; Blau and Scott, 1962; Etzioni, 1961; Geogropoulos and Mann, 1962; Goffman, 1961), with managerial requirements (Durbin and Springall, 1969; Mauksch and Tagliacozzo, in press; Pfiffner and Sherwood, 1960), or with the system's efficiency (*Operations Research Quarterly*, 1968; Hage, 1965; Kast and Rosenzweig, 1966), and relationship to its human resources (Argyris, 1957; Crook, 1965; Levinson, 1959). Attemtps also have been made to synthesize the institutional process on a systemic level (Bertalanffy, 1951; Boulding, 1956; Howland, 1963) and on a personal level (Crook, 1964; Goffman, 1961; Jelinek, 1969; Strauss *et al.*, 1963).

One could simplify the institutional process as a dynamic that moves from input through process to output. The predominant proportion of the literature stems from viewing organizations from the vantage point of process or of input (Durbin and Springall, 1969; Kast and Rosenzweig, 1966; Miller and Rice, 1967). Institutional analyses seeking to explore the organizational properties which appear when output becomes the focus of observation are more rare, probably because most institutions do not have a product that suggests itself as a worthwhile point of departure for investigation.

The present contribution is a result of the lack of conceptual resources that can be applied to study the hospital in an explanatory manner. I am not sug-

*Paper presented at the Conference on Hospital Organization Research, May 22-23, 1970, Institute for Social Research, The University of Michigan, Ann Arbor, Michigan. Hans O. Mauksch, Ph.D., is Professor of Sociology at the University of Missouri. The author wishes to state that the paper started as an attempt to add to a systematic organization of the relevant literature but finally became a statement of a personally derived professional point of view. For this reason it is not steeped in an exhaustive search of the literature. He also wishes to acknowledge a theoretical debt to the interactionist approach, particularly to Erving Goffman and Anselm Strauss. (Some modifications of the original paper have been made by the Editor.)

gesting that there are no attempts in the literature to examine the quality of the hospital's product, i.e. patient care, but the very difficulties which those who seek to do so have encountered may well indicate a knowledge gap between the existing understandings of the hospital and its product. An attempt will be made here, therefore, to present a somewhat different approach from the conceptual schemes previously applied to the study of hospitals.

This paper examines the hospital centering on the output of the organizattion—patient care—as the vantage point from which to try to understand the institution. Two major assumptions, or observations, underlie the proposed approach. The first of these is the assertion that the output process of the hospital is not merely, or even primarily, the direct consequence of management and authority processes translated into an output flow, but rather that patient care is a "negotiated order" which represents the results of interaction between relatively discrete systems operating simultaneously within the social entity called the hospital (Bucher and Stelling, 1969; Goffman, 1961; Strauss et al., 1963).

The second observation is also dictated by the perspective of patient care. Most analytic schemes treat the subsystems of the hospital as subordinate and dependent upon the total system. Viewing the institution from the output point of view, however, suggests that these subsystems and other categories subordinate to the total institution should be viewed independently from the overall institution and examined as they affect each other in the process of yielding patient care (Mauksch, 1966).

A Conceptual Framework for Organizational Analysis

Three conceptual constructs are here suggested as important: the "worlds," the "process systems," and the "stages." These, it is proposed, represent crucial components of those processes which determine the actuality of patient care and the characteristics with which the institution reveals itself to its clients. These three constructs do not represent phenomena that exist distinct from other aspects of formal organizational and institutional processes. They do, however, provide a different way of structuring data and of organizing potentially predictive models of behavior.

Several social structures exist within an institution, each involving its own functions, norms, and role expectations. Occupants of positions within the formal hierarchy may belong to one or to several of these structures. Although the same person may participate in several systems simultaneously, his behavior, adjusted to the structure within which it is performed, may vary considerably. Such inconsistencies of behavior need not be experienced as role conflict, although conditions of stress and conflict may produce inconsistencies in role behavior.

Looking at the university as an example, one must define it as an institution exhibiting a modicum of formal bureaucratic unity and organization.

Simultaneously, the university is a federation of systems which, in an important sense, are not subsystems of the university; as enclaves of various disciplines they can be profitably viewed as subsystems of disciplines and professtions. The university must also be understood as an umbrella for an aggregate of individuals who are socialized to operate as autonomous individual systems, managing individual careers, concerns, and purpose-production dynamics.[1] Faculty members in the university are members of all three systems, and a fruitful approach to understanding universities should include the hypothesis that the designation of the appropriate system as reference framework is necesary to explain apparent inconsistencies and diversity of individual or collective behavior.

The hospital too can be identified as subsuming several such systems. By contrast with the relatively insular separation of the university community, however, the processes of the hospital are characterized by greater interdependence. In the university the student penetrates the components of the federation through his course registration, declaration of major, and faculty contacts. Thus he does not, in his role of work product, force the parts of the federation to move out and encompass him, thereby significantly interacting with each other. The teacher who assigns homework does not have to consider the work which the student is expected to accomplish for other instructors. Professors or entire disciplines are proponents of viewpoints and theories without being restrained by possible conflict that the student may experience as recipient of conflicting and diverse forms of knowledge. On the contrary, this condition is thought to contribute to the learning process, to the intellectual independence and critical capacity which is one of the objectives of education.

While the student is perceived to be an active and interactive factor in the institutional output of the university, the patient is seen as the passive recipient of services. Patient care is supposed to be a flow of planned, integrated, and coordinated events in which all resources are interdependent. Furthermore, the patient in the hospital is relatively stationary except for such special islands as the operating room or the x-ray department. Therefore, if the assumption of separate systems can be substantiated, a process of interaction, negotiation, and integration between the system components can be anticipated.

Two characteristics are suggested as being peculiar to the hospital and differentiating it from the university: (1) the centripetal and integrative consequences of a stationary work product which requires the convergence of institutional components; and (2) the social process implications of functional interdependence among the organizational components of the institution. These two assertions are not sufficient to analyze the processes of patient care as the vantage point for hospital organization. Three further considerations also must be taken into account: (3) the highly developed level of

---

1. To examine the social function of certain individual statuses as microinstitutions might prove useful in an endeavor to understand complex social systems. Certain social roles are sociologically "incorporated" and involve most of the characteristics typically applied to institutions.

specialization and division of labor in the hospital; (4) the strongly developed and continuously proliferating professionalization of the components of the hospital output system; and (5) the absence of a formally legitimated integrative status at the locus of institutional output.

These characteristics imply that the events of patient care result from encounters between institutional resources. These encounters are necessitated by the integrative requirements of patient care; however, they are not rigidly programmed by the prevailing organization of the institution. Three conceptual constructs are suggested as means of analyzing the process of patient care. The first, that of hospital "worlds," is not unlike the federation model of the university. The second construct—the "process systems"—seeks to articulate the system consequences of institutional diversification of objectives and authority. Finally, the construct which seeks to encompass the encounters themselves is here called the "stage."

The hospital is composed of subsystem entities which have various degrees of autonomy, variously distinct norms and objectives, and variable linkages to institutions situated outside of the hospital. These will be labeled here the "worlds," suggesting degrees of symbolic autonomy or social membrane formations which serve as border formations for communications, norms, and role developments. The notion of "insider" is crucial to the determination of the symbolic territory of such worlds, whether it is the medical staff, the serology laboratory, or the medical records unit in the hospital, or whether it is the academic department in the university.

While the concept of worlds is clearly applicable to other institutions, the notion of "process system" is more peculiar to the hospital. As will be stated below, it stems from the division of authority which has been considered a characteristic feature of the hospital. The third construct—the "stage"— is based upon the observation that worlds and process systems meet at various points of the institution where they interact, negotiate, and develop modes of accommodation. In the hospital one of these stages provides the environment for the main product of the organization, i.e. patient care. The notion of the stage is different from the well-known proposition that the full development of the division of labor requires the functions of management and coordination. Beyond the coordinated integration of specialized work products it is proposed that other problems of synthesis arise from the relatively autonomous drama enacting the encounters among hospital systems.

The Worlds

In order to articulate the peculiarities of the stage properties of patient care, it might be well to take a closer look at the worlds of the hospital. Status structures and departmental organization have been predominantly used to conceptualize the territories and barriers which exist in the hospital (Blau, 1959-60; Hall, 1962; Julian, 1966; Mechanic, 1967; Price, 1968). These factors have been shown to be related to problems of communication and lack of unity in purpose, priorities, and performance among the various components of the organization. It may be fruitful to treat status, departmental identity, and occupational characteristics as dependent variables and to examine the hospital as a host agency. This agency supports several more or less well-defined social subentities, generally but not necessarily synonymous with occupational and departmental divisions. These worlds are characterized by a sense of identity, by a common definition of purpose, and by a prevailing system of internal formal and informal communications.

The obvious examples of these hospital worlds are medicine, nursing, dietetics, and the other professional groups whose functioning supports the formation of the "world" phenomenon. The business office, the maintenance shop, and the operating room also manifest significant characteristics of worlds. The occupation-linked characteristics of most hospital worlds are a probable and prevailing, but not a necessary, phenomenon. The psychiatric and the pediatric setting in general hospitals occasionally show rudiments of world formation which cut across occupations, thus incorporating patient care as a focal point of the world. This is in contrast to the above stated observation that patient care in the general medical and surgical patient care unit involves interworld stagelike encounters.

Just as the worlds of the hospital vary in the degree of self-conscious identity, they also vary in the degree to which their conduct is governed by intrainstitutional and extrainstitutional reference systems. One could distribute the worlds of the hospital along the cosmopolitan-local continuum (Gouldner 1957, 1958). In many hospitals medicine is likely to be cosmopolitan, even though the term would need to be redefined. It may encompass the profession as a national institution, or in other localities the extrainstitutional frame of reference may be the local medical society. The business office might be one example of a hospital world which is primarily based on an intrainstitutional system.

From the point of view of a patient-care based analysis, the key issue of the world phenomenon is the degree to which world membership overrides institutional identity. This could be profitably tested by examining the existence of a world perspective in various types of hospitals. The small hospital, where the lack of numbers makes the development of world identities unlikely, would display a greater sense of institutional cohesion. The large institution, rather, is likely to be the seat of the worlds. Identity with segments of the institution is likely to provide the feeling "we," characteristic of the world phenomenon. Thus the concept of the world is interposed between the alternatives of an institutional community and the mass society. What may appear to the manager as anomie may in fact be a federated cultural system.

The Process Systems

Based on the prevalence of multiple lines of authority, which characterizes the hospital, we propose that these lines of authority can be viewed as process systems (Bucher and Stelling, 1969). This view has been previously formulated by this author (Mauksch, 1966) but is now integrated into a more comprehensive position. The assertion that the processes of cure and care have different although overlapping and interdependent objectives is merely a starting point. Emanating from these objectives are identifiable decision-making processes and the mobilization of activities.

One difference between a university and a hospital lies in the peculiar characteristic of the hospital that the processes of cure and care cut across its worlds, while the teaching and research processes generally are synonymous with the world organization of the university. Although interdisciplinary research and education programs are being developed in universities, the difficulties such programs encounter merely support the organizational assumptions presented here. The one process observable in the university which is not dissimilar from certain phenomena of the hospital can be identified as the management process. In the university, however, the functionaries who devote their time to institutional self-maintenance are distinct and almost segregated from those who produce the institutional output.

The above discussion of the care and cure process systems implied that institutional self-maintenance is subsumed under care. There is some reason, however, to separate the process system which is institutionally self-oriented from those events which are output-oriented. To maintain the alliterative game, the system devoted to self-maintenance could be called "core."

While the worlds of the hospital represent self-contained subcultures, the three process systems (care, cure, and core) involve continuities which are sometimes covert and sometimes manifest. Unlike other institutions the hospital places many of its functions into positions in which they participate, sometimes simultaneously, in more than one of these process systems. The characteristics of these three process systems within the hospital are of significance because they represent objectives, processes, and role expectations which converge at the site of patient care. Like the worlds, care, cure, and core tend to become components in the negotiating process, which in the position taken in this paper represents one essential view of the social organiztion of the hospital.

The processes of care and cure can be conceptualized as systems of functions and role obligations which assume certain properties of organizational collectivities within the hospital. Some members of the institution may assume roles in only one of the three process systems suggested here. Many functionaries, however, occupy simultaneous statuses in two or in all three of these systems. It can be documented that functionaries in the hospital, such as physicians and nurses, behave as inconsistently as the aforementioned professors within the multiple structure of the university. It must be repeated that the inconsistencies need not be experienced as role conflicts. The physician who voted as a member of a policy committee for a given procedure will not hesitate in his clinical status to disregard or circumvent it. The role of the nurse has been of special interest to this author because of her participation in all three systems and the institutional expectation that she absorb and reconcile their inconsistencies in translating these systems into patient care.

The Stages

The assumption that patient care is the product of sound management of

resources and people is not a sufficient one for understanding hospital organization. The suggested constructs of the patient care processes and of the
hospital worlds imply that the work product of the hospital, called patient
care, involves a negotiated order which encompasses the meeting grounds
between worlds and between process systems.

Although this paper is primarily concerned with the analytic consequences
of looking at the hospital from the vantage point of patient care, the stage as
a sociological phenomenon exists throughout the institution. It describes all
those situations in which contacts between worlds and process systems
involve netotiations, encounters, and role presentations. Thus interdepartmental committees, administrative planning, and patient care
conferences serve as stages, each containing institutionalized expectations of
appropriate representations for those who speak for worlds or for process
systems. It can be said that the hospital, as an organization, is beset by many
of its problems because the input processes on the management level as well
as the output processes on the patient-care level are set in the framework of
stages rather than worlds. The university president and his administration
represent a world which negotiates with the worlds of academic departments.
Hospital management as a process, however, has no world of its own. Thus
the pattern of negotiation of entities rather than merely of positions and
persons describes the stages of the hospitals.

We can now turn to an examination of the stage which denotes this domain
of the hospital where patient-care encounters occur. The theatrical analogy is
chosen because the stage represents the process of negotiation between performers, thereby yielding, in more or less dramatic ways, the product for the
client. For purposes of analysis and future research this suggests that the behavior of physician, nurse, dietician, or maid may be significantly different
when observed within the confines of their respective worlds than when
observed in the interchange and negotiation of the stage. One logical implication of this assertion raises questions about the scope and generalizability of
much research conducted in hospitals. Although extrapolation of behavior of
hospital functionaries from one site to another is obviously valid, the intra-
cultural or intercultural conditions prevailing in the three suggested systems
(worlds, process systems, stages) might well flavor the reality and meaning of
conduct. Thus studies of attitude about intrahospital relationships or about
norms and realities of patient care may need to be interpreted in terms of the
context in which the data were obtained. Inconsistencies of actually observed
behavior might be interpreted in terms of its reference to the appropriate role
location, be it world, process system, or stage.

Levels of Observation and Analysis

The processes of intersystem encounters within the hospital can be studied
in many ways. Three of the most fruitful levels of analysis are the focal points
of objectives, roles, and tasks. Some of the current literature (Bucher and
Strauss, 1966; Crook, 1964; Levinson, 1858; Perrow, 1965; Schullian, 1969)
reports studies on these levels, even though studies of tasks as symptoms of

social processes are least frequent. Most difficult to specify as directly related to the worlds and the three process systems are the various objectives which may complement or conflict in the synthesizing process of patient care. These conflicts or convergences become visible if they are identified with different actors representing different priorities among goals.

The scheduling of surgical intervention may conflict either with care-oriented judgments of patient needs or with core-oriented restraints imposed by hospital resources. One can sometimes observe conflict between the physician's judgment that the tasks of cure have been met and the patient is ready to be discharged and the consternation of the nurse or social worker who feels that the objectives of care have not yet been fulfilled. The dilemma between the pressure for beds and the requirements of continued hospitalization occurs sometimes within the framework of confrontation between worlds. It is less obvious when conflict between institutional objectives is resolved by a single individual rather than by negotiation between role incumbents or departments. Not infrequently, such diversities of objectives are part of the day-to-day decision-making, internalized by the phsycian or by other hospital functionaries. Yet examinations of interviews have suggested to this author that some of these intrapersonal decisions represent not only choices between priorities but also between role identifications in the described system.

Essentially, the institutional process can be analyzed from the vantage point of the differentiation and articulation of objectives, identified either with division of labor, institutional worlds, or cross-organizational process systems. There is a difference between objectives peculiar to medicine, nursing, or social work, and those which are identified with care, cure, and core. The latter have the capacity of cutting across the organizational and subcultural identities of the hospital. Either way, at the point of delivery of patient care—on the stage—we find the locus of negotitation and/or decision-making which resolves conflicts between objectives and negotiates priorities or accommodation.

The second level of negotiation taking place on the patient care stage occurs in relation to role incumbency: behavior, expectations, and assertion. This use of the stage is primarily an interaction between worlds, even though the process systems are obviously involved. It has been apparent to many researchers that the occupational groups of the hospital hold intragroup opinions and expectations of other occupational groups which are sometimes signficantly different from the overt behaviors manifested at the various stages of the hospital.

Stage behavior occurs at all of the established meeting grounds between worlds and process systems. Different stages, however, may produce different behaviors, particularly on the level of role interaction. Thus the norms of the physician's world may involve expectations of the nurse's role that are radically different from what is projected to nurses, patients, and others when the physican is acting on the patient care stage. This exchange of role expectations at the patient's bedside is again different from statements the physician is likely to make while participating in the drama of policy-making which takes place on a different, administration-oriented stage.

On first thought, one is tempted to think of the stage as the primary place where role behavior serves as a representation of world or process system interests. This is frequently the case. The nurse's attempt to project the authority of hospital policy through the vignette of the nurse's role frequently results in the physician responding to her role rather than to the legitimacy of the core system. This does not mean, however, that role behavior within the worlds is of necessity "backstage" behavior (Goffman, 1961)—less subject to role strain than behavior on the stage. Intraworld role expectations may also be experienced as a strain, such as the currently not infrequent dilemma for physicians who wish to foster interdisciplinary teamwork but have to cope with intraworld sanctions even though the stage may offer rewards.

The third level of analysis can be applied to the orchestration of tasks. Tasks have a special property. They are tangible products and not readily identifiable with all their antecedents. Patient-care tasks are simultaneous properties of all three systems suggested in this paper. The choice of tasks, the mode of their execution, and the criteria applied to their qualitative worth reflect a sometimes indeterminable mix between the systemic forces which have given rise to them. At the same time tasks are the manifest output of the system. If properly analyzed, tasks can be used as sociological benchmarks for institutional priorities, normative criteria, and style.

The use of task as an analytic tool for the understanding of behavior models is suggested as a fruitful approach to the vexing problem of the dilemma between professional and bureaucratic norms which compete in hospitals and other institutions of complex nature. The structure of task performance lends itself to categorizations which show the respective influences of the norms representing the hospital systems here discussed.

Task Models

Cursory examination of task behaviors in hospitals suggests that the bureaucratic and professional models may not be sufficient to account for all task orientations. The same task may also be judged by different criteria when viewed by different actors, at different times, or within different contexts. Six task models are presented here as an example of an analytic framework which, at this point, does not pretend to be exhaustive of all probabilities. These models, summarized in Chart 1, are suggested as ideal types; realities will rarely show pure versions. They are: the professional model, the bureaucratic model, the craft model, the technical model, the service model, and the entrepreueurial model.

The professional model. If we forget the identification of occupations as professions, paraprofessions, or nonprofessions, tasks could be examined regardless of who performs them. The professional model involves obviously the assumption of responsibility for the conduct and consequence of the task. It is also directed toward the needs of the client as interpreted by the performer. The professionally performed task does not preclude delegated activity, provided responsibility is transferred to the performer. The transfer

CHART 1
A PARADIGM OF MODAL TASK ORIENTATIONS

Model	Target	Expected Outcome	Criterion
Professional	Client needs	Reduction of client problem	Appropriateness, principles
Bureaucratic	Institutional integrity	Satisfaction of job requirements	Policies
Craft	Task itself	Product appearance, esthetic quality	Beauty, elegance
Technical	Specific task purpose	Task completion	Efficiency
Service	Client demands	Client satisfaction	Compliance
Entrepreneurial	Task performer	Profit	Selling maximization

itself can be a point of conflict or negotiation. The client's needs represent the major orientation of the professional task, principles of knowledge are the criteria of conduct, and the goal of the professional task is the reduction of client problems. Rewards for professionally performed tasks are consequence, satisfaction, and peer approval.

The bureaucratic model. Following the well-documented descriptions of bureaucratic behavior, one can observe that certain tasks are performed in such a fashion that the organization itself, or its integrity, is the target of the activity. The policies of the institution are the criteria of performance, and the satisfaction of more or less formal expectations is the expected outcome of the task. Bureaucratically performed tasks are performed within the context of institutional resource manipulation rather than within the system of client needs. They are performed within the framework of requirements and frequently involve the obligation of reporting and recording. Approval by superiors represents the source of rewards.

The craft model. The preoccupation with bureaucratic and professional conflict has resulted in an oversight of the fact that actual behavior can be guided by other norm orientations. Participating in doctoral examinations of students in mathematics, I was impressed with the frequency with which a student's dissertation performance was described as meeting the criteria of "elegance" and of "beauty." The esthetic characteristic of the task itself and the pride of workmanship were thus considered. This same set of criteria is also observable in the actual flow of patient-care performance. Whether it is the admiration for the diminutive and neat surgical incision, the impeccably made bed, or the elegance of the physician's self-presentation at the patient's bedside, the importance of the craft component in the synthesis of patient care should not be underestimated. As a special area of interest, it can be observed that a large proportion of the almost traditional criticisms of dietary output fall within the craft model.

The target of the craft model is the task itself. Its criterion is elegance and beauty, and the outcome is the esthetic quality of the product. Admiration rather than approval describes the flavor of the appropriate reward.

The technical model. To the extent that technology involves the processes of technique selection, application, and assessment, and to the extent that technique application has been institutionalized and ritualized, the performance of the techniques themselves tends to shift from a level of professional, judgmental, and artistic behaviors to the technical sphere, i.e. the expert performance of thoroughly rehearsed, competently performed tasks placed into a larger functional context by initiators and assessors. The term "technical" is used here to describe those activities governed primarily by a means-end relationship between a determined task objective and the task resources. Target is the immediate objective of the task itself, the criterion is efficiency, and the outcome is task completion.

The technical model can be observed in all aspects of patient care. Performance of physicians and nurses includes behaviors which are governed by the technical perspective, even though the repertory of the so-called technician leads us to expect these functionaries to resort more typically to the technical model. The technical task involves direct dependence on the superordinate functionary who initiated the request for the task and whose approval represents a reward.

The service model. Integrated into the sequence of patient care activities are tasks which are the direct result of patient demands. These tasks are sometimes performed without the interposition of stage judgments. The service model has the client's demands as its target. It seeks client satisfaction, its criterion is compliance, and it is rewarded by client approval. Although the service model is more likely an appropriate framework for tasks performed by certain personnel categories, it is by no means absent from any level of status, including physicians. The prevalence of the service model in certain exclusive accommodations of prestige hospitals might be a fruitful tool of assessment in differentiating patient care in various settings. Furthermore, the client orientation of the service model is possibly a clue to the different degrees of interaction potential inherent in the nature of task performance.

The entrepreneurial model. Even though the hospital is not an expected site for entrepreneurial behavior, this reference syndrome represents an important task guidance system since it does occur in the practice of medicine, particularly outside of the hospital. Yet it does occur within the institution, and not only among physicians. There are times when procedures, tests, or even drugs are "sold." There are ways of suggesting posthospital resources which approximate entrepreneurial behavior. Of all the models suggested here, this one is least supported by the institutional system and is frequently associated with questionable behavior. Nevertheless, some departments in the hospital pride themselves as being revenue-producing units. The target of the entrepreneurial model is the interest of the task performer, the outcome is profit, and the criterion is selling. The rewards of the entrepreuneurial model lie in the economic sphere.

Implications and Conclusion

The constructs suggested in the previous pages are admittedly imprecise and, at this time at least, at best heuristic devices. They succeed, it is hoped, in presenting a picture of movement, interaction adaptations, and receptivity to ever-changing forces. The function of these constructs is to move perspective and emphasis from institutional operations to the conditions of institutional output. While this shift of emphasis is presented as scientifically required and justified, this concern with the institutional setting from the client's point of view also seems to fit other current trends.

One reason or explanation for this shift can be provided within the framework of the sociology of knowledge. The mood of our society is shifting from examining the forces which support the effectiveness of the establishment and the power of the executive to preoccupation with the objects of institutional control and the recipients of services. It is plausible therefore that sociological analysis follows this trend. The cries for concern with the fate of the client, be it the student, the inmate, or the patient, are a powerful and persuasive voice in the choice of sociological perspectives.

Related to this shift in social climate is the demand for relevance of the disciplines. Associated with the far-reaching dissatisfaction with the effectiveness of social institutions are the emerging traces of a social mandate which is being imposed on the social scientist. There is some evidence that increasing segments of society look to the social scientist for realistic and relevant answers. The flavor of the questions asked of the social scientist has significantly moved from requests for understanding and prediction to intervention and improvement. This begs the age-old question of pure and applied research. Implicit in the approach taken here is the assumption that the distance between pure and applied research is inversely proportional to the quality of the research itself. At the level of the best scientific product the distance could be zero.

This paper represents a somewhat groping attempt to combine a continuing commitment to the integration and accretion of scientific knowledge with a shift to client-oriented application and formulation of data. In synthesizing existing research, the questions must be asked about the extent to which the currently existing framework will serve the institution or its client.

We are witnessing the increasing inroads made by technology into the inner workings of the hospital. Computerization of patient-care events is likely to result in reduced degrees of freedom for negotiations and modifications among the encounters involved in patient care. Increased prescriptions and rigidity could conceivably enhance the efficiency or even effectiveness of patient care greatly, provided certain assumptions are met. One of the assumptions, to be tested, is the reality level of a wholistic system capable of thriving under conditions of reduced ambiguity. If the suggestions in the preceding pages are valid, prior questions need to be raised. Is it conceivable that the optimal utilization of technology is dependent upon a fundamental reorganization of hospital processes? Is the "stage" essentially an artistic environment which will wither with ritualization and prescription? Should we create a "world" environment for the site of patient care with all of the implications of unity of communications and the development of social identity before changes in procedure can be beneficial?

In closing, it should be noted that the foregoing discussion does not include the relationship of the patient himself to the institution; nor does it raise questions of patient response and patient experience. The main purpose of the paper was to present a conceptual-analytical framework for the study of hospital organization from the perspective of system output and patient care. The discussion suggests that an analysis of existing literature, and the much needed endeavor of establishing conceptual schemes with which to synthesize accumulated research, should not be confined to the implicit assumptions which have traditionally characterized such research. On the contrary, the remarkable repertory of knowledge which has been accumulated should be examined for lacunae of coverage, for phenomena not adequately described within prevailing approaches, and for areas of importance which have not received their share of attention. Our discussion suggests, moreover, that under the conditions of complexity which characterize the hospital traditional research techniques may not be adequate. Synthesis of analytic schemes and propositions may need to lead to carefully controlled experimental approaches which can test the phenomenological validity of different conceptual schemes.

References

Anderson, T. R., and Warkov, K. Organizational size and functional complexity: a study of administration in hospitals. *American Sociological Review,* 1961, *26,* 23-28.
Argyris, C. *Personality and organization: the conflict between system and the individual.* New York: Harper, 1957.
Bertalanffy, L. General systems theory: a new approach to unity of science. *Human Biology,* December 1951, 303-361.
Blau, P. M. Social integration, social rank, and processes of interaction. *Human Organization,* 1959-60, *18,* 152-158.
Blau, P. M. and Scott, W. R. *Formal organizations.* San Francisco: Chandler, 1962.
Boulding K. General systems theory: the skeleton of science. *Management Science,* April 1956, 197-208.
Bucher, R., and Stelling, J. Characteristics of professional organizations. *Journal of Health and Social Behavior,* 1969, *10,* 3-15.
Bucher, R., and Strauss, A. Professions in process. In W. R. Scott and E. H. Volkart (Eds.) *Medical care: readings in the sociology of medical institutions.* New York: Wiley, 1966.
Crook, R. K. Role differentiation and functional integration: a structural model of a mental hospital. Doctoral dissertation, Princeton University, 1964.
Durbin, R. L., and Springall, W. H. *Organization and administration of health care.* St. Louis: Mosby, 1969.
Etzioni, A. *A comparative analysis of complex organizations.* New York: Free Press, 1961.
Georgopoulos, B. S., and Mann, F. C. *The community general hospital.* New York: Macmillan, 1962.
Goffman, E. *Asylums: essays on the social situation of mental patients and other inmates.* Garden City, N.Y.: Anchor Books, 1961.

Goffman, E. *Encounters: two studies in the sociology of interaction*. Indianapolis: Bobbs-Merrill, 1961.

Gouldner, A. W. Cosmopolitans and locals: toward an analysis of latent social roles, part I. *Administrative Science Quarterly*, 1957, *2*, 281-306.

Gouldner, A. W. Cosmopolitans and locals: toward an analysis of latent social roles, part II. *Administrative Science Quarterly*, 1958, *2*, 444-480.

Hage, J. An axiomatic theory of organizations. *Administrative Science Quarterly*, 1965, *9*, 289-320.

Hall, R. H. Intraorganizational structural variations: application of the bureaucratic model. *Administrative Science Quarterly*, 1962, *7*, 295-308.

Howland, D. A hospital system model. *Nursing Research*, 1963, *12*, 232-236.

Jelinek, R. C. An operational analysis of the patient care function. *Inquiry*, 1969, *6*, 53-58.

Julian, J. Compliance patterns and communication blocks in complex organizations. *American Sociological Review*, 1966, *31*, 382-389.

Kast, E. F., and Rosenzweig, J. E. Hospital administrative and systems concepts. *Hospital Administration*, 1966, *11*, 17-33.

Levinson, D. J. Role, personality, and social structure in the organizational setting. *Journal of Abnormal and Social Psychology*, 1959, *58* 170-180.

Mauksch, H. O. Organizational context of nursing practice. In F. Davis (Ed.) *The nursing profession*. New York: Wiley, 1966.

Mauksch, H. O., and Tagliacozzo, D. The patient's view of the patient role. In E. G. Jaco (Ed) *Patients, physicians, and illness*. New York: Free Press, 2nd ed., in press.

Mechanic, D. Sources of power of lower participants in complex organizations. *Administrative Science Quarterly*, 1967, *12*, 349-364.

Miller, E. J., and Rice, A. K. *Systems of organization*. London: Tavistock, 1967.

Operations Research Quarterly. Decision-making in hospitals. *Operations Research Quarterly*, 1968, *19*, 52-54.

Perrow, C. Hospitals: technology, structure, and goals. In J. G. March (Ed.) *Handbook of organizations*. Chicago: Rand McNally, 1965.

Pfiffner, J. N., and Sherwood, F. P. *Administrative organizations*. Englewood Cliffs, N.J.: Prentice-Hall, 1960.

Price, J. L. Impact of departmentalization in interoccupational ccoperation. *Human Organization*, 1968, *27*, 362-368.

Schullian, S. J. M. A study of management by objectives systems. Masters thesis. Xavier University, 1969.

Strauss, A., *et al*. The hospital and its negotiated order. In E. Freidson (Ed.) *The hospital in modern society*. New York: Free Press, 1963.

8

ISSUES AND DISCUSSION
OF PART THREE

Professionals, Work Technology, and Organization:

Presentation Highlights: W. R. Scott

In some ways what I am trying to do in the paper fits somewhere in between the work of Neuhauser and Andersen, i.e. the comparative-structural studies of hospitals, and the Mauksch approach, if that is possible. And perhaps it suffers from the errors of both types of approaches.

I begin by discussing some general trends. One of these is this trend that we are all very aware of, moving from case to comparative studies. It very seriously concerns me that as we begin to move from case studies, where there is a fairly good descriptive material gathered from sizable samples of respondents, to comparative studies, we move to the polar opposite of basing our organizational study on the reports of one respondent or one set of statistics that some assistant to the hospital administrator was good enough to send out. This scares me very much. I think we as a profession have to begin to develop standards for reliability and for validity, and so forth, just as we developed these when dealing with samples of respondents. It seems that we need to begin to think very hard about what kinds of valid data can we really expect to collect from certain types of respondents. The use of informants, as opposed to respondents, in comparative structural studies is becoming an increasingly critical issue in my opinion.

Also I had a comment on the fact that a good many of the old case studies and comparative studies continue to rely on samples of respondents or sometimes on the total population. But I see very little tendency in this work to begin to try to weigh the answers given by the various respondents. Somehow one doctor is just like another doctor when we begin to add up satisfaction scores, or other scores about what is going on, when everything we write in all the other pages says that one respondent is not like another. In fact, there are enormous variations across respondents in terms of their information, their influence, their commitment, and so on. It seems to me that it really is time to become somewhat more sophisticated in even the old survey techniques as they apply to organizations.

Next, I made some comments on the general move from the use of closed to open system models. I think it is hard to be very clear about what is going on because these new open system models are new, just at the stage where they are nothing more than a kind of promise, raising questions about previous perspectives without being terribly clear, particularly about methodological implications. But one of the implications is that we have to take seriously, more seriously than in the past, the effect of environmental variations on structural systems.

The focus on intrastructural variation as though one could talk about intraorganizational variation in hospitals without taking into account the environmental setting of those hospitals raises serious questions. Clearly, there is a serious charge leveled against really everything that has been said up to this point about structure. There is such a powerful and neglected set of variables there, representing environmental variation, and the question arises as to whether we know anything or not at this point about intraorganizational variation. I think this is a question that we should take very seriously.

As I try to interpret and understand the message of the open system theorists, it seems to me that they are trying to say something about different levels or different types of structure, and characterize this as different degrees of tightness or looseness of structure. One of the things that they are telling us is that maybe some of the categories we use in order even to begin to talk about structure may be inappropriate, given certain kinds of problems. It may be that it is absolutely absurd for us to be sitting around here talking about hospital structure as though a hospital was a meaningful unit of analysis. Perhaps what we really should be talking about is health-care systems rather than hospital structures. The hospital plays a certain kind of role in certain kinds of health-care delivery problems, but it may be that we cannot take that out and look at it as though it were a system because it is just a part of a system—the total health-care delivery system. For a large number of problems that we think we are studying this may be a good criticism.

The third trend that bears very directly on my paper, I wish I could more completely understand it too, is that I begin to hear distant rumblings of gradual dissatisfaction on the part of my colleagues with the entrepreneurial model as an approach to professional organizations. It is a model that we have long used, a model that certainly I have used and a good many of my friends have used, but I think it may be an image and a model that very much gets in the way of our seeing what in fact is going on in these complex structures. We may be just years and years behind the times in still trying to apply this model to these completely new and different work settings.

As a way of getting at some of these new work settings I focus very much on the variable of technology,* I think because of its critical importance for the way in which work is organized. This is also very much in line with Freidson's comment that the work setting and the place in which work is carried out probably have a great deal more to do with what, in fact, happens in terms of activities and interactions than do the kinds of skills and professional characteristics or standards of the trainees who come into these settings. It seems to me that one of the serious problems that we have is that our socialization

---

*Editor's note: the reader should keep in mind that Dr. Scott uses the term "technology" in a broad sense, to include not only the physical but also the social technology of work.

settings continue, among other things, to inculcate this entrepreneurial professional model, which ill suits people to come into these work settings and
play an effective role in them.

I very quickly suggest, in a rather apologetic way, several kinds of ways for
looking at the dimensions of technology. None of these are new; they all have
been used in one place or another. Specifically, I focus on: (1) the uniformity
and nonuniformity of inputs and outputs; (2) the efficacy or the extent to
which the transformation strategies of the organization are or are not
rationalized—that is, the extent to which there is a cause/effect kind of
relationship built-in such that the effects or the results are replicable and
people can be trained to carry out these techniques; and (3) the variations in
the social importance attributed to both inputs and outputs. One of the
reasons why I focus on these three is that it seems to me that they tend to
move in opposite directions, particularly as it affects the organization of
hospitals and the care of patients.

The emphasis on the nonuniformity of inputs and outputs, which is very
much reinforced by the clinical orientation and the physicians, and the social
importance attributed to the objects worked on, together move toward the
production of certain kinds of structural characteristics that emphasize
uniqueness, individualized attention, and customizing of the work process.
But the other major variable, efficacy, or the increasing reationalization of
these transformation processes, very much pushes in the opposite direction,
toward a division of labor and then, given labor divided, toward mechanisms
for coordinating and for directing that work. It seems to me, therefore, that
we have two different kinds of critical dimensions by which we characterize
the patients, and the technology of the organization very much presses in
opposite directions at this point—on the one hand toward customizing, and
on the other hand toward increasing specialization and division of labor.

Along with the recent trend toward the comparative perspective, the other
very important trend in organizational research is toward the emphasis on
technology and its relationship to structure. It is for this reason that I tried,
in my paper, to raise a number of problems that I see in attempting to move
directly from technology to defining characteristics of inputs, outputs, and
the transformation process, and to studying the characteristics of the structure.

If we focus just on the professional side of the hospital (and there are other
kinds of work going on in a hospital), for example, or on the care and cure
structure in Mauksch's terms, certainly the degree of efficacy varies
enormously across the different professional groups. Even if one looks at a
particular group, such as physicians, Straus and others remind us that in fact
there is a very uneasy union of a whole range of competing and conflicting
groups with different skills, different interests, and different efficacies associated with their technologies. Even if we just focus on the individual practitioner, we see that there are a whole range of tasks, some of which are highly
routinized, others of which are not routinizable, and some of which are highly
efficacious while others are not. Given the variations that are in fact present
in the kinds of tasks being carried out, and the kinds of skills that are

brought to bear on those tasks, it is a serious question as to what you say about the technology associated with a complex organization such as the hospital.

But even more important than any of these complexities (and in the paper I suggest one or two ways perhaps of dealing with some, for example focusing on core tasks) is the fact that if we are not careful we are likely to fall into a technological determinism in our approach to these problems. It would be a mistake to believe that there is something called technology which is there for everyone to see and which somehow is a real thing that can be measured and objectively evaluated. The more I look at what goes on in structures such as hospitals, the more I am convinced that social definitions and social conceptions play a critical role in terms of how technology is viewed. With respect to the three dimensions I have talked about, for example, it seems to me that it is possible, depending upon how you emphasize things, to see high uniformity or nonuniformity in the very same phenomena. It just depends on whether you emphasize the characteristics that are similar or the characteristics that differ among the task options. Even efficacy is very much a social definition; it depends in part on how we define and how we view the end product. I consider this to be a great victory for the sociologists—in a sense we reclaim this for our own—because in these terms the study of the work technology in relation to organizational structure and functioning becomes again sociological instead of economical or Marxian or whatever you like.

Even the technology presents a kind of "now you see it, now you don't" problem because of these enormous differences. One way to get a handle on this problem is to look at some of what is going on by asking, "Whose conceptions are we talking about?" Incidentally, this kind of simple-minded question comes from and relates to lots of other important questions, like the question of goals: "Whose goals?" Somehow we organizational theorists do not ask this question often enough.

In asking this kind of question, one way in which you can view some of what is going on in these complex structures is to begin by saying that very often there are certain managerial conceptions about goals, tasks, technology, etc. That is, there are certain people in organizations who define what the task is, and who have a responsibility for setting up a structure to achieve it. Very often there is some kind of calculus involved in their conceptions, such as "given this kind of work, then these are appropriate arrangements." Just to relate this to the paper, what I have in mind here with respect to managerial conceptions are things like views of uniformity/nonuniformity, efficacy/nonefficacy, and social importance. What I have in mind with respect to structural arrangements are things like the division of labor, the extent of formalization, the degree of bureaucratization, the kinds of evaluation of arrangements that are set up, and so on. One can talk about what tasks are appropriate and what they may lead to, or are consistent with. This is simple enough, perhaps, and here is where most of the work has been done.

But I would like to suggest that in addition to the managerial conceptions of tasks, performers too have conceptions of the work they do, and these are very much affected by the structural arrangements in the organization. That is, your conception of the task you do is affected by how the work is given to you, whether you are given an order or whether the work is delegated to you, by the way in which your work is evaluated, and the like. All these things give some clue as to the way in which your work is viewed. In other words, task arrangements, particularly those mediated by evaluation and allocation structures, affect very much what the performer's conception of the work is.

Particulary in professional organizations such as hospitals, there is another very important source of these performer conceptions, the external reference groups of performers, especially the professional institutions themselves. These socializing institutions in a sense are a part of what this group is all about. They try to inculcate into the performers certain conceptions about what the core task is; about what it is that you are trying to do; what it is that you are here for; and what kinds of skills you should have. And this is very much mediated, if you like intervening variables, by the orientation of the particular performer to his reference group—does he or does he not look to this group for these kinds of standards and these kinds of views of his work?

The conceptions of the performers in turn have certain kinds of impact on the managerial conceptions. The impact is largely mediated by variables of power and power dependency relationships—are these people dependent upon these people, or are they dependent upon those? In the case of physicians, because of the administrative-professional dependency relationships here, the performers' conceptions are such that physicians in effect are able to impose their conceptions of their work, and appropriate arrangements for that work, on the administrators, the people who set up those tasks. Other professional groups, such as social workers, nursing groups, and so forth, are not in similar positions, and in these cases it is the managerial conceptions that are in effect imposed upon their work. As a way of studying this, and I am trying to study it as a matter of fact, one can say that these performer conceptions of work give rise to preferred organizational arrangements or structures: "If I am doing this kind of work, I should have this kind of structure."

One can then look at the discrepancy between the actual structures and preferred structures in order to make certain predictions about instability, dissatisfaction, or whatever. This kind of model (which is a messy paradigm—I am not trying to pass it off as a great path diagram) or set of variables, it seems to me, both gives you a way of looking at any one system at a point in time and also says something about the way in which these systems are really changing. For example, we are studying teachers now, and one of the things happening is that teachers, partly because of their school training and because of the new sort of militant professionalizing attitude of the schools of education, are beginning to develop new conceptions of themselves. They are beginning to put new pressures on management, and management is beginning to take new views of what the teaching task is, how much autonomy a teacher should have, how much curriculum can be simply directed down toward them, and so on. One would expect then, as one measures the degree of discrepancy between the preferred and the actual operating arrangements, to get an indicator of what is going on in this system.

This model also helps with the old problem of whether there is really a conflict between professional and organizational arrangements more generally. In the case where the professionals are in a position to dominate and dictate the structure, I think the answer is no. In the case where in fact that structure is imposed upon them, then the answer is yes. There is going to be a lot of tension, conflict, and dissatisfaction in that structure.

Let me just say one or two more things about these changes in technology and the effects that they are creating on the division of labor. Regarding specialization, simply because of increased scientific knowledge, a professional now has to choose to be an incompetent generalist or a competent specialist. And, as we know, they are all choosing to be competent specialists. Therefore, they get involved in organizational structures and a division of labor which has some need for coordination and integration of their activities. And, although I agree very much with Eliot Freidson and others that there is just an enormous lack of control in these structures, I am beginning to see the beginning signs of structural arrangements there for coordination and control. In this sense I agree very much with Etzioni, in his comparative analysis book, who indicates that more and more of the actual operation of professional control has moved away from the professional community as such and into the professional organization.

There are three different kinds of structures that one can isolate here that are beginning to exercise this control function in an appropriate way, allowing for the clinical problems and for some individualized treatment. One of these is the so-called peer group process, using peer group in a very loose sense. I think Freidson is right that in the old-fashioned sense probably the peer group is a creation of the professional public relations men and the sociologists who happen to have a certain kind of model. As you know, he looked in the clinic and did not find any sign that this system was working. But I would like to suggest that a least my own observations in the Stanford hospital suggest that, if you define peer group broadly enough, you can see peer group processes going on in some of these working group arrangements. These groups, which very often are called teams, can be analyzed as temporary structures which, in fact, exert an enormous amount of quality control on the work being conducted. I am very impressed by the amount of criticism, the visibility and possibility of control, and the actual control that is exerted in informal ways within those teams. It seems to me that we would be neglecting a very important part of the control process if we did not look at what is going on there.

Also I think that in addition to this peer group phenomenon within all these organizations there are very important distinctions (I think I would refer to them as differential peer group control), particularly the tenure versus nontenure distinction, and between finished and trainee kinds of distinctions. Again, there is a good deal of control going on there, a different level of control, as well as training.

Third, and this is nothing new, is the actual bureaucratization of the professional group. And this, I think, is an important and a fitting place to close on. Goss, for example, in her discussion of authority and influence in a hospital, looks at that and finds a very specialized kind of control structure where authority is influenced in one area and influences in another. I look at her data and think "This group has gone a long way toward bureaucratization of the control arrangements where certain people, certain specific members of the medical-care team, are now charged with the right to sample performance. They are charged with the right to appraise performance, and they are charged with the right to make suggestions which have to be taken into account. Whether or not their suggestions are followed is immaterial, or rather it is not an issue. They have to be reckoned with, and if they are not followed you have to be able to explain why you did not follow them. It seems to me that this really moves an enormous amount in the direction of organizational control over these kinds of performances, and in a way that is appropriate because of the qualifications of the people holding these positions.

Discussion

Question: Do you see any input from the managerial conception of the task into the professional institutions down at the bottom? I think one of the great problems in our system is that the professional institutions down at the bottom are not accountable in any way and that there must be some input from the managerial conception of the task to drown these professional institutions in reality.

Answer (Dr. Scott): You know there is, and you are absolutely right. But one of the nice things is that the discrepancy of conceptions may be small. We have corollary studies, for example, which show that where managerial conceptions were involved in the transitions of diploma programs in hospitals, there was very little discrepancy between these conceptions and those of the nurses. In the diploma programs where you had a really independent unit, on the other hand, there were great disparities leading to conflict. Where they have some influence, the discrepancy is much reduced.

Comment: I do not agree with what you say.

Answer: Let us hear about that because I thought that that was a great study. What happened?

Response: Some of the data were expressions of conversions when, in fact, some of the data show that the behavior was very different and showed discrepancies which are very real in the diploma program. There are some very good things about the study, but this is one area where I felt it missed. If you recall, some of the data appeared in various journals simultaneously, and if you combine them all you can see certain behavior aspects which would suggest that there are many more real differences.

Comment: But there are other factors apart from conception disparities that would go into that. There are self-selecting factors, the provincialism of the hospital school of nursing where the students do not have interaction with other professional students on campus to get a professional ethos, and other kinds of structural variables that cause the attitudinal set.

Comment: The model you have proposed strikes me as being closer to the current goals of national spokesmen and political and social leadership than anything else I have heard discussed this afternoon. I think because of this that there are some implications in this which are worth your discussing here. There is a possibility that, in fact, as you said in your opening statements, hospitals are not the center of the health-care system. The hospital is really a badly defined and also rapidly varying piece of a much larger system. Once you enter the hospital per se, you are raising all kinds of questions about role conceptions which perhaps you ought to avoid just like the hospital administrator or the nurse ought to avoid.

The next point is that the concept of the move to bureaucratization and the notion of bringing more components of the system under control strikes me as the central focus of effort in the health-care system for the 1970s. From a pragmatic viewpoint, the system is now clearly out of control in almost every aspect, and the whole job of the next decade will be to try to bring decision-making and control processes to rational levels which are responsive to community notions. As an administrator, I know of no other way to formulate my professional job. This means, perhaps, that you have to abandon craft models and professional models and turn to much more bureaucratic models in describing the organizations which will result. Certainly that is the way it would appear to me. And that gets us to the contribution that you can make, on a practical level, toward understanding the dynamics of these kinds of changes. What are the dynamics involved, for example, in taking a highly integrated profession like medicine or nursing and imposing upon it goals that are quite external to its profession, and having to do it first by alteration of the educational system and simultaneously by changing the attitudes of a range of professionals from age 25 to 65?

Comment (Dr. Scott): I do not know exactly how to respond. Let me just say a couple of things. One is that I do think that increasingly these arrangements are being bureaucratized in hospitals, and I think in a pretty intelligent way. That is, it seems to me that there is an awful lot of coordination and integration that can occur in a quasi-hierarchical way, by feedback and by plan, rather than by directive. And this is the way in which this kind of work is appropriately coordinated. I also think that we really need to understand much better how these transitory and temporary teams in fact operate and function. In those cases where bureaucracy is the model, as opposed to hospitals, I am impressed with how much we have to get outside of that framework in order to get anything done. In those cases we create ad hoc committees, task forces, and teams, and this is how and where the real work gets done.

Comment: And the reason for this may be the nature of the bureaucracy. Because the bureaucracy is a very bad bureaucracy and the rules are stupid and they do not make any sense in terms of the technology, you have to create such task forces and committees. But if you had a bureaucracy that made a little sense, in terms of the changing of rules, you might have much less need for this kind of activity, which in fact is costly.

Answer: There are different kinds and degrees of bureaucracy. But I also think that, regardless of how benevolent or how intelligent and intelligible the bureaucracy is, there are problems with the organization of work that simply come from the routinization of that work. In this connection I recommend that you all take a look at Miles' article. Some of his comments are very important, those on the peculiar advantages of a temporary system, in terms of a sharply focused range of activity, in terms of immediate goals that people can actually see they are making progress toward, and in terms of breaking through status barriers where all the people are working together and making contributions to these things. It seems to me that there are reasons why you go outside even the best, most intelligent structure. There are reasons why you want to keep enough flexibility to be able to form and reform groups within the overall mold. In fact, we act this way all the time in our universities and in our government, but no one really pays any attention when we become theorists.

Comment: Nobody would disagree with that. It is a question of where the problem is, where the crisis is, or where the focus should be.

Comment: The crisis is not at the level of the solution of the specific problem. It is clear what the problem is, and this is where the transitory team is a beautiful model. But it is not a very good model in terms of the broader objective, in which case the bureaucratic model is more appropriate. The two have to be brought into some concordance with each other, however.

Comment: I do have trouble with your model. I do not think that you emphasize enough the consumer, the outside conception. I cannot emphasize too much how I feel, at least as a physician, the fact that the center of gravity is moving away from the administrator, away from everyone else, and into the hands of those who are asking that these instruments, these hospitals, be put to certain purposes that they see. I think your model has to take this into account. Perhaps it does vaguely, but it does not say what to watch for.

Question: Who are these people? You mean the consumers? Patients?

Answer: Yes to both. You cannot ignore, for example, what has happened in the last seventy years. What do you think is the genesis of Medicare and Medicaid? What do you think is the genesis of Regional Medical Programs or Comprehensive Health Planning programs? These are vaguely perceived.

Comment: Not from the consumer.

Answer: Wait, who is it then? Is it the legislature? Well, these are consumers making their demands through their representatives. Whatever you want to call them, let us say these are forces outside. Why do you have trouble with this? I really think this is the most important part of the process, and I am concerned that it has not come sufficiently into any of the considerations here. The legislation is a way the public, the consumer, all consumers, are saying to us, all of us, and you are included in this, "What is the system for?" "We want it to be used for certain things." They perceive that there is no planning, be it group planning or comprehensive health planning. But in a vague kind of way they attempt to get some planning and input into the system.

Comment: Right now you find disagreement as to who the consumer is.

Answer: Let us not get lost in this kind of thing. I am talking about the people outside of medicine, generically speaking the public or whatever you want to call it. It is the public, it is the voters, and it is the Congress. They are feeling the pressure of unfilled needs.

Comment: Yes. It is handled in a political arena through the voters and through legislation. But it is also handled in an economic sense.

Question: Is this not a social force to be accounted for? That is what I am asking here.

Comment (Dr. Zald): Since my topic is the social control of institutions, I would ask you to look at my paper again because we did not talk much about this. I agree with you, but I think there is a terminological problem which is very important. When most people use the word "consumer," they are talking about somebody getting the direct output. If you are talking about the political game involved in creating Regional Medical Programs, for example, it is very important to make a distinction between political forces which have not a consumer game and the entrepreneurial game of political symbol-makers. It is very important for us, as social scientists, to remember that when we talk about outside forces we do not just mean the guy who just had a heart attack. He is not demanding anything other than the solution to his own problem. The process by which we get legislation is a much different process than the process you would conceive of if you focused upon the demand of an individual. It is very very different, and the whole shape of our institutions is caught up in this process.

Comment (Dr. Pellegrino): I would like to respond to that. I think that you are misinterpreting the force of an action which you attribute, let us say, to policical symbol-makers. I think that is to be blind to what has been happening in the past decade. If you talk to legislators as I do, trying to get support for health sciences centers, they are reflecting what the people are saying. If you do not want to call these people consumers, that is a different matter. I happen to regard everybody as a consumer of health care, everybody who is deeply concerned with this now. These people *are* making these needs felt. And I submit that you are doing a fine job of analyzing within the system, but unless you put this into your system as an extremely potent force in control, I think you are missing an important factor. That is all I am saying. You mentioned it, but you do not account for it in your model.

Comment: Let us move back to the model here. We do have the problem of boundaries in the system, and Scott brought that up. You always have to draw the boundaries arbitrarily, and the question is how you weigh them. So let us accept this as a hospital. Now a very interesting thing that he alluded to was the business of power.

Comment: Excuse me, except it is a hospital that brings in the training institutions and outside pressures.

Comment: You are right; it is a hospital as an ongoing system at least. But what is very interesting to me is that you can account for most of those things except that you glossed over power, and this is directly relevant to what Pellegrino is saying here. I am sure you have given it attention, but I am not quite sure to the extent that you maintain it. What has happened recently, and the real impact of this on the hospital has not yet been felt, is that the doctor who previously by legislation had responsibility for the patient and, therefore, had power because his commitment took precedence, no longer enjoys this position. The legal commitment is going to the trustees who are going to be ultimately responsible for the patient, so that we get power now gradually transferred as trustees realize their responsibility under the law. This will have a fantastic impact. As to the matter of Regional Medical Programs and related health programs in the country, I think hospitals have wonderful abilities, as do other organizations, to transform any of these inputs and use them for their own ends. Obviously certain hospitals have increased in size and have taken on new kinds of functions. But I wonder how much effect this has had on the system.

Comment: I agree with you about the effectiveness of outside forces to date. I was simply trying to signal, as I think you have, that there were indications of a shift in the center of gravity of the forces impinging on the system that can throw the whole system out of its orbit. Regarding the matter of power and the role of the board of trustees, again I agree with you. I think that, more and more, the relationship between craftsmanship and bureaucracy, and the related conflict of aims and objectives, very frequently has to be resolved in a new way. I happen to think that the appropriate resolution would be to put the professional in the role of expert witness but not in the role of setting the goals. The boards of trustees probably will be the instruments in society for bringing this whole system into some conformity with the outside world.

Comment: I think there is a very important case in support of the role of the consumer, and the politicians are only in the act now because they represent the consumer like never before. Congress turned down several Medicare bills under President Truman because then the American Medical Association could knock these off, and there was not enough support from the consumers to countervail the professional obstacles. The situation now has changed. A beautiful case of how the consumer dictated to the medical staff what kinds of medical service they are going to provide occurred recently in Seattle. The medical staff refused to provide psychiatric services and physical rehabilitation until the board of trustees (there they elect their own board from the membership of enrolees in the health plan) said: "You doctors are going to bring in psychiatric service or we are going to go out and get it someplace else." And the physicians then provided psychiatric service, provided physical medicine, and provided long-term care service. If they had their way, they would not be providing these services to the consumer. Power is a fantastic organization whereby the consumers can get some of the services that they want. Comprehensive Health Planning legislation now requires that a portion of the board must be consumers as opposed to providers of health care, and the consumers must outnumber the providers. They even have a ratio in there, 51 percent.

Comment: We have not even begun to see the role of the consumer because he is prepaying. But now he has got power. The board of trustees of old never even had any sensitivity to consumer wants. When it was made up of wealthy donors and prominent individuals, it provided services in a paternalistic fashion. This is definitely changing, however, because the economy is changing and the quality and character of trusteeship is changing in the whole health care picture. In all this the government now is just symbolic, I think, as the consumers rise in power.

Comment (Dr. Mauksch): I do not think Scott's model is necessarily exclusive of this; as was presented, I think it is only part of it. As a matter of fact I think his comment earlier startled me a little bit, because he saw it as a set of simple dimensions while I was listening to, observing, and seeing that it was a nice diagram of the real complexity. I would like to try, if I may, a sort of marriage between the concepts that I presented and Scott's. Let me just deal with Pellegrino's point. Here is the notion of the performing groups, and here is the notion of the performing standards. Now obviously there is also the board of trustees, and they represent one kind of input. In addition, there are funding programs and funding agencies, and these too represent an input. But whatever it is, you have external power sources which serve also as financial power sources and as vehicles for input of power. These themselves contain another set of these preferred structural norms, more or less explicitly.

I would like to complicate this model by suggesting that even these performing groups within the hospital—there are really about fifteen of them—are simultaneously negotiating. The matter of power is, of course, one of degree, and these various groups are negotiating. As they are negotiating they are subject to change. I think Peter Blau's notion of power and exchange is very apt here because, as technology makes the manager more powerful, since you cannot get the kidney machine in your private office, there is an exchange involved here. The system becomes more complicated because there is negotiation and exchange between managers and professionals, among professionals, and among the various other groups. The old story that the hospital manager is no exact fit is, of course, true. He is really a mediator between different worlds and an expert in foreign relations and a negotiator in that sense. This is really what I think your model suggests to me.

Question: Could you just add one box—unions—that is half way between the performing groups and the outside power centers?

Answer: No. The union is half in and half out.

Comment: So is the professional group.

Comment: To carry this a little further, and I do not know whether this muddies the water or ties the two groups together even more, let me add a comment here. The activism we have in society just did not suddenly spring upon us. It has been growing by increments over quite a period of time, whether we became aware of it suddenly or not. The growing old-age population that got Medicare, the black power movement that got these neighborhood health-care centers, and other societal forces did not spring up suddenly. There is also another movement that has been growing within the health professions and changing their orientations from those of an efficient treatment of illness to those of health maintainence and illness prevention. This makes everybody a perpetual client of the health-care system because the whole concept of keeping everybody well, which Kaiser Permanente has emphasized, is becoming central in the system. Within the health-care system those who have been looking toward the whole evolution of a new system are saying that everyone is a full-time client all the time, and this makes everybody a consumer willy-nilly.

Comment: Could I just add one more comment to yours? If you take the union as being partly in, then I would say that a professional society also can be partly in. If the external source happens to be the local medical society— and the local medical society is a powerful force very much like the union is— then it too would be considered as being partly in, and I am not sure that we would want to do that.

Comment: I mentioned the half in and half out because of a rather strong feeling that, as we talk about internal control and social control, it is terribly important to remember that these are simplifying assumptions and that it is awfully hard to make the distinction whether they are in or out. What we are really talking about is conflict of power.

Chairman: Much of this discussion illustrates very well the point that Scott made earlier about the open system approach, namely the importance of looking at the inputs, the transformations, and the outputs when studying social systems. Only very recently has the inputs side become so critical with respect to looking at the internal structure of organizations, and the systems approach would emphasize this. But this particular need to look at the internal structure of the hospital and the impact of the environment upon it has received quite a bit of attention here today. Zald talked about the importance of social controls residing outside the institution, for example, and Neuhauser and Andersen talked about the importance of the environment of hospitals, except perhaps that they did not elaborate as much as did Zald. And Scott has talked about the importance of technology, although his definition of technology is a social-psychological one rather than one representing what conventionally is referred to as technology. For example, the technology that Woodworth discusses is not quite the same. This is why, perhaps, social definitions are very critical in the technology Scott is talking about. And I agree with his conception.

A related comment that I would like to make at this point is that, in the case of hospitals, the importance of the inputs is becoming increasingly critical with respect to internal structure and behavior, partly because of a more general movement in the health field to approach the broad task of patient care not in terms of treating patients and disease, but in terms of ensuring and maintaining a high level of health for the population. What we are seeing is a major shift in goals and approach. From what initially was a mainly corrective approach (i.e. one aimed at correcting the health-related problems and dysfunctions of patients), and then a regulatory approach (i.e. one aimed both at correcting dysfunctions and restoring the patient to some minimal level of functioning or equilibrium), the system has begun to move more toward a preventive approach (i.e. an emphasis on health maintainence and disease prevention, and on preventive medicine and community-oriented medicine). The next likely step in the process will probably be a further shift toward a promotive approach wherein health care, and the promotion of health levels, rather than disease prevention, is the main target.

Partly because of this major shift in approach and focus, the hospital is becoming more other-oriented and less inner-directed. As a consequence we even see people who are members of the institution become much more sensitive to the impact of external forces than in the past. The younger physicians, the interns, and the medical students, for example, now take a much different view of the outside world and of the social responsibility of the hospital than did their predecessors a few years ago. We are dealing with something more, and perhaps more pervasive, than the matter of power. We are dealing not only with external and internal groups that are exerting power to alter the structural arrangements of the hospital and get changes in the preferred arrangements, but also with shifting goals for the organization and a new system of expectations, simply social-psychological expectations, which promotes and reinforces this behavior, and which poses new demands on the institution and the health care system. These intervening variables may be just as important as power and bargaining. And I was very much impressed by the fact that Scott emphasized the importance of social definitions in relation to technology. I would like to underscore his statement that the impact of technology upon the social structure of the hospital, at least its more proximate impact upon behavior, is mediated by social definitions and performer conceptions, or by what I would prefer to call the social-psychological expectations and role conceptions of the participants. In his paper, Mauksch makes essentially the same point with respect to task models, and Jaco makes a similar point in his paper about the impact of the ecology of work on behavior in the hospital.

I would therefore raise the issue as to what kind of research models would be especially appropriate for handling the complexities that we have been discussing. Broadly speaking, it seems that we more or less accept the necessity of using open system models that point to relevant inputs from the environment as well as to internal structure and process and to particular outputs. But, strategically speaking, from the point of view of proper emphasis and economy in organization research, what sorts of models should we adopt at this juncture of our work? For example, should we follow an ever-expanding model which suggests that we go out to the environment and the community and look at all the variables which seem important to us and then have these factors brought into the hospital system as inputs in a reductionist way? Or would it be more promising to focus instead on the intervening variables that we have been discussing and their relationships to the outcomes of the system? And, in any case, how complicated do we have to make our research models in order to synthesize our knowledge in some meaningful way?

The second issue that our discussion raises for me has to do with the implicit recognition in our models of the crucial role that interdependencies play as a determinant of behavior. We talk about coordination, integration, the interdependence of worlds on the patient care stage (see Mauksch), the interdependence of task conceptions, the interdependence of the staffs, and so on. If we accept this idea of interdependence seriously, in view of the great complexity of the hospital as an organizational system, do we really do ourselves and the field any justice by continuing to focus on single variables rather than on patterns of variables or on profiles and syndromes of variables? I think that the systems theory would move us in the direction of looking at patterns rather than on single variables. Earlier we talked about the importance of total layout, for example, as against the importance of particular dimensions of the physical setting of the patient unit. What are the implications of this for theory and methodology? Do we continue to look at single variables, controlling for a number of other single variables, or should we shift and look at patterns, creating the necessary methodologies that would be required by such a task? These kinds of questions, it seems to me, may be critical both from the point of view of future research and from the point of view of the practical implications that they entail.

Would you comment on the two issues that I raised, Dick?

Answer (Dr. Scott): I will comment, particularly on the second point because it worries me. This kind of conference does give one a heady feeling that one has got the power to shape the work of the coming decades. And I personally would be very loathe to decide, by some kind of resolution, to follow one kind of approach rather than another; I would like to not be bound by that kind of consensus. One can talk in a general way about where the greatest payoff is in the next few years, but I really think it is a payoff for what, for whom, and for what kind of purpose. And, certainly, from the standpoint of making recommendations to planning groups and administrators, it seems to me that we have to develop much more complex models than we have been dealing with. But I am also impressed at how quickly we get trapped in the mazes of our ingenuities, and the more complex we get, the more general and kind of useless we get in some ways. So on one hand, yes, on the other hand, no, is my response.

Question (Dr. Pellegrino): Do you not see the possibility, however, of a short-circuiting that I tend to see, a short-circuiting between this force outside the system and the point at which the clinical decision-making is being made, cutting through all the intervening steps. That is a possibility I think I do not know if you want to research it, but do you not see it as a possibility?

Comment: Talk more about it; what do you mean by it?

Answer: Yes. For example, a board of trustees or another group representing the community (and I want to come back to that always as the determining agent) determine, let us say, that they are not interested in open heart surgery. They have learned enough to know that if we apply the prudential decision-making principle to, say, the proper treatment of a sore throat, this is more consonant with what they want out of the health care system than fixing up a damaged valve in a person 40-55 years old which costs many dollars. I see that kind of decision being made, and that is a short-circuiting that goes beyond the managerial conception of tasks, which is of no consequence there.

Comment: I see it being made, but I do not really see it being implemented very readily.

Answer: Yes, but it can be implemented by this very signal that we gave you of the dollars. It is going to be done. These are precisely the kinds of questions that must be decided at a level other than the professional. These are value questions. What do you want to do with the resources? We are avoiding these questions. Yet the system is only secondary to that.

Comment: You are right that some of these things will happen. Yet this is still a base. I think that Georgopoulos' really crucial questions suggest that, yes, policy decisions will be made, and some of them will be made for reasons a little different than previous ones. But they will not be based on the kinds of scientific knowledge and validated knowledge for which I think we are groping. Complementary to what will happen and complementary to this question, I feel we have one way in addition to this kind of continuous intelligent groping that I think Scott is describing. At some point we, as social scientists, must more meaningfully get into experimental controls and experimental approaches.

Comment: No doubt. As a scientist myself, who still works in the laboratory, I cannot disagree with you at all. I simply am trying to signal, from the point of view of someone who feels the pressures in a way which you do not, that there is a short-circuiting effect which you have got to build into your investigations and into your questions, or at least take into account. That is all I am saying.

Comment: I just want to add something about Pellegrino's short-circuiting and see if it holds. There is also another short circuit that I think may affect the health-care system, and that is the tremendous change going on in the education of the health-care professions. As you well know, the education of the physician seems to be shortening to some extent, while the other health professions are expanding their education and getting much more clinically oriented. Somewhere there is going to be a merging of knowledge, and it is going to be a different kind of power orientation about decision-making. Decisions may become much more rational, if there is such a thing, based on the application of science to the practice represented by such a merging of knowledge. This in itself may be a hidden short-circuit and, certainly, no one is looking at it right now.

Comment: I agree with you, but I almost think that some of the things you are talking about are in the realm of axiology.

Comment: There is another factor here, speaking of education, the impact of mass education—what I call the *Reader's Digest* phenomena—on the behavior of the general public vis-à-vis health ideas. My favorite example is the 1954 pressure to divert what was to have been a research project involving gamma globulin and polio to a mass application with the significant result, incidentally, of freezing the supply of gamma globulin and making it unavailable for use on measles and hepatitis. This comes back to a point Pellegrino is making, and that is that we are expecting, not so much in terms of the hosptial as in terms of other aspects of the health-care delivery system, a very profound impact of public pressures in response to growing sophistication of medical ideas, but also often in response to simply premature or inaccurate information about medical innovation. I think we need to be prepared to consider this variable as it begins to reach the hospital; and it is just around the corner.

Comment (Dr. Scott): I would like to respond to your comment in two ways. First, if there are outside pressure groups here, then they undoubtedly are affecting the managerial conception; they will say how this is going to operate and what the goals of it are, and so forth. I think this is going to have an effect on the practitioners—the kinds of arrangements you set up, how you evaluate performance, how you divide the work, and so on are going to be affected.

Second, I suggest that we should never underestimate the power of the professional groups to reinterpret and to redefine what the goals really are, to attempt to gain control over their own work process, and to get themselves organized to do what they were trained to do. There is going to be tension under these circumstances. You may be right that for the next ten years the balance of power is going to be with the various outside groups because they are going to be backed by dollars and by public demand, and that the apparent dependency relationship is going to shift with the medical group being less powerful and these other groups being more powerful. If so, I would say that this probably will be temporary, because one of the characteristics of all professions is that they care very much about having control over what they regard as the central conception of their work and having some say in the kinds of work arrangements that are devised to carry out that work. I do not think we are disagreeing. In fact, I think that you are within my model.

Comment: I have much the same feeling as to the impact of consumer groups. Hospitals are not as involved in this right now as are other parts of the health-care system. But with the introduction of such things as the legal decision for trustee liability for quality of care, which has already been mentioned, the prospective payment of financial arrangements, and comprehensive health planning, the hospital will become deeply involved. Somehow, we have to build a management solution which is neither a bureaucratic model, because that is inflexible and fails to recognize the inevitability of some of the things Scott said about the professions, nor a professional model, because that has created the mess we are now in. The hospital will have to be organized in a way in which consumer opinion and the rights of professionals, both as consumers (because they have this characteristic) and as professionals, all get taken into account in the decision-making processes that determine the structure.

Comment: One reason why these kinds of things are best studied in the professional organization is because it is specifically a characteristic of professional groups that they care about their work.

Perspective for Hospital Organization Research

Presentation Highlights: H. O. Mauksch

I think it would be appropriate to say that in my paper I deviated from the original purpose of this conference. Rather than synthesizing existing knowledge, I am really groping for a shift in perspective concerning the validity of various kinds of perspectives for studying the hospital. Perhaps this is a justification, but it really has implications for what we are trying to accomplish here. My approach was motivated by a number of things, some of which have been already mentioned earlier. A number of things are happening in the hospital—somebody very appropriately, for example, said that unionization is coming in, has come in, and is increasing—which have important implications for research. Let me mention four things, all of which in effect will have as a consequence a decrease in the flexibility of negotiations within the system. This is basically the premise with which I would like to start.

Unionization is one. Another is the increasing inroads of technology, including the computerization of various aspects of hospital functioning whether these be in the area of diagnosis, in record-keeping, or in administrative decision-making. These also will have as a consequence a decrease in options for deviation and negotiation. Similarly, the new careers that were mentioned will provide less and less space, less and less living room for negotiation. And, lastly, the whole cultural era of our day will move into the hospital with the result that what might be called the increased politization of the interaction between component parts in the system is also likely to diminish negotiating potentials and negotiation.

It was because of these factors that I started to be concerned with the very nature of the sociology of knowledge in the hospital field—with the kind of research that has been done and the way we have looked at the institution. In the process I became conscious, or somewhat aware at least, and concerned about the fact that much of our past research is, in terms of the new radicals, "establishment research." It deals with the establishment as a given thing. It deals with the manager, and it deals with the view of "papa," even though more recently we have moved to the other extreme, namely to the client area. Within this formulation I tried to see to what extent the various studies really do constitute an impressive accumulation of knowledge that we can witness. Do we have integrated knowledge or does this knowledge lend itself to different interpretations using possibly the same data, and what else can we say about it?

As a point of departure I took the moment of the coming together of the various processes which in the hospital have to be segregated as part of the division of labor, specialization, and departmentalization, and tried to examine what happens at that point. And I have suggested that possibly what we need is several concepts which are parallel to, rather than substitutes for, existing concepts of total systems, of formal organizations, and of managerial or institutional kinds of dichotomies.

What I would like to suggest, with a terrible degree of apology, is that the scheduling of opportunities to present something is not necessarily correlated with the intellectual processes of those who participate. What I have moved to bring out here is essentially a cake that has been in the oven much too short and is only half-baked at this point. I am not comfortable yet, and this is something that has bothered me and I would like to grope with here. Obviously you can see in this paper that I have a considerable intellectual debt to the interactionist approach; I have some Anselm Strauss and some Erving Goffman. Although I did not mention it in the paper, I should have also indicated that I am somewhat influenced by phenomenology, the methodology of looking at a thing as it is seen by those who experience it.

There are three kinds of conceptual constructs that I would suggest as being useful in explaining the hospital, and possibly also useful in terms of the mission of this conference for reexamining the implications and utility of much of the recent research. The basic assumption underlying these constructs is that no human organization is subject to the laws of physical science which say that only one object can be in one place at one time. On the contrary, in social structures there can be simultaneously concepts and constructs, with actors participating in several diverse systems which need not be interpreted as role conflict within the same Newtonian scheme. Sometimes, participation in nonsynchronized role systems, where role conflict only occurs under conditions of stress, may be latent but not necessary.

One of the three concepts I propose represents the development within systems of what I call the worlds. The worlds, and I do not particularly hold with the term I chose, refers to the notion that within institutions of a high degree of specialization and institutions that have all kinds of preconditions, or a breakdown of communication, subcultural units develop with their own communication and norm systems. These represent what I almost would like to call conditions of social membrane formation—social membrane formation which sometimes may be permanent and sometimes may be transient. These formations, in fact, determine and influence much of the role behavior that we see in an organization. In an institution like the hospital, moreover, these worlds meet, react, and negotiate under certain conditions.

In our institutions we occasionally behave as members of the overall institution, without seeing the conflict, and sometimes we behave as members of the subworlds, with rather different behavior implicit. All of us have seen that faculty, let us say the members of a department, vote one way as department members, and then on the very same issue vote in a different way when the whole faculty meets as a group. There are different kinds of latent identities that are called forth by the two situations. Essentially, the concept of the worlds is seeking to juxtapose a different view on the structural or formal organizational view.

In the hospital, medicine or nursing is conceivably one world. Some of it, however, may engage in discussion of the business office as involving relevant world aspects. It is interesting to note that the worlds are not necessarily synonymous with particular groups, subsystems, or units. I think that this is implicit in Bob Straus's point about reorganizing patient care. There are rudiments of the capacity of developing worlds that are interdisciplinary, for instance, in such units as the lonely pediatric unit in the general hospital. It may be that by virtue of the entire group's position, the pediatric unit develops a world phenomenon which unites these people against other nurses, other doctors, etc., but the world is the world of pediatrics. Obstetrics sometimes also has this character, and psychiatry certainly does except that discriminatory practices rather than self-selection enforce a world in this case.

Let me leave the world for a moment, I mean the concept and not our world because you can not leave the world now, and move on to the second construct. This, which again has been referred to earlier, is the construct of the process systems. The notion of the division of authority within the hospital along two lines I think is relevant at this point. I would say, however, that very little has been done with it as a means of explaining institutional processes or as a means of explaining the kinds of things that Bob Straus talks about—the conflicts and controversies and negotiations that occur at the patient's bedside or, let us say, within the patient's area.

Some time ago I used the terms "care" and "cure" as describing, on the one hand, the process which is in the domain of medical intervention or medical responsibility (in the social mind of the physician) and, on the other hand, those things which are supported by the system in the area of patient care (there are certain kinds of autonomous components among the components of care). Because I was also getting into what might be called the dimensions of self-management and institutional maintenance, in order to keep the alliterative game flowing, I called this additional aspect the "core." But these, i.e. care, cure, and core, are distinct processes, and they do conflict, and they do involve the same people. The nurse has been very much studied as being the person who becomes the negotiator and acts inconsistently, depending upon whether she acts in the capacity of the care system, the capacity of the cure system, or occasionally as a manager.

The main point is that I see all of these as fluid, as negotiating, as interacting systems, with the actors continuously moving between these worlds and processes depending upon what kind of role they are taking. In the final analysis, therefore, the patient or the product itself becomes a "negotiated order" out of representations and negotiations which are *not* the direct translation of a managerial process that the manager is priviledged to perceive. The manager is not able to perceive these simply because they take place within a perspective that is not within his purview when he sits on the top of the institution. There are many studies which, though they have not given this as the reason, have shown the existence of differing perspectives within the hospital arrived at from varying points of view.

The third construct, that of the stage, is a way of sociologically defining the points or the platform at which the worlds negotiate and the process systems interact. I have referred to this as the stage, obviously borrowing from Goffman here. The stages are the places where the representatives of the different worlds and the process systems negotiate with each other and interact with each other. Contrary to the situation in other institutions, however, including practice in the factory system, the peculiar tantalizing thing about the hospital is that the patient's bedside is in fact a stage where all of the subsystems of the organization negotiate with each other. In the university, on the other hand, the student tends to move from world to world. If I teach an undergraduate course I have no obligation whatsoever to consider the compromises of load and demands that, say, the course in philosophy or the course in statistics has on the student. He is within my domain, the domain of my course and of my department, and the obligation of fit or continuity which is part of the patient-care picture is missing in the case of teaching (except that it may be coming very fast as a change on the scene).

I would say that the same thing holds true for the upper level of hospital organization, because of the division between care and cure authority, the obvious managerial dichotomy already mentioned. I would suggest that if you really look at the management process in the hospital, you will find that it is unlike that of the university or a factory. You will find that hospital management is not a world which negotiates with the various worlds of the operating units in the organization, but in itself it is a stage. And, if my model has any validity, herein lies one of the real issues of hospital effectiveness, because we have a system where the input instrumentalities as well as the output instrumentalities are themselves identified with negotiating necessities.

In my paper I also squeezed a somewhat different kind of concern for which I had a prior desire to design a table. In trying to study stage behavior, I have been impressed with the fact that we have been so preoccupied with the old dichotomy between professional and bureaucratic models that we have forgotten that we may not be able to account for it all on this basis. And when I really started to look at stage behavior and the norms which govern stage behavior (some of this came up today and has some relevance to Zald's paper as far as control is concerned), it became apparent to me that there were a number of different models which were operative. I describe six such models here that I believe are important to understanding stage behavior in hospitals.

I am suggesting that there is such a thing as a professional model, which incidentally is the most difficult one to study from the point of view of quality control of task performance. I am talking not about the professional role or a profession—at this point I could not care less whether medicine is a profession, nursing is a profession, or elevator operating is a profession—but about whether the tasks are performed expertly. If I may refer to a target expected outcome and a criterion of quality paradigm, with a client's needs as determined by the professional and the expected outcome being the reduction of the client's problem, appropriate professional behavior is very hard to measure.

The bureaucratic behavior model, on the other hand, is easier to measure. This task model involves the target of institutional integrity policies. Policies are the criterion, and satisfaction of job requirements is the expected outcome. Both of these have been much discussed here today.

Another important task model, and one that governs much of hospital processes and negotiation, is the craft model. And yet in the literature you do not find much about it. Certainly when we talk about the real kinds of concerns and rewards that are given among surgeons or among nurses, for example, an important one is the beauty or the elegance of task performance—the task itself is the target. The elegeance and appearance of the product have a tremendous value in the set of performance norms that we find in hospitals. In interviewing patients it became very clear to me that even much of the criticism of hospital food is within this craft framework.

I discuss three more models. One of these is the entrepreneurial model, obviously. Though this model is relatively alien to hospital norms, it does exist. Its concern is for profit and with selling. Next there is the technical model, which I think is increasingly encroaching on the hospital scene, and which relates to the problem of increasing hospital costs. This model deals with the means-end relationship and with the ritualization of procedures through technology which, incidentally, may deprofessionalize those affected. Finally, there is the service model, which is concerned with meeting the patient's demands. In some hospitals the behavior of physicians, for example, may show more service-modeled task behavior than in other hospitals.

Let me summarize what I have tried to do in this paper, which is admittedly personal, highly exploratory, and groping. I almost feel that as social scientists we are constrained to try to look at the perspective through which we have looked at social phenomena in the past. But I am suggesting that there are other perspectives which may be useful. In a sense what I tried to do was to see if we could approximate shifts in social values by shifting also the sociological lens of our vantage point. And, as I suggest, our subject matter does look different when we do so.

Discussion

Comment: You skipped over the entrepreneurial model a little too fast.

Answer (Dr. Mauksch): In a sense entrepreneurial behavior is profit-seeking and profit maximizing behavior. Let me give you an example. An element of entrepreneurial behavior came up when we analyzed the exit interview between the attending physician and the patient. There was, and sometimes this was not very easily determined, a difference between the physician's clinical judgment of what this patient ought to be doing in the future and the occasional opportunity, or at least unutilized opportunity, of "keeping this patient with me for some time." The behavior of the pharmacy and x-ray, which are the two departments in many hospitals that are the profit-making departments, often is entrepreneurial in nature. Many of the acts performed by these departments are within the orientation of "we are a selling department."

Comment: That possibly explains why in x-ray and the lab often you have huge lines of patients waiting to go through. There units are aiming for high profit, no matter how much discomfort it is for the patient. Patients may wait in line for an x-ray for any number of hours, despite all other neglect of their care, even though the x-ray might be done upstairs if a process orientation prevailed. To give you another small example, we recently had an industrial engineering firm study the x-ray department and its effect on the rest of the hospital. The study indicated a tremendous unit effect, showing that while it was maximizing profit it was doing the rest of the hospital terrible harm.

Comment: The situation is more complicated than that, though. Hospitals cost account for the profit they get off of the lab and x-ray. Hospitals use these profits to keep room charges uniform and as low as possible, because room charges vary in terms of what it costs the hospital to provide its different patients with room and board. If hospitals lose money, they can make it up in the lab, the operating room, or the nursery charges, etc.

Comment: I just want to finish the industrial engineering study example. They presented their findings to the x-ray department and, of course, there was a big blowup. The x-ray department refused to accept any portion of the report. What we had to do then was go out and get another industrial engineering firm to restudy the same thing. They too came up with exactly the same findings. Now the problems are looked at a little more dispassionately with regard to how the x-ray department disjoins the rest of the organization and what the real costs are for the rest of the hospital.

Comment (Dr. Mauksch): I would suggest that, as a methodology for our research from the point of view of a patient-care framework, one would almost need to assume a research approach that differentiates between an analysis of tasks performed, of role orientations, of manifest functions, and of projections. And, I would say, whatever comes afterwards, what we find when we synthesize all these in terms of convergence or divergence is a subsequent matter which should not be assumed.

Questions: I would like to ask a question on your models, Dr. Mauksch. Is there any indication or implication that some of these models for the performance and evaluation of specific tasks may be in conflict if they reside in the same role incumbent?

Answer: Without having the data, I would say that there are conflicts. There is an integrity to each of these models, and my point is that I do not want to deprecate any of these models because it is their fullest integrity which may produce the conflict that you are suggesting. The elegance of task performed, for example, sometimes becomes almost a compulsive aspect that may be interfering with either the filling of policies as far as the bureaucratic model is concerned or the meeting of the patient's needs and providing service for the good of the patient.

Comment: I too am concerned about the variety of tasks performed within this thing we call a hospital, and about the variety of appropriate work arrangements for doing this kind of work in the hospital. It seems to me, continuing on this issue about conflict, that it is possible in these very complex organizations to develop various insulating mechanisms, I think you referred to as membranes. It is possible to develop devices whereby, in effect, one technology is in a sense protected from another technology. But such arrangements would be appropriate, or effective, from the point of view of the people who practice that technology. As you pass patients through the hospital, however, you know that patient's problems unfortunately do not come in neat technological packages. And as you pass patients through these things, expectations differ, the treatments of patients differ, and so on. I think that at the organizational level and in terms of stability or the amount of conflict within the structure, these things can be moderated somewhat. But for the people who are the recipients of the service, it seems that the effectiveness of insulation mechanisms and protective devices is quite a different matter. And that is where I think the real problem is.

Comment (Dr. Mauksch): I agree. This is why I said, is it not startling in the light of this that we put it on the stage, where the various inconsistencies are bound to occur, instead of within the confines of what I call the world? I totally agree with you.

Comment (Dr. Pellegrino): I would like to support the notion of investigating all of the models, but with particular emphasis on the craftsmanship model. I hope you take that with good humor, but, in all seriousness, the great defects we are encountering now that are of most concern to me as a practitioner and educator relate to a failure at the craftsmanship level. And I would like to see, from the standpoint of approach and methodology, that craftsmanship be measured only partially in terms of the craftsman himself. I would like to see craftsmanship defined and measured in terms of the job being well done, measured in terms of prudential decision-making for individual patients. The reason is that there is a difference between an operation beautifully done, which will give the operating team an intense sense of visceral excitement, and the feeling that this has been a successful day, and an unnecessary operation which had no relevance to the patient's needs, however beautifully it might have been performed.

Comment: It is at that level where conflict can occur.

Answer: There is a conflict, of course; the conflict is obvious. As far as I am concerned, however, we ought to explore the professional model, but I would say, again apodictically, that model has to disappear into this craftsmanship role. If you get into the craftsmanship model, please do not measure it only in terms of a surgical job well done or a medical job well done as seen by me.

Question: What do you mean when you say the failure of craftsmanship? Are you talking about some recent breakdown or has this always been the case?

Answer: It has always been the case, but let me emphasize one point. When capability is such that we can alter the natural history of disease, the gap between capability and performance is, in my mind, very disturbing. Out of my own personal experiences as a teacher, as a clinician, and as an investigator, I say to you that underlying much of the unrest about medical care, even though it may come out in terms of medical cost, is the nagging feeling on the part of the patient that the things he came to get resolved, first, have not been resolved, and yet a lot of money has been expended, as well as time and energy, and, second, that the patient did not get the full value from this contact of the medical institution or personnel. In the patient's mind is the question, "Have I really tapped into what is possible for my needs?" This is what I mean by the gap, and I think this is a very serious discontinuity.

Question: Do you think that this gap may have come out of something that Mauksch described in some of his earlier work when he talked about care being so splintered that now there is no way to fix blame or responsibility, and people somehow are gliding along under that umbrella?

Answer: That is one factor, certainly. I too have been concerned and have written about the new ethical problems of the care team working together. This is a new realm of ethics. We have to talk about ethics of health care as opposed to medical ethics, for example. But that is another consideration. I am really concerned about the competence and the ability to deliver what we can deliver, given our present capability. The difference between capability and actual performance is very big.

Comment (Dr. Mauksch): I am torn between fully agreeing with you and having a little nudge there that bothers me. I also have become very fascinated with what I would almost call the crisis of craft in much of our professional behavior. Even there, however, I would distinguish between the professional task model, which is really client-oriented, and the craft model. If you move craft too far, the beauty of the thing itself becomes the point of contention, and this then diminishes the point that you are making.

Answer: I think that we are in agreement on this.

Comment: Let me play the devil's advocate, as an anthropolgist and an arguer against ethnology. The differential use of models is one difficulty that we have with the age-old problem of professionalism versus bureaucracy, and we have been through that. I think we get certain kinds of insights about social processes as we look at these ideal models or as we look at simulation games in which we have gotten rid of a lot of the complexity. But if we are interested in analyzing an organization, it seems that the analysis of what you are pointing to, at least what I get out of it, would yield criteria for evaluation. What you have here are different people, or different actors, using different criteria, and to the extent that these become operational then you can attach values to them.

Comment: You know, there is a beautiful example of this very dilemma, the problem of craft or the asceticism of doing a fine job, in the field of dentistry. I did a study years ago and found that dental students were mad and agitated at the criteria that the dental school faculty used to grade their performance. The criteria revolved around how good or how pretty was the mold they made, how good a filling they did was, and how beautifully they did a particular task. The more humanistic dental students thought this was demeaning to the profession of dentistry. To put all this emphasis on the mechanics of dentistry and ignore rewarding the dental students who could put a patient at ease before he went grinding away in his mouth was demeaning. The latter, these students thought, was more professional in the patient-dentist relationship, but they got no rewards for it in the grading system by the dental faculty, who did not recognize that.

Comment (Dr. Mauksch): In the same vein, I would make an extremist statement that one of the tragedies with the patient's chart is that, while it is intended to be within the care system it in fact has ended up with the core system of institutional maintenance, recording, and reporting. This means that the rewards for the nurse, for instance, are in giving a bath because it has to be charted (for those hospitals where this is still the case). And, next door, the patient who is desperately looking for somebody to talk to and to listen to can find no nurse. In other words, to a large degree care in the hospital has no legitimizing devices and much of it is attached to a low prestige group, nursing.

Comment: I think that your description is very accurate when you refer to bedside as a stage and to the world of management as a stage rather than a force. But I feel that this is something which is not inherent at all in the technology of hospitals. What has happened is that the whole technology of hospitals has changed tremendously. As hospitals have gotten larger and more complex, they have begun to face an increasingly unstable environment and the organization has lagged behind the technology. In other words, I feel that you can organize in terms of centralizing in one locus the responsibility for care, cure, and core at the unit level of the hospital. If hospitals were structured differently, i.e. if they were organized differently, these problems would change. And, in fact, the technology is compelling changes in hospital design and organization.

Comment: This provides an additional argument in support of much of the discussion that Straus initiated. What we do need is rigorous, carefully designed experimentation on the organization of care and experimentation with different forms of organization. To paraphrase Sigmund Freud, let world be where stage was. Let us create unity and communion in all those things that are the key issues. I believe this would be possible. I do not think, however, that it can be done by a policy committee. It has to be done through research and experimentation.

Comment: I would like to get back to the craft model briefly. I think it represents an important notion. Everybody in this room, in one way or another, probably has commented on what I am going to talk about in this connection, except perhaps that they do not appreciate the intensity of the way clinicians understand it. My point is that the too much overspecialization of task activity at every level in the hospital is destroying craftsmanship, because now if you take the physician, as an example, he may be an expert on catheterizing the right side of the heart but he does not know anything about the left side. The cardiologist cannot be a complete cardiologist, the nurse cannot be a complete nurse, the social worker only works with certain kinds of incidents and other social workers handle others, and the whole thing is broken up into little tight categories of tasks which hit the patient randomly but none of which are organized with scientific intent. And the patient only gets good care by random chance. Now these things gel around the patient by some intuitive set of circumstances rather than by definitive planning. As a consequence, the patient often gets good care only at random or by chance. This is a major problem.

Comment: We also have certain climates which actually deemphasize craft. In some of the social sciences, for instance, if you are too good a lecturer, you are slightly suspect, at least at some universities.

Comment (Dr. Zald): Let me play devil's advocate number 2—Paul White was devil's advocate number 1. What is the use of this to me as somebody who is trying to change an organization? Where does the stage and world view concept take me?

Answer (Dr. Mauksch): Obviously this is a very important, almost a key, question. What I am really groping for here is a translation of an essentially social-psychological concept within an organizational framework, and this is insanity in some ways. But I believe it has to be done. The point this leads me to is that a certain synthesis of intellectual frames of reference will only be meaningful when we are able to experiment with them. In other words, I would say that the next step from this concept would be an actual experimental setting in which this can be tested by examining the extent to which social-psychological perceptions and experiences are in fact organizational reality. As I point out in my paper, one must also recognize that the questions asked of social scientists have significantly moved from the quest for understanding and prediction to intervention and improvement.

Question: Even if you get what you want, how can you use it? I have difficulty in applying the task models too. I see each of them more as an elegant model rather than something you could use as an administrator to change your organization.

Answer (Dr. Mauksch): You are touching on a matter of faith here. Let me just say that I believe that in any science the dimension of pure versus applied research is usually forgotten. This dimension turns out to have the quality of an intervening variable, and I believe that the distance between applied and pure research is negatively correlated with the quality of the research. In response to your question, which I think is rather crucial, if what I am suggesting has any value as a model, then at some point it must be the multiple in some experiment.

Part Four

Part Four

9

HOSPITAL ORGANIZATION FROM THE VIEWPOINT OF PATIENT-CENTERED GOALS*

Robert Straus

Among the many complex problems facing contemporary society is a widening gap between the potentialities of medical science for protecting health and treating disease and the actual quality, quantity, and distribution of health care being delivered to the public. Public concern for this problem has been intensified by the popularization of medical knowledge. In the last few decades the public has become more sophisticated regarding the nature of medical advances and increasingly expectant and demanding that the benefits of medical science be available to all. Since hospitals are a major resource in health care delivery, the ability to produce results which are in keeping with both their technical potentialties and their patients' expectations is central to the broader issue.

Organizational Goals and Functions

Hospital goals can be defined in many ways. These include organizational efficiency, medical excellence, social purpose, and the well-being of patients. This paper is concerned with hospitals in terms of their patient-centered goals, the results they produce in the form of patient care, and the processes involved in defining goals and achieving results.

Many very basic questions need to be asked about the hospital in relation to its patients. What are the medical goals of the physician? What are the goals and expectations of the patient for himself? What are society's goals? What are the specific goals of various categories of people who work in hospitals? What should be the hospital goals in terms of optimal result of hospitalization for the patient? What, in its totality, does the hospital do for and to the patient? How does this end result coincide with the phsycian's

*Revised version of paper presented at Conference on Hospital Organization Research, May 22-23, 1970, Institute for Social Research, The University of Michigan, Ann Arbor, Michigan. Robert Straus, Ph.D., is Professor and Chairman, Department of Behavioral Science, College of Medicine, University of Kentucky. Here—the author wishes to point out—he presents a personal professional position and not a systematic review of the relevant literature on patient care. Some selected references to monographs and collections of readings pertinent to the experiences of patients in general hospitals are appended. All of these and others not mentioned, together with the suggestions of numerous colleagues and students, have influenced the writer's thinking in this area.

goals, the patient's goals, the goals in terms of the patient's optimum benefit? To what extent does the process of hospitalization—the interaction of hospital norms, people, techniques, apparatus, and activities—contribute to or interfere with the fulfillment of these various patient-centered goals?

An Historical Note

For most of history man has known relatively little about how to protect himself from illness or injury or to promote recovery. Most events related to his health have been ascribed to the supernatural. Man's earliest physicians were magicians and some of his earliest hospitals were temples. Because illness and injury were usually ascribed to evil spiritual forces, many early societies isolated or ostracized the sick or injured in order to safeguard the healthy. Therefore, early hospitals were often places where sick persons were forceably incarcerated until they recovered or died. Because of the high rate of death associated with childbirth, many societies had places of "confinement" for pregnant women approaching full term; they were released if and when they survived the crisis of delivery. Often laboring women and the dying were assigned to a common retreat. As time went on, the same or similar institutions were provided for persons who were mentally disturbed or destitute.

The purpose of this overly simple historical note is to emphasize that our modern hospitals are in part descended from institutions established to protect the healthy from people who were considered a threat to the well-being of the larger society. This reasoning and response pattern was reinforced by early knowledge about infectious diseases. Even with the emergence of patient-centered humanitarian goals, hospitals remained primarily institutions for the indigent sick, the terminally ill, the disturbed, and other rejects of society. Patients were essentially prisoners, and to a considerable extent the patient's status in contemporary hospitals reflects this historical practice.

It should be noted that the modern hospital, like modern medicine, has experienced a major transition from spiritual to scientific conceptions of disease, primarily during the last century. Scientific breakthroughs, initially in the areas of asepsis and anesthesia and later in techniques for surgical intervention and chemotherapy, have made the modern hospital the center of complex medical care primarily concerned with treating and rehabilitating patients and returning them to their homes and societies. As the potentialities of medicine have advanced, the expectations placed upon hospitals and other medical facilities have expanded. The techniques performed, apparatus used, and activities engaged in by people in hospitals have become increasingly complex and diverse. The roles of people who work in hospitals have expanded and become more specialized and stratified, and hospitals have developed elaborate distinct patterns of internal normative behavior.

With the change in the primary function of hospitals from that of protecting society from patients to that of treating patients and returning them to society, the stated goals and expectations have changed accordingly.

The status of patients themselves, however, has remained ambiguous. Although the primary goal of hospitals is now defined in terms of what they do to and for the patient, the patient's role in influencing this outcome is not well defined.

Throughout the history of hospitals it appears that the position of the patient as a sanctioning agent and his ability to influence the behavior of others has been weak. This has in part been due to the incarcerated nature of his situation. It has been perpetuated by his imposed dependence. For the modern patient, whose hospital stay may be relatively brief, his transiency in the system also deprives him of the opportunity to mobilize sanctioning power. A letter received in March 1970 from a patient who was in the fifth week of hospitalization for myocardial infarction told of various efforts to improve his comfort and ability to rest which had "not yet been taken seriously." He added, "I'm a transient, and probably capable of assembling only a few patients as picketers in my last days here, so my effectiveness [as a change agent] I rate as nil."

Hospitals as Factories

Hospitals have sometimes been compared to factories for pusposes of organizational research. This warrants a brief comment. Factories are created to produce an inanimate product or products. The human beings served by the product of the factories lie outside of the factory itself, and their personal involvement in the system is expressed indirectly through their demand for and acceptance of the factory's output. Modern factories are designed specifically for their production function. If the product changes, old buildings tend to be abandoned or their interiors completely redesigned. Efficient factories tend to be directed by a single line of command, their organizational charts are clear, and there tends to be delegation of authority commensurate with responsibility and accountability commensurate with authority. Because profit is the ultimate goal of a factory, economic forces demand modification of the system to produce maximum quality and quantity at minimum cost. Although historical heritage and personnel with entrenched power act as forces resistant to change, such forces can generally prevail in a factory only as long as they maintain profit in the face of competitive economic forces. Compared to a modern hospital, most factories have relatively simplistic goals and functions.

Hospitals, as often noted, operate according to split authority and have two or sometimes three separate lines of command. It is common to find people with responsibility but no authority and even some people with authority but no real responsibility. This confusing organizational pattern for medical, nursing, and administrative functions may be permitted to persist because most hospitals, unlike factories, are operated on a nonprofit basis. Although there are strong economic pressures on hospitals to avoid deficits, the responsibility for cost accounting and fiscal management are generally assigned to administrators who are given no control over the type, quantity, or quality of production (patient care), and who often can extract responsibility from only a small and insignificant number of their workers. The products of hospitals are their patients, and these are human beings who enter the hospital and become directly involved in the system only for the duration of the "production." Physicians have responsibility and demand authority over the patient's medical care, but they themselves are transient and only present to exert their authority for short periods of time. Nurses are left with much delegated responsibility and often assume authority.

Because they seldom experience directly competing economic forces, hospitals frequently permit their physical plants to become obsolete and inefficient and, in the absence of profit motives, relatively little is invested in research on hospital design. Despite rapid changes in the technology of medical care and the number of complexities of functions performed, hospital designers have provided few really imaginative, innovative, or experimental ideas. (There are some exceptions such as recovery rooms, intensive care units, rooming-in units, and a few experiments with circular wings to permit more effective patient supervision.)

It is interesting to note that some factories have found it useful, in the interest of quantity and quality of production and thus profit, to try to "humanize" their product. They have adopted various devices designed to help the workers identify with the finished product or some clearly delineated part thereof. A large corporation, in establishing a new factory to produce typewriters, recently experimented with various types of production ranging from the assembly line where each worker performed one or two small tasks to the opposite extreme where a single worker produced an entire typewriter. Although the latter method led to surprisingly good quality and quantity performance, it could not be implemented because no efficient method could be devised for delivering each of the parts of a typewriter to each worker. The system finally adopted retains the element of personal identification between the worker and his product by having each worker assemble identifiable components. The workers receive immediate feedback on the quality control of their product, and advancement and pay raises are based on earning the assignment to assemble more complex and demanding components.

Many other devices have been tried by industries in an effort to individualize their products. Automobile assembly lines, for example, may intentionally interspace various models and vehicle specifications rather than send a group of identical products down the line all in a row. Other factories give human names to products or use animated types of instructions. Ironically, while some factories have been trying to individualize or humanize their inanimate products, hospitals have been doing the opposite. Numerous observers of the patient care process have identified a tendency on the part of hospital personnel and practices to organize patient care on a production line basis, to dehumanize and subvert the individuality of their patients, and to treat them as categories of diseased entities rather than unique human beings.

A Unifying Concept of Behavior

For an understanding of the unique human being who is the hospital patient, and of the many interrelated factors which impinge on the experience of the patient, a frame of reference is proposed which assumes that all human behavior involves interaction among the following components:

Biological: Man the organism
Psychological: Man the personality
Environmentl: Man in his physical milieu
Social: Man's roles as a member of his society and its various social
   systems
Cultural: Man responding to his normative and material culture
Temporal: Man's orientation to the dimensions of time.

Biological components of behavior include the anatomical structure and physiological functions of the human body as well as characteristics of body chemistry, the impact of heredity, and the body's way of relating to microscopic and cellular organisms. Biological characteristics have a certain stability but most are subject to change throughout the life cycle and in response to the other major components of behavior. At any particular time the biological characteristics of the human organism establish potentialities and limitations for human behavior and determine the degree of relative resistability or vulnerability of the organism to outside stress.

Most patients in general hospitals are suffering from disbalance or trauma of one or more of the basic body systems. Their problems may be structural, functional, chemical, congenital, or a combination of these. For most patients their condition reflects vulnerability to some source of stress, perhaps to a physical trauma, perhaps to a concentration of infectious agents or allergens or other environmental contaminants, perhaps to changes in their own cellular or biochemical status, perhaps to biological manifestations of emotional stress. In any event, because human biology is part of a larger unified system of behavior, stress experienced at the biological level will inevitably elicit adaptive responses at psychological, social, or other levels— some of an accommodating nature, others perhaps compensatory, and still others antagonistic.

Psychological components of behavior comprise the personality—man's characteristic ways of feeling, thinking, acting, relating to others, and evaluating himself. Many psychological characteristics reflect and are, in part, determined by biological factors. People with unusual stature, weight, or other physical features which single them out often reflect in their personalities a sense of feeling "different." Short men may become overachievers in areas of behavior where their stature is no handicap; very tall women may develop personalities reflecting their effort to avoid being conspicious; or very stout people may deny their stress by engaging in Falstaffian behavior supporting the fallacious stereotype of the "jolly fat man." Biological status at any particular time—chamical, nutiritional, functional adequacy—helps determine how a person feels about himself and the amount of energy he is able to invest in relating to others. Such psychological characteristics as intelligence, anxiety level, and stress threshold also determine the individual's potential capacity and impose limitations on behavior. Like most biological traits, psychological characteristics have both basic consistencies and the capacity for change, especially in relation to major transitional periods in the life cycle. Psychological stress in individuals is often reflected in their biological processes as in psychosomatic diseases.

Because of medicine's primary preoccupation with organic disease, the psychological components of disease have been relatively ignored. They are identified in the literature, acknowledged in the general sense, and may even be recognized in the individual patient, but despite this they tend to receive relatively little attention in the actual process of hospital care. Yet there is reason to suspect that the experience of hospitalization may for many patients inflict much added psychological stress which is deleterious to the patient's well-being, thus negating some of the benefits of organic treatment.

Environmental components of behavior include such general or natural factors as climate, topography, fauna, flora, mineral and water resources, and the concentration of allergens, infectious agents, and other toxic substances. They also include the characteristics of communities, neighborhoods, housing, and the immediate environment of the moment. It has been frequently demonstrated that changes in such factors as lighting, sounds, temperature, the ratio of people to space, and the nature and arrangement of furnishings can profoundly affect the way people feel and behave. Consider the difference between a large well-lighted, well-ventilated, attractively furnished, quiet hospital room and one which is crowded, dimly lighted, meagerly furnished, dingy, dirty, foul smelling, and constantly assaulted with such typical hospital sounds as the squawk box used for paging, carts with misaligned wheels, employees gossiping, or physicians discussing the intimate details of a patient's problems.

The external environment of the patient can have numerous profound influences on his biological and psychological status; it may have contributed directly to the problem he brings to the hospital, and the environment to which he will return may be a crucial factor in his ultimate recovery. But of more immediate relevance while the patient is in the hospital will be the degree to which adaptations to the hospital environment impose unnecessary or deleterious stress of sufficient proportions to compromise his hospital care. For example, many hospital patients identify their inability to control the temperature of their room and the constant, but often irregular, strident and shocking array of noises as sources of considerable frustration and stress.

Social components of behavior derive initially from the total dependence of the human newborn on society in order to survive. This is basic to the nature of man as a social creature and to the development of a complex system of human activities which are specialized according to sex, age, biological, and intellectual attributes, and a broad spectrum of learned and cultivated skills and roles. The family is a basic social group found in some form in all societies and concerned with procreation (a biological function) and with nurturing, teaching, and supporting children to their point of maturation. Early personality development begins shortly afer birth and takes place within a family context. Family living initiates patterns of personal interaction with others, and provides acclimatization to a particular kind of environment. Within families, children and parents and husbands and wives develop intimate personal patterns of interrelationships and dependence. In contemporary societies people have a large number of significant social relationships outside the family including churches, schools, age peers, factories, and fraternal organizations. There are also neighborhood, community, state, regional, and national social identities.

All of these groups and others to which an individual belongs or with which he identifies are called reference groups. The behavior of other members of the group is an important force in establishing a point of reference for the individual's personal attitudes, values, beliefs, and practices. Within each group, depending upon its ultimate function and his own status in the group, an individual assumes certain specialized activities, duties, or responsibilities which are called his roles.

The roles an individual can play are in part determined by his biological equipment, especially when these call for or can be performed with greater effectiveness by persons of a particular sex, stature, or vitality. Roles are also partly determined by the limitations or potentialities associated with psychological traits. In turn, the opportunity to perform in certain capacities may contribute to or impede either biological or psychological development. Many roles are determined by the requirements of coping with features of the physical environment. They may be concerned with modifying the environment and must often be adaptable to changes in the environment.

Human beings are generally engaged in fulfilling several roles at the same time. The husband is a lover, father, provider, companion, and teacher within his family; he fulfills one or more roles within his area of employment; he fills additional roles in his community, religious, social, and political life.

When people require hospitalization they are forced to relinquish their usual roles for varying periods of time and accept instead the role of being a patient. They are cut off or restricted from their usual social contacts and are required instead to relate to a large number of strangers. A primary requirement of the patient is that he accept a dependency status, submit to the ministrations of others, relinquish control of his environment, and assume an identity based primarily on the classification of his primary organic problem. The first three of these requirements are often justified by hospital personnel on the grounds that surrender is therapeutically essential; the last reflects primarily a hospital bias which assumes that all aspects of a patient's identity and behavior are quite secondary to his organic disease.

Cultural components of behavior comprise the aggregate of customs, attitudes, laws, values, expected ways of behavior, together with the knowledge, techniques, artifacts, and material apparatus that characterize the behavior of a particular social group at a particular time. The normative aspects of a culture encompass the conventional or expected ways of acting. Sanctions in the form of group approval or disapproval, rewards or punishments, tend to coerce the individual toward conformity. Norms vary in the degree of importance attached to them and the degree of formality with which they are expressed. Norms or customs which are considered proper but not essential are sometimes called folkways; those which are so important that their violation threatens the well-being of the group are called mores; either folkways or mores which are codified and supported by specific sanctions are what we call laws.

Each patient brings to the hospital a life pattern of normative behavior reflecting his unique configuration of family, ethnic, religious, educational, community, racial, regional, occupational, and social class identities and the attitudes, values, beliefs, and sanctions associated with them. Everyone who works in a hospital also brings in his own outside culture; but, in addition, hospital personnel engage in behavior reflecting a distinctive internal culture. Some aspects of this culture are peculiar to hospitals in general while other aspects reflect the specific hospital. Most people who work in hospitals tend to become acculturated to the expected normative behavior, integrating it into their personal behavior patterns. Patients, on the other hand, are thrust so suddenly into a setting with new and radically different expectations for their behavior that they may well experience culture shock. This is quite comparable to the experience of people who move from one country to another, from the South to the North, or from rural to urban living. For the hospital patient, however, culture shock comes at a time when, because he is sick or injured, his capacity for adaptation is compromised. In addition, he is generally deprived of the support of relatives or friends and thrust into a totally alien social setting. Culture shock provides another form of potentially severe stress imposed on the already weakened capacity of the patient to engage in effective adaptive behavior.

Along with normative behavior, culture also encompasses the technical and material products of man's behavior. Modern medicine employs a broad range of techniques and devices to compensate for biological impairment. The surgeon's instruments represent extensions of his hands and fingers, the medical record is an extension of human memory, pharmacological agents permit modification of body chemistry, a pacemaker supplants an essential function of a vital organ. The material culture of a hospital represents another source of newness and strangeness for many patients; strange apparatus, strange sights, sounds, and smells; strange and often frightening or physically distressing diagnostic or therapeutic procedures. All these require getting used to at the very time when the patient is apt to be experiencing pain, weakness, or anxiety.

Finally, there are the temporal components of behavior. These include historical traditions which heavily influence contemporary cultural norms; the timetables of human growth and development which are reflected in the characteristics of the patient's organism, personality, and social roles; the individual's personal biological timetables of rest and activity, eating and elimination; the time orientation which is part of personality, dictated by social organization or prescribed by cultural norms; the impact of prior experiences with hospitalization; and the patient's expectations regarding the duration of his hospital stay.

People vary enormously in the extent to which time regulates their lives, in their adaptability to changes in the scheduling of daily functions, and in the extent to which they are oriented to the past, the present, or the future. Hospitalization for many patients requires the adaptation of schedules involving their basic body functions to the daily hospital routine and to the timetable of their particular periods of hospitalization. Patients who give little heed to time are less apt to follow reliably therapeutic procedures based on time intervals. Those who are oriented to the past or the present will be less responsive than future-oriented patients to the preventive aspects of health care. Finally, many people who work in hospitals believe that they rarely have enough time to do everything they are required to do. This may reflect reality or it may be a rationalization for avoiding certain activities, such as taking time to establish more than incidental or superficial relationships with individual patients. Adequate time for effective communication is often a crucial missing variable in the whole process of patient care.

In summary, this section has suggested that studies of hospital organization as it impinges on the patient should encompass a unifying concept of behavior. This assumes that both the responses of patients to hospitals and the responses of hospitals to patients reflect the interaction of biological, psychological, environmental, social, cultural, and temporal factors, all of which impose limitations and determine potentialities for behavior. This framework will now be applied to some further considerations of the experience of being a patient.

The Experience of Being a Patient

Both public and medical expectations for the contemporary hospital include the utilization of the knowledge, skills, techniques, and apparatus of medicine in applying the full potential of modern medical science and technology to the treatment of sickness and injury, the prolongation of life, and the rehabilitation of the diseased or disabled patient. Yet the experiences of hospital patients suggest that good "medical" care is not always good patient care. Often the requirements of the hospital or of its medical, nursing, or administrative subsystems impose on the patient deprivations or demands which are contraindicated by the requirements for his care or are in direct conflict with his total health and well-being.

There is a growing body of literature which describes hospitalization in terms of the patient's deprivation of his normal roles and identity, the stripping away of all that is familiar, and the imposition of a new "sick role" involving enforced passivity and dependency. This process has been justified as often essential in order to make the patient receptive to a medically prescribed regime. It is important here to differentiate between medical care, that is, the activities which are concerned directly with the patient's illness or injury and are often focused almost exclusively on the organ system with primary pathology, and patient care, or the process concerned with the broader administration to the patient's total health, including his comfort and peace, of mind and his investment in his own recovery and rehabilitation.

The experience of being a patient in a particular hospital will invariably reflect the convergence of several established forces, each of which is itself complex and influences the nature of behavior we call patient care. These include characteristics of the patient, his illness, the external culture of the society outside the hospital, the internal culture of the hospital, and such factors as communication, prejudice, hospital routine, and enforced dependency.

The Patient

A conceptual approach to the consideration of factors significant to the behavior of the patient himself has already been suggested. His unique characteristics have contributed to the etiology of his problem and they will determine his response to his illness and to the hospital. His characteristics and behavior will also help determine the responses of physicians, nurses, and other hospital personnel toward him. He is a unique organism with his own structure, function, body chemistry, and genetic traits. He is a unique personality with his own way of feeling, thinking, believing, and acting. He has had unique life experiences shared with a unique combination of reference groups whose beliefs, attitudes, values, and customs have significantly influenced his own behavior. The patient is young or old, male or female, dark or light skinned, rich or poor; he has ethnic, religious, educational, intellectual, and emotional characteristics, each of which helps determine his behavior and also the way in which others—in this case hospital personnel—will respond to him and his problems.

The patient has a life style with well-entrenched habits regarding such factors as eating, elimination, activity, rest; he has a well-established concept of time—both in terms of the scheduling of events and in terms of past, present, or future orientation; he has a concept of space and dimensions, he has established habits regarding the comfortable temperature of a room, the hardness of a bed, the impact of noise and smell, the need for solitude or for companionship. Perhaps most significant of all, he has had prior experiences (or *no* prior experiences) with illness and hospitalization, and from these has either preconceived expectations or the anxiety of uncertainty or both regarding himself and his current hospitalization.

The Illness

The nature of the patient's illness and its requirements constitute another major variable in the experience of the patient. The patient's medical care— the diagnostic tests run, apparatus employed, treatments prescribed, and in some instances the area of the hospital in which he is confined—is in large part determined by the nature of his major presenting symptoms. Within illness categories it has been found by numerous investigators that many options for diagnostic and therapeutic intervention are sometimes selected on the basis of socioeconomic or personality variables rather than strictly medical criteria. These choices are dependent upon the responses of hospital personnel to the patient. In addition to his personal and social characteristics, responses of others to the patient may vary, depending upon whether his illness is perceived as life-threatening, painful, severe, disfiguring, disabling, or whether it is seen as transitory, mild, and subject to total cure. They will vary depending upon whether the patient is perceived as the innocent victim or as a contributor to his own disease. Responses will also vary if the disease is infectious or otherwise perceived as a threat to the well-being of others.

The External Culture of the Hospital

Just as the patient's personal characteristics reflect the culture in which he lives, hospital behavior is strongly influenced by the social and cultural influences of the community from which a majority of its patients and staff are drawn, and by the physical characteristics of the neighborhood in which it is located. Hospitals historically were sponsored by various religious denominations, private philanthropy, or governments. Such affiliations still prevail and contribute to the overall charter and philosophy of organization and service within which the hospital operates. Staff, too, may be drawn primarily from certain ethnic or religious or other sociocultural backgrounds and may reflect certain biases toward medical care, or toward certain kinds of problems or procedures and certain kinds of patients. All such factors, of course, will impinge on the hospital experience of the patient.

The patient brings to the hospital numerous expectations derived from his sociocultural milieu. he may consider himself priviledged to be admitted or may feel that he has a perfect right to occupy a hospital bed. He may come with dread of death, pain, or fear of the unknown, or he may look with optimsim on his anticipated care and cure. He may anticipate the drama and excitement suggested by countless contemporary novels and television programs which exploit the hospital as a setting for depicting adventure, romance, and crisis. He may feel repugnance for sickness in himself or in other patients or he may welcome new companionship and a chance to express compassion for others. He may idolize physicians, nurses, and other health personnel or he may see them as his exploiters and tormentors.

The Internal Culture of the Hospital

The social structure, organization, and internal culture of the hospital affect patient care in many ways in which the patient is merely an innocent participant. Most hospitals today operate at or beyond the capacity for which they were designed. They are under constant pressure to implement new and increasingly complex medical techniques. They suffer shortages of personnel at almost every level of training and responsibility. There is always the pressure of inadequate time, and in the face of this hospitals have become oriented to emergencies, critical illness, and to a constant tone of busyness.

Within hospitals there are almost always two and sometimes three distinct lines of authority, each concerned with different functions but with many overlapping and ambiguously defined relationships. The medical staff has ultimate responsibility for the welfare of patients and undisputed authority with respect to medical care. Yet many functions which are essential components of total patient care are under the authority of hospital administration. Nursing may constitute still a third line of authority or may be simultaneously responsible to the sometimes conflicting concerns of the physicians and the hospital administrator. Other essential services such as dietetics, social service, pharmacy, and housekeeping may be similarly divided in their allegiance.

As medical care and patient care have become more complex, responsibility has become increasingly fragmented. In the course of even a brief hospital stay a patient may be seen by, and have to relate to, several different medical specialists and a small army of different people, each performing distinct specialized functions. In this respect the modern hospital has indeed come to resemble the modern factory for, like the factory product, the patient's care is sometimes produced in assembly-line fashion. Like the assembly-line factory worker, the hospital employee contributes to such a small part of the total care of an individual patient that he or she rarely has the satisfaction of knowing his patient and identifying with his treatment or recovery. Thus the hospital worker can become alienated from the ultimate goal of the hospital—patient care.

Depending upon outside influences, personnel characteristics, and the outcome of struggles for influence and power within the hospital, varying priorities of hospital operation have their impact on the experience of patients. While some hospitals must operate on a balanced budget, others have alternative resources of financing. Hospitals also vary in the extent of absolute power invested in physicians and the relative power delegated to nurses, administrators, and others. They differ in their orientation to patient needs and comfort versus administrative tightness and housekeeping orderliness (these need not be in conflict but often are). They vary in terms of the emphasis placed of such functions as teaching and research, the frequent concomitants of patient care. These variations are so great that knowledgeable people sometimes characterize particular hospitals as "administration oriented," "physician oriented," "teaching or research oriented," or even "patient oriented."

Communication and the Patient

An essential ingredient to patient care which is often given short shrift is effective communication. This includes communication both with and about the patient. Two factors already identified, shortness of time and complexity of organization, contribute to this deficiency.

Much communication between members of the medical team is limited to notations in charts which have themselves become obsolete anachronisms of an earlier, simpler form of hospital organization. Despite the development of an ever-increasing number of technical diagnostic procedures, direct communication with the patient remains an essential component of accurate diagnosis. The course of a patient's treatment and the patient's involvement in his own recovery and health maintenance depend primarily on effective communication to him concerning the nature of his illness and the implications of measures prescribed for his care.

While some aspects of medical care, such as the administration of tests, surgical intervention, and the application of some therapy, can be performed on a relatively passive patient, the provision of total patient care requires the patient's involvement. It is in the area of patient care that a breakdown of communication—staff with staff, patient with staff, and staff with patient—can prevent fulfillment of the hospital's goals. For patients who are worried and expectant of information about themselves, the silent treatment from physicians, nurses, or other staff, or their thoughtless use of nonverbalized sounds such as "um huh," "ah hah," or "tich tich" during or following an examination may induce acute anxiety or distress. Ironically, although patients are often given very little direction, and discouraged from asking too many questions of hospital personnel, they are expected to know their appropriate role. The classification of patients as "good" or "bad" and the rewards or punishments accorded by staff often depend on whether or not they behave "as patients should."

In a recent pilot study Roland P. Ficken (1970) interviewed fifteen patients who had been admitted to a general hospital for the first time to solicit their perceptions about their own problems and the reasons for their hospitalization. Four of these patients had very different perceptions of their problems than those held by their physicians. Ten had no idea of what to expect from their hospitalization. One patient under treatment for a stomach ulcer was sure that he had cancer. In his lonelieness and anxiety he persistently paced the floor. Yet so inadequate was communication with this patient that a nursing note reported that his walking the corridors was a sign he was feeling well.

Inappropriate communication is as serious a problem as the absence of communication. Several patients told Ficken of the distress they experienced when hearing physicians talking about other patients, and one reported hearing two physicians discussing their uncertainty about the course of therapy and one facetiously suggesting to the other that they flip a coin. Although anyone who spends any signficant amount of time in a hospital and listens can report numerous incidents of seemingly inappropriate communication, there has been little or no systematic study of the impact of communication or the lack thereof on patient care.

My own favorite observation took place in the corner of a public hospital lobby. A uniformed lady called a gentleman's name and when he approached her she held out a paper container and said rather loudly, "Can you give me some urine in this?" To his look of amazement, which she apparently interpreted as failure to hear, she repeated the request in a voice so loud that fifty people were now watching. Only a quick recovery by the lady prevented the gentleman from literally complying with her request.

Prejudice and Imposed Routine

A major impediment to effective communication in hospitals is prejudice. Within the social structure of the hospital many personnel become so preoccupied with their own special function that they fail to see it in the perspective of total patient care. Categories of personnel compete with each other for status and prerogatives. Misunderstanding, bitterness, stereotypes, and prejudice ensue. These are reinforced by the fact that the hierarchy of responsibility and status within the hospital is frequently based on educational, occupational, and other social class criteria which reflect and are reinforced by the forces of caste and class prejudice which prevail in the outer society.

Although the patient brings his own potential for prejudice toward hospital personnel, this is often mollified by the patient's feelings of helplessness and dependency. But no such factors inhibit the physician, nurse, or aide from classifying patients as good or bad, according to social as well as medical criteria, or as uncooperative simply because the physician has failed to communicate effectively with them. Nor is prejudice limited to discrimination of upper against lower class, the educated, or the majority against the minority, as witnessed by the neglect or even punitive treatment which service personnel may accord to a patient they perceive to be overdemanding or condescending.

A more passive but equally malignant form of prejudice can be found in the imposition of relatively inflexible medical or organizational procedures on the hospitalized patient. While often justified in the interest of providing efficient care for the majority of patients, hospital routine as applied to the unique needs of the unique patient may include elements which are in direct conflict with the goals of both medical care and patient care. An illustration can be found in the experience of patients with respect to sleep or rest.

There are many conditions for which medical goals include maximizing opportunities for physical rest in order to facilitate recovery. This is true for most surgical procedures, serious injuries, and severe infections, and is considered particularly important for patients with myocardial infarction. In recent years the liabilities of prolonged continuous bed rest have been increasingly recognized, but the belief prevails that most hospital patients can benefit from an opportunity for more than an average amount of sound, uninterrupted sleep. This medical goal is symbolized by the commonly seen street signs denoting a "Hospital Zone of Quiet."

Yet ironically many factors inherent in the social structure and organization of a modern hospital converge to make rest more difficult for all but the heavily sedated patient. Far from being restful, patients report great difficulty in acquiring uninterrupted sleep in most hospitals. The patient is often awakened to meet the convenience of hospital routine. His personal biological timetable is upset. There is considerable noise engendered by the comings and goings of a large number of people, the movement of equipment, and the urgent voice of the hospital page. Most hospital patients must try to sleep in close proximity to other patients whose personal habits, periods of wakefulness and sleep, desire for entertainment, and requirements for medical attention may vary from their own.

The Patient Is Lost

One aspect of the modern hospital that seems evident from personal observations and available literature is the tendency for an individual patient to become lost in the complex organization. The patient himself begins to feel that no one knows him or is familiar with every ramification of his illness and his hospital course, and often this feeling of the patient reflects quite accurate perception. At a given time and place in a hospital today it is not at all unusual to find no one who really knows the patient. It is even possible that no one will know where a given patient is at a particular time.

Ideally the attending physician knows the significant facts about his patient or at least the facts which he accepts as significant. But many physicians are constantly fighting the battle of time and rarely seem to be able to devote enough time to become thoroughly knowledgeable about an individual patient. Even significant information in the medical records of patients is sometimes not seen by the physician.

The distribution of nursing functions among a large number of people with various special skills and statuses has deprived most nurses of the opportunity to know very much about any one patient. For example, a nurse whose special assignment is the distribution of medications to sixty or more patients will often be able to make no connection between the patient's problem and the medication she is administering. Yet without such knowledge the nurse is unable to detect errors which she or the physician may be making.

Others have corroborated my own experience as a patient on a sixty-five bed floor of a voluntary community hospital. Although my admission was primarily for total rest, I met more than fifty new and different people during the first twenty-four hours. During my two-week stay about thirty-five different people entered my room every twenty-four hours (not counting those who came while I was sleeping). Most of these people performed one or at most two functions, with a different person performing this function each eight hour shift, swing shift people covering two days out of seven, and no consistent assignments even within regular shifts.

From the entire experience the only four people I distinctly remember are a nurse whom I had to prevent, on two occasions, from giving me the wrong medication (my rare physician had explained to me what he was prescribing, why, and what it should never be taken with); a cleaning lady who told me some of *her* life history (she was about the only person I saw consistently at least five days a week); a laboratory technician who seemed somewhat of a sadist (he later made the news for assaulting a young lady): and an EKG technician who, on three separate occasions while her machine was recording, managed to say something with emotionally loaded overtones ("Is this the first time you've ever had a heart attack?" "They don't know what's wrong with you, do they?," and "Did you hear about that coed who was raped and murdered last night?"). My total rest was not facilitated by the fact that the door to my room was opened with little or no warning between fifty and sixty times each day and, in response to my physician's request that I be weighed (once), I was awakened at 5:30 each morning for a week and asked to stand on a scale (it took several days for communication cancelling that order to become implemented).

Dependency

A final aspect of the experience of being a patient has been alluded to earlier. This is the status of dependency which is imposed on the patient from the moment of admittance until discharge. It has been suggested that the dependent status of patients has historical roots; that early hospitals were primarily conceived of as places in which to confine the sick in order to protect the well. This reasoning continues to be functional for a small number of highly contagious diseases. In addition, many patients are temporarily dependent because of their illness or injury. Much of the hospital routine imposed upon *all* patients, however, involves forcing them to be needlessly dependent upon the institution. Basic necessities such as food, "clothing," and shelter are prescribed and provided. The expression of initiative is limited or punished. Many patients find themselves cut off when they have the temerity to ask questions about themselves. Medications are administered by others. A routine is established and enforced. Social interaction with the outside world is restricted; personal privacy is invaded; the patient's body is given up to the ministrations of others; and the territory he occupies is subject to invasion by numerous strange people at any time of day or night.

Although the imposition of dependency status upon the patient is sometimes justified as therapeutically indicated, a consideration of the patient's experience from the perspective of a unifying concept of behavior will raise many questions concerning the contribution of dependency to the patient's total well-being both while in the hospital and in the transition back to family and community living. The degree of dependency imposed on hospital patients and the uniformity with which dependency is imposed on all patients raise questions concerning whether this process is primarily responsive to the therapeutic interests of patients or to the needs of the hospital and its various personnel to maintain control over patients. Similar questions apply to the other experiences of being a patient discussed in this section.

On Inquiry and Experimentation

This paper will conclude with a few thoughts and suggestions regarding research on patient care in hospitals. Despite the insightful observations and important documentation now available in the literature, most efforts to study patient experiences in hospitals have thus far been compromised by the fact that hospitals are reluctant to be studied. Much of the available research has been achieved in spite of the barriers imposed rather than because of the facilitation provided by key hospital personnel. Ironically, resistance to permitting research on patient care has often been justified on the grounds that the rights of patients must be protected. Research strategies can, of course, be developed which meet the demands of scientific rigor and compromise neither the personal rights of patients nor the quality of medical care.

Of primary concern is the study of the impact of hospital organization on producing patient care which is reasonably compatible with goals and expectations. First, there are a whole host of basic questions which must be asked. Before some of the relevant questions can even be identified, there is need for in-depth study of the "life history of patienthood." Detailed profiles of individual patients and their entire hospital experience must be recorded. It is assumed that numerous patients can be found who represent a cross-section of the patient population and who will be willing and may even find it diversionally therapeutic to participate actively or passively in such studies. Active participation would involve the patient in maintaining detailed records of his experiences with hospital personnel and procedures. Passive participation would require the patient's willingness to have his experience recorded by human observers or electronic monitoring devices or both. Human observers should be no more of an imposition on the privacy of a patient than a roommate.[1] Monitoring arrangements should be not nearly as traumatic as many on-line devices now used to monitor various physiological functions.

Parallel to the study of individual patients there is need for recording in comparable detail the activities of various categories of hospital personnel which involve doing something to or for patients. Parallel studies should also be focused on particular hospital functions such as food service, the admission and discharge processes, the x-ray and laboratory functions, and the perscription, administration, and use of pharmaceutical items.

This kind of thorough documentation is needed to test the tentative kinds of notions expressed in this paper and in the available literature. It is basic to the generation of hypotheses and to answering such questions as: How are the needs of patients being met? Where in the hierarchy of other needs in the hospital do needs of patients fall? How does the relative hierarchy of needs vary among different hospital functions? To what extent do the roles of various categories of hospital personnel, and the fulfillment of various kinds of hospital functions, reflect recognition of a unified conceptualization of the patient's needs and behavior? What in its totality is the impact of hospitalization on the health and well-being of the patient, and that of his family, and on the patient's capability for assuming his posthospitalization roles?

A second strategy which must be applied to patient care research is that of experimental design. This involves creating experimental and control situations in which the impact of particular procedures on patient care can be measured and compared. Experimental design is commonplace in medical

---

1. A project using human observers who record for computer analysis data on every interaction between patients and the hospital system has been described by Daniel Howland.

research and applied to a whole variety of situations involving particular diagnositc and therapeutic techniques. Although some studies involving experimentation with the patient care process have been undertaken, the idea of structuring an experiment in a hospital in which variations are introduced in the organization or routine of patient care has been commonly resisted. It has been argued that it is not morally right to deliberately withhold from one group of patients some service which might affect their wellbeing. Yet in the absence of such research hospitals have no valid guidelines for evaluating their organizational effectiveness or the relative efficacy of many specific services or modus operandi they now provide.

In closing I would like to suggest two specific proposals for experimentation in the delivery of hospital care to patients, both of which could be studied on a controlled basis. My first suggestion is stimulated by the experiments of a typewriter factory alluded to earlier. For many years hospitals have been involved in a one-directional trend toward greater specialization and fragmentation of what used to be known as nursing care. The "old fashioned" nurse used to perform most nonphysician services for each patient under her care. With more and more specialization, the modern hospital nurse may perform at most only one or two functions for each of sixty or seventy different patients. One RN may dispense medications, another may record selected vital signs, an LPN or an aide may record other signs, a laboratory technician may collect blood, urine, or stools, a dietician may discuss food, a maid deliver means to the room, and an aide place the tray before the patient.

Just as the typewriter factory asked whether the extremely fragmented assembly line was conducive to the best production of typewriters and experimented with various models of production between the assembly line and the one worker/one typewriter extremes, so it seems timely that hospitals ask whether the assembly-line approach to patient care is indeed functional in terms of producing the greatest quality and quantity of patient care at the least cost. It is suggested that experiments be established in which fewer people each be assigned to do more things for a given group of patients. [2] Several models should be designed and each of these should be studied in comparison with control situations in which traditional hospital organization is maintained for a group of comparable patients. The outcomes of the experiment and control must both be measured in terms of their total impact on the patient; on his disease; on his physiological, psychological, and social responses to his care; on the communication process; and on the responses and satisfactions of hospital personnel.

My second suggestion is for an experiment designed to compensate for the fragmentation of patient care and the ambiguity of the patient's role by the creation of a new professional role to be known as the patient advocate. Informally and on a highly selected basis this role already exists. A private group of physicians who cater to an upper-class clientele employ an attractive

---

2. An experiment of this kind is currently being conducted at Vanderbilt University. Personal communication from Dr. Luther Christman, Dean, School of Nursing, Vanderbilt University, Nashville, Tennessee.

hostess to serve their patients whenever they must be hospitalized. This woman arranges for admission, greets the patients at the hospital (or transports them to the hospital), and endeavors to expedite every step of the patient's hospitalization, mimimizing inconvenience, discomfort, and anonymity, and maximizing the patient's sense of self-identity and his identity with others. In many hospitals specific physicians or specific departments have come to rely on someone to perform a similar function for their own selected patients. This may be a secretary or a social worker or a nurse, but the common denominator is that of coordinating and facilitating the normally fragmented bits and pieces of a patient's hospital experience. For experimental purposes it is suggested that the role of patient advocate be formalized for certain patients and that their total experiences be compared with those of appropriate controls. The impact of the patient advocate would of course have to be measured not just in terms of the patient's experience but also in terms of its impact on the behavior, attitudes, and effectiveness of other hospital personnel.

Conclusion

In summary, this paper has offered some reflections on the impact of hospitals on patients. It has been suggested that the study of hospitalization can be facilitated by examining the impact of processes within the hospital on goal fulfillment and by employing a unifying concept of behavior. Research on patient care requires both intensive observation, monitoring and recording of the individual experiences of being a patient, and experimental designs to permit measuring the impact of innovations as compared with controls. As possible models for innovation in patient care, it has been suggested that there be more experiments in which fewer people each do more things for fewer patients, and in which new roles such as the patient's advocate are introduced and tested. It is hoped that, over time, research of this kind can contribute to a narrowing of the gap which now exists between the great potentialities of medical science and the fulfillment of patients' needs by hospitals and the nation's health care delivery systems.

References

Apple, D. (Ed.) *Sociological studies of health and sickness.* New York: McGraw-Hill, 1960.

Bloom, S. W. *The doctor and his patient.* New York: Russell Sage Foundation, 1963.

Brown, E. L. *Newer dimension of patient care.* Parts 1, 2, and 3. (The use of the physical and social environment of the general hospital for therapeutic purposes; Improving staff motivation and competence in the general hospital; and, Patients as people.) New York: Russell Sage Foundation, 1961, 1962, 1964.

Burling, T.; Lentz, E. M., and Wilson, R. N. *The give and take in hospitals.* New York: Putnam, 1956.

Cartwright, A. *Patients and their doctors: a study of general practice.* London: Routledge & Kegan Paul, 1967.

Coe, R. M. *Sociology of medicine.* New York: McGraw-Hill, 1970.

Duff, R. S., and Hollingshead, A. B. *Sickness and society.* New York: Harper & Row, 1968.

Ficken, R. P. Patients' expectations and perceptions of hospitalization. Unpublished paper, Department of Behavioral Science, College of Medicine, University of Kentucky, 1970.

Freidson, E. *Patients' views of medical practice.* New York: Russell Sage Foundation, 1961.

Freidson, E. (Ed.) *The hospital in modern society.* New York: Free Press, 1963.

Freidson, E. *Profession of medicine.* New York: Dodd, Mead, 1970.

Howland, D. Toward a community health-system model. *Bio-Medical Computing,* 1970, *1,* 11-30.

Jaco, E. G. (Ed.) *Patients, physicians, and illness.* Glencoe, Ill.: Free Press, 1958.

King, S. H. *Perceptions of illness and medical practice.* New York: Russell Sage Foundation, 1962.

Knutson, A. L. *The individual, society, and health behavior.* New York: Russell Sage Foundation, 1965.

Koos, E. L. *The health of Regionville.* New York: Columbia University Press, 1954.

Macgregor, F. C. *Social science in nursing.* New York: Russell Sage Foundation, 1960.

Mechanic, D. *Medical sociology: a selective view.* New York: Free Press, 1968.

Mumford, E., and Skipper, J. K., Jr. *Sociology in hospital care.* New York: Harper & Row, 1967.

Parsons, T. *The social system.* New York: Free Press, 1951.

Roth, J. A. *Timetables.* New York: Bobbs-Merrill Co., 1963.

Scott, W. R., and Volkart, E. H. (Eds.) *Medical care: readings in the sociology of medical institutions.* New York: Wiley, 1966.

Simmons, L., and Wolff, W. G. *Social science in medicine.* New York: Russell Sage Foundation, 1954.

Skipper, J. K., Jr., and Leonard, R. C. (Eds.) *Social interaction and patient care.* Philadelphia: Lippincott, 1965.

Taylor, C. *In horizontal orbit: hospitals and the cult of efficiency.* New York: Holt, Rinehart and Winston, 1970.

Zborowski, M. *People in pain.* San Francisco: Jossey-Bass, 1969.

10

ECOLOGICAL ASPECTS OF PATIENT CARE AND HOSPITAL ORGANIZATION*

E. Gartly Jaco

The physical setting and design of the hospital has received much attention in terms of efficiency and function from the architectural perspective. Very little research in the usual sense of the term has actually taken place, however, concerning the effects of physical design on the care of patients by nursing and medical staffs, on patient and staff satisfaction, or on the organization, structure, and function of the hospital itself. The main purpose of this chapter is to provide an appraisal of the available research.

Some reasons for the lack of controlled studies in this area may be: historical development of the hospital as an institution in which the esthetic and social psychological comfort of the patient took a lower priority to meeting his acute medical needs; general lack of funds to permit the hospital architect to design what may be regarded as luxuries into his Spartan-like plans; the late involvement of the social and behavioral sciences in the hospital and health care fields; and the general lack of theoretical and secure knowledge of the potential relationships between spatial, temporal, and distributional aspects of the physical environment and human behavior. Nevertheless, it appears that an increasing recognition of the need to examine these relationships, as well as of the need for more effective collaboration between architects, engineers, and behavioral scientists, is indicated.

Before such collaboration can begin, however, existing problems of communication between these fields need resolving. One problem is the different use of similar concepts and perspectives, as succinctly described by Sommer and Dewar (1963, p. 320): "When architects and social scientists talk together, they are likely to use certain key words in different ways. For example, it may be unclear whether space refers to the floor or air space and how its boundaries are defined . . . . In common speech 'space' refers to the absence of something, while in architecture it refers to something very tangible such a floor space or ground area. Architects are trained to an aesthetic

*Revised version of paper presented at Conference on Hospital Organization Research, May 22-23, 1970, Institute for Social Research, The University of Michigan, Ann Arbor, Michigan. E. Gartly Jaco, Ph.D., is Professor of Sociology at the University of California, Riverside. The author wishes to acknowledge with thanks the kind assistance of Professor Hans O. Mauksch in suggesting several important bibliographic sources, and of Professor Edward T. Hall, Dr. David K. Trites, Madelyne Sturdavant, and Mr. Stanley Lippert for their cooperation in providing materials and reports of their studies reviewed herein. (Some modifications of the original paper have been made by the Editor.)

appreciation of space per se, and discuss the proportions and scale of their air-filled volumes that may overlap, intersect, interweave, and so forth."

Early Works on Ecology and Behavior

Man's use of space has long been a topic of interest to social scientists. Simmel (1921, p. 350) in the nineteenth century regarded "locality, or the place and soil on which the group lives," as a basic "element of the continuity of group life." Geographical space and its human use has long concerned economists, geographers, and particularly early American sociologists who established a specialty label "human ecology" (see Hawley, 1950; Quinn, 1950). The sociologist Sorokin (1943) differentiated between psysico-geographic and sociocultural space, with the latter being directly determined by the structure and culture of different societies, and thus having divergent meaning in various societies. He then emphasized the "distributional aspects" of society in sociocultural "space," such as its stratification system and social structures. These studies may be viewed as being primarily concerned with macrospace—such terms as "territory," "community," "locality," "natural areas," "settlement pattern," and the like reflecting an orientation toward the larger aspects of man's use of the physical environment.

Behavioral scientists have been interested in the human use of microspace, and in the perceptions of and responses to the individual's surroundings. A classic experiment by Mintz (1956), after studying the effects on subjects of an "ugly" and a "beautiful" room, found that the former room caused such reactions as monotony, fatigue, headache, sleep, discontent, irritability, hostility, and avoidance of the room, while the latter brought about feelings of pleasure, comfort, enjoyment, importance, energy, and a desire to sustain activity. He concluded that "visual-esthetic surroundings can have significant effects upon persons exposed to them."

Hall (1968), in particular has studied cross-cultural divergencies and cultural interpretations of uses of personal space and territory, labeling such studies as "proxemics." He reports how Americans in Arabic countries when conversing with the natives would back away, regarding Arabs as standing "too close," which offended the Arabs who regarded the Americans as cold, aloof, or distant. Hall also draws heavily upon Osmond's (1957) descriptions of two basic types of microspace: "sociopetal space," space and furnishings which pull people closer together; and "sociofugal space," surroundings which keep people apart, divided, or separated.

Osmond's (1957, 1959) and Hall's (1963a, 1963b, 1968) works have stimulated several studies by Sommer (1959, 1966, 1967a, 1967b), Sommer and Dewar (1963), and Sommer and Ross (1958) on specific aspects of "personal space" and "territorial defense of space" in various settings. Following Osmond's concept of sociofugal space, Sommer found that such space in a library reference room "tends to be large, cold, impersonal, institutional, not owned by any individual, overconcentrated rather than overcrowded, without opportunity for shielded conversation, providing barriers without shelter, isolation without privacy, and concentration without cohesion" (Sommer 1967, p. 655).

Another approach to the study of the relationship between environment and human behavior in terms of "behavioral settings" has been formulated by Barker (1968) and his associates who label their emerging specialty "ecological psychology." A theory of "eco-behavioral systems" is formulated according to which such behavioral settings provide "inputs with controls that regulate the inputs in accordance with the systemic requirements of the environment, on the one hand, and in accordance with the behavior attributes of its human components, on the other. This means that the same environmental unit provides different inputs to different persons, and different inputs to the same person if his behavior changes; and it means, further, that the whole program of the environment's inputs changes if its own ecological properties change; if it becomes more or less populous, for example" (Barker 1968, p. 205).

Thus Barker disagrees with such earlier conceptions of the environment and behavior by Lewin (1951) and Brunswik (*International Encyclopedia of Unified Science*, pp. 656-750) that both are independent parameters, that environmental factors occur independently from the behavior of inhabitants in the environment. Rather, Barker (1968, p. 186) states: "According to behavior setting theory, the ecological environment of human molar behavior and its inhabitants are not independent; rather, the environment is a set of homeostatically governed eco-behavioral entities consisting of nonhuman components, and control circuits that modify the components in predictable ways to maintain the environmental entities in their characteristic states . . . . This means that the ecological environment varies systematically from inhabitant to inhabitant." Studies of what Barker terms "undermanned" and "overmanned" behavioral settings, in terms such as population density and related factors, support his conceptualization of the interdependence of environment and behavior rather than independence.

Implications for Hospital Research

Nearly all of the above studies encompass a variety of phenomena other than the hospital and health care areas. Only recently have studies been conducted on certain aspects of the work environment in hospitals, particularly dealing with the impact of physical design and spatial arrangements on patient care and on the activities of hospital personnel such as nursing and medical staff. Furthermore, the few studies that have been undertaken did not seemingly benefit from the theoretical and conceptual formulations of the preceding ecological perspectives in other fields. Most have attempted to assess what impact, if any, the physical setting of the hosptial might have on reactions, utilization, activity, or the satisfaction of patients, nursing, and medical staffs.

Investigations of the effects of physical environment on patient care are still remarkably sparse, nevertheless, since the bulk of patient studies have concentrated more on interpersonal relationships between hospital staff and patients. Only a very few investigations have focussed on the physical setting and its shape in relation to patient care, leading Sommer and Dewar (1963, pp. 319f.) to comment: "Most research dealing with hospital patients has stressed the patient's relations with other people, especially nurses, doctors, other patients, and visitors. Much less has been written about his reactions to the physical environment. This field has been regarded as almost exclusively the province of the architect and the interior designer."

This dearth of research possibly reflects the lack of similar studies of social organization from the ecological or morphological perspective in the social and behavioral sciences in recent years (Duncan and Schnore, 1959). Robinson's (1950) methodological criticism of "ecological correlations" also has cast some doubt on the general validity and utility of analyzing and predicting behavior in terms of areas and spatial dimensions. Nevertheless, the notion still persists that the environment, physical or otherwise, has some valid significance for the behavior and responses of human beings. While the old saw about igloos never being constructed in the Sahara desert nor refrigerators being found among the Eskimos is rarely heard today, Winston Churchill could still make the observation that "we shape our buildings and then they shape us" in urging that the House of Commons be rebuilt in its original form after being destroyed in World War II, holding that changing the building might alter the character of Parliament (Cf. Hall, 1963b).

A few studies have reported the significance of ecological, or spatial and temporal, factors in hospital activity. Examples of these include: Coser's (1958) study of decision-making on two hospital wards as related to specific spatial patterns; Thompson's (1955) study of patient preferences for a four-bed ward in a general acute hospital; Pace's (1957) study of the intrusion into the personal space of hospitalized mental patients; Freidson's (1960) study of patient location in the referral system; and Wilson's (1954) observations on timing and rhythm essential to teamwork in the surgical operating room. But spatial and temporal factors in these investigations were only a small part of the total inquiry, in which other factors were given equal or greater attention.

Ecological Studies of Hospital Care

One of the more recent studies in this area was conducted by Rosengren and DeVault (1963). It was concerned with the effects of the physical layout of an obstetrical service in a large general hospital. Such factors as the spatial distribution of activities in the delivery service of patients, the segregation of behaviors in which persons of differing status would perform differently in varying places, and the rhythm, tempo, and sequences of behavior in this service were studied. The researchers concluded that much of the activity in the OB service was at least partially a function of the kinds of spatial, symbolic, and physical segregation that set each area of the unit apart from each other. Futhermore, the degree of spatial segregation was related to the value put upon those activities in the area involving the basic objectives of the service. Physical segregation was related to status differences among hospital staff members. Symbolic forms of segretation between areas were related mostly to the communication of organizationally appropriate attitudes and values. That is, many of the normative components of the physician-nurse and physician-patient relationship were modified by the physical location in which such interaction ocurred in this service, particularly in the interstitial areas of the unit. Moreover, "both the spatial and the temporal organization of the service seemed to be geared to cast the incoming patient into a role and mood that would allow the personnel of the service to behave in ways which they had learned to expect that they should. The staff members themselves—residents, interns, and so on—seemed to be subject to the same proscriptions that stemmed from the morphology of the hospital" (Rosengren and DeVault, p. 290).

Rosengren and DeVault are critical of posing ecological and behavioral parameters as "either-or" propositions, and propose three conceptual models: (1) the ecological or physical setting is viewed as the prime factor in the social behavior occurring in it; (2) the behavior system of an organization manipulates the environment to conform to the norms of the participants; and (3) the normative patterns are only compatible with—limiting and limited by—the facts of the physical setting. In the first model behavior is controlled largely by the setting; in the second the individuals control or direct the environment; and in the third model neither the participants nor the environment is altered appreciably by the other.

These researchers further contend that in all three situations a condition of unstable equilibrium or minimal accommodation prevails. Thus they do not feel the need to choose between either a strictly ecological or a behavioral approach. Rather they believe that studies can best proceed jointly from three perspectives: the possible independence of the ecological complex, the possible independence of the normative system, and the possibility of a condition of unstable adjustment between the normative and ecological factors. We therefore note a similarity in the conceptual position taken by Rosengren and DeVault and that of Barker's (1968) eco-behavioral theory.

Rosengren and DeVault's study concentrated almost entirely upon the effects of the physical design of the obstetrical unit upon the interrelationships of the nursing and medical staff rather than upon the patient. Since the primary purpose of the hospital is to care for sick individuals, i.e. "patients," a major need is to study the impact of the physical setting upon the welfare and therapeutic functioning of patients as another factor contributing toward the recovery of the patient from his illness. The effect of the physical design upon the *patient* may be more significant than it is upon the hospital staff; the physical setting may enhance or impede the care of patients. Other than the comment that "the staff was in agreement that the patients seemed to 'behave better' while in labor under the quieting effect of the gray decor of the rooms" (Rosengren and DeVault, p.276), this study reported more aspects of patient care as affected by the staff's *behavior* than by the physical environment of the unit.

Some insights into the effects of hospital furnishings upon patients are presented by Sommer and Dewar (1963). These investigators, for example, report on the rearranging of chairs. Chairs that were ordinarily located around the walls of a corridor and used by patients and relatives when visiting would be rearranged into smaller groupings so that visitors could converse more comfortably. But rearrangement of the furniture never occurred in the wards where only patients interacted, and patients would often put back chairs along the walls after the researchers had attempted to rearrange them into smaller groupings. Sommer and Dewar (p. 332) concluded that "the moral was clear that the friends and relatives were arranging the geography to suit their needs, while the patients were *being arranged* by the geography." They further observed: "This is typical of institutions of all kinds, including general hospitals. Patients, dispossessed from their homes and familiar landmarks, keep aloof from their physical surrounding by remaining in bed or sitting in the corner of a room, afraid to tamper with the physical environment. Removed from their territories and defined as sick or helpless by those around them, the patients adapt to the hospital instead of changing it to suit their needs" (p. 333).

The arrangement of furnishings in hospital units is more likely due to facilitating the maintenance of the hospital than to meeting patients' needs. As Sommer and Dewar (p. 335) suggest: "The patients prefer a stable ward environment, while the nurses admire the neat appearance of a ward with rows of chairs arranged shoulder to shoulder. *It is usually true that if function does not determine structure, then structure will inevitably determine function* [italics added]. If the staff do not arrange the furniture to facilitate social interaction they may find that the chairs will arrange the patients to minimize social interaction." The use of space by patients was also studied. Patients in large groups in which they felt to be strangers tended to prefer to sit against the walls away from the others. Patients preferred "private places" they could retreat to in their wards and other places in the institution. Patients who remained in the hospital for a lengthy period tended to "nest" into the ward and hospital, complained less about the facility, and probably had more blunting of their sensory mechanism due to their longer institutionalization than shorter-term patients.

Sommer and Dewar's study was conducted in a mental hospital. They believe, however, that many of their findings would apply to general hospitals. They stress the importance of such concepts as "personal space" and "territory" of patients, and suggest that patient complaints about lack of privacy may reflect intrusions into the patient's personal space, while comments about the impersonality or coldness of a hospital may indicate the patient's inability to acquire a territory within the institution. Finally, they point out the dearth of research on how the physical setting of the hospital affects the condition of patients.

While the researches of Sommer and Dewar and Rosengren and DeVault are valuable contributions to many facets of the impact of physical surroundings upon patient behavior, their results are derived more from selected observations and impressions than systematic statistical findings, and without related research controls that are truly needed in order to arrive at valid and reliable generalizations. Impressions and observations of patient and hospital staff behavior are subject to innumerable biases, distortions, and transitory illusions. Patient activity and the atmosphere of hospital units change markedly during the 24-hour day, day of the week, and season of the year. Nursing activities differ on the day shift from that of the relief and night periods of duty, as does patient behavior. Surgical units vary from medical, obstetrical, pediatric, and psychiatric services by virtue of having different needs of patients to attend as well as divergencies in the demographic, socio-economic, and personality characteristics of patients placed in these areas of the hospital. Therefore, unless appropriate steps are taken to sample these parameters of patient and staff "worlds," the risk of inaccurate recording of such activities remains high. Needless to add, adequate replication of research findings in different settings, an urgent need, is further reduced when systematic and controlled observations are lacking.

Design Efficiency Studies

Moving from the preceding "eco-behavioral" studies to what might be termed "design efficiency" studies, we note some interesting developments. This category of research tends to focus upon the manner in which the nursing staff utilize the nursing unit in providing care for patients occupying the unit. The emphasis usually is on the shape of the total layout or design of the unit, and on the amount of travel between various points in the unit required of nursing personnel, such as frequency of trips from the nurses' station to patients' rooms, from rooms to rooms, etc.

One particular study by Pelletier and Thompson (1960) developed the Yale Traffic Index as a measure of the efficiency of such hospital units. This index has been used in many studies of nursing unit efficiency. These researchers question traditional architectural yardsticks of design efficiency, such as number of beds per ten running corridor feet, distance of the farthest bed from the nurses' station, number of beds per unit of area, and area per bed. They contend that all measures of functional efficiency of nursing units are reducible to "how far staff members travel in caring for the patients." Their index is based upon "links" of travel by nursing staff between two specific areas or spaces within the unit, such as between patient rooms (the nurse traveling from one patient room to another patient room), between the nurses' station and patients' rooms, utility room to patient rooms, nurses' station to utility room, patient rooms to elevator lobby, and so on. These "links" are regarded by these investigators as the prime determinants of unit efficiency.

The index in question is based upon two major assumptions: (1) activities performed by nursing staff are relatively uniform throughout the nation; and (2) with similar facilities, traffic links will assume the same importance independent of plan configurations. It should be noted that there is some question about the full validity of both assumptions. Pelletier and Thompson computed their index for 19 different types and sizes of nursing units, including radial, angular, and T and X shapes, with single and double corridor variations.[1] They rank-ordered these 19 designs in terms of their index scores and then compared them with more traditional architectural measures of efficiency, including distance from nurses' station to the farthest patient's room, and number of beds per 100 square footage of the unit. They suggest that the results from their index did not correlate very well with these other indicators, although there was some fairly high association with the distance from nurses' station to the farthest patient's room. They conclude that inpatient unit efficiency is not related to the size of the unit, but contend that the total design or layout of the unit is the key factor.

Some other investigations using the Yale Index include architect McLaughlin's (1961) analyses of radial and rectangular nursing units. Employing a modified version of the index, this investigator concluded that the latter design was more efficient than the former. In a subsequent article, McLaughlin (1964) used a modified Yale Index to evaluate eight different physical designs, included estimated construction costs involved, and measured distance to the bedside.

Results with the Yale Traffic Index apparently have not convinced many architects of the need to revise their traditional methods or approach in designing inpatient units. For example, this measurement was given only casual recognition in a recent architectural textbook by Wheeler (1964, p. 72), who pointed out the tentativeness of the results with the index and disposed of it with the remarkable comment: "They were qualitative but not yet adequately quantitative." Wheeler supports the measure of the distance from the nursing station to the door of the most remote patient room in planning such units and adds such items as: the shape and size of the floor plan, the "working reltionships of the departments, and the amount of space devoted to stairs, corridors, and elevators in relation to the net assignable space." He considers the latter two factors more important than shape in appraising the functional efficiency of a unit (p. 71).

Others who are also critical of the Yale Index are Freeman (1967) and Lippert (1969). Freeman criticizes the index for ignoring the requirements of patients receiving nursing care; lack of probability statistical tests for observed differences between nursing services being measured; artificiality of certain measures; and the omission of any relation of traffic distances to traffic costs or unit construction costs. Lippert points out that the Yale Index measures distance only to the door of the patients' rooms, and should be extended to the patients' bedside. This extension, he suggests, would add more precision, be more sensitive to variations in the number of beds per patient room, and give a more precise assessment of time in nursing staff movement to the bedside.

---

1. The index is computed as follows: the number of links is first established for the unit to be measured, with the authors suggesting that 14-16 links are a typical maximum per inpatient unit. The actual length in running footage is measured for each link in the unit and multiplied by its appropriate weight. The weight of each link is determined by work sampling observations of the nursing staff traveling in each link and the percentage of time the total staff is observed in these links. Then the products of this multiplication for each link are totaled, this final number comprising the index score—the larger the number the less efficient is the unit.

Following Freeman's suggestion, Lippert has offered an expansion of the "link" concept of the Yale Index by suggesting "tours" of nursing personnel within the unit as a better basic measure of traffic. A "tour" starts when the nurse departs from the nursing station to visit a patient's room or other area of the unit and ends upon her return to the station. He proposes equations wherein the major theoretically possible types of tours are measured, encompassing maximum tours including visits to patients' rooms located at the extreme distances from the nurses' station in the unit, ordered tours when the nurse visits several patients' rooms in one tour, and random tours where specific patients' bedsides are attended. He also proposes other variations of these basic tours in which visits to the utility room are included in the tour with or without patient-room visits, and partial tours. Lippert and his associates at Tufts University are continuing their studies. Lippert regards his analysis as superior to the Yale Index in assessing travel time of nursing personnel in terms of the physical shape or geometry of hospital units. He further suggests that an assessment of travel demands of nursing units is needed prior to any behavioral studies of nursing activity in such units, in order to be able to control for such differences when studying nursing behavior.

The foregoing works obviously are directed toward the development of precise quantitative assessments of the physical layout of hospital units. They focus on physical measurements, tend to employ algebraic models, linear measurements, and deductive reasoning in their evaluations, and also omit almost entirely any considerations of behavioral and social factors as possibly affecting their models, variables, and related concepts. Indeed, some of the investigators who employ these approaches regard physical features as independent or unaffected by behavioral factors. In their view, personal differences between nursing personnel, patients and their needs, staffing patterns, occupancy levels, modes of nursing and medical practice, and the like have no effect on use of the physical environment of the hospital units. The constants in their equations are not altered by such behavioral and organizational variations, they contend.

Sociobehavioral Studies

Studies of the above kinds are of more value to those hospital designers and administrators whose interest gives higher priority to physical efficiency and cost than to patient comfort and welfare. They tend either to ignore or disregard the social-psychological impact of the physical environment on patients' satisfactions, nursing and medical staff responses, and the overall human benefits of patient-oriented hospital design. Consequently, they do not satisfy behavioral scientists and others in the hospital and health care fields who are more sensitive to human patient needs.

There are, however, other hospital researchers who either tacitly assume or overtly assert that the physical design of a unit conditions the activities of people in such settings. They are interested in testing hypotheses about the potential relationship between various aspects of the physical setting and

organizational and related behavior of individuals interacting in such surroundings. Studies of this kind are extremely rare to date, however, despite the
potentially enormous contributions to hospital organizational behavior and
patient care of such research.

One series of studies attempting to determine if a particular design of a
hospital unit would differentially affect the activity patterns of the nursing
staff, and the "satisfiactions" of patients receiving care, was conducted at
Rochester (Minnesota) Methodist Hospital by Sturdavant, Trites, and their
associates. One type of design, the radial-shaped unit, arranges patient
rooms in a circle around the nurses' station located in the center of the area.
This allows constant observation of patients by the nursing staff without
having to enter the patient rooms, and also reduces the travel distance
needed to visit the rooms from the station, in contrast to the traditional
single-corridor unit.

Some hypothesized effects of a radial design, in theory at least, were that
the reduction in travel time made possible by it would: reduce fatigue of the
nursing staff by reducing the amount of walking to attend patients; reduce
tension and anxiety by permitting continual direct observation of the patients
from the nurses' station at a minimum of effort; and bring about more direct
bedside care of patients by nurses freed from the usual physical demands of
the traditional angular-shaped layout. The patients supposedly would also
benefit from the nursing tasks being made easier, and would feel more secure
in having any critical needs attended to by the nursing staff who could readily
observe them at all times with a minimum of effort.

The use of a circular shape was clearly based upon the premise that hospital physical design could be altered deliberately to improve performance of
nursing tasks and functions (and be more functionally efficient) which, in
turn, would enhance favorable responses on the part of patients benefiting
from improved nursing service. The circular design was thought to be of
more value to caring for the critically ill patients and was thus initially
employed for intensive care units.

The first Rochester study (Sturdavant, 1960; Sturdavant et al., 1960) was
an effort to test some of these hypotheses for surgical patients needing
intensive care. A radial unit was compared to a rectangular unit for such
factors as types of nursing care, use of the unit by the nursing personnel, and
reactions to both units by patients hospitalized therein and by nursing and
medical staff. Although some of the results were ambiguous, the researchers
concluded that the radial unit was superior to the rectangular unit in more
effective use of nursing time, and greater satisfaction of patients, their relatives, nurses, and surgeons in the service. They credited the shape of the
radial unit, which brought about less travel distance and high visual contact
between patients and nursing personnel, for the results. The investigators
also appropriately qualified their results as pertaining only to intensive care,
small-sized units, and units containing only private rooms. Regardless of the
relative merits of the circular over the rectangular shaped hospital units, this
study clearly substantiated the assumption that the shape and arrangement
of the unit had an impact on the behavior and responses of staff and patients.

The study stimulated sufficient interest and support to construct an entirely new hospital facility in which reasonably comparable units of different designs were built into the new structure. Three basic physical designs were constructed in the new hospital: the radial, double corridor, and single corridor. This permitted a unique opportunity to evaluate such designs under more reasonably comparable physical conditions than in the initial study, and to compare differently shaped units, although the radial units were smaller in area than were the other two designs in that hospital.

A study of the comparative effects of these three designs upon nursing performance, use of the units, and subjective feelings of the nursing staff was conducted in inpatient units, four each in the radial, double-corridor, and single-corridor units. Variations in visual and auditory contact systems existed in these units, so these factors could be studied. Intervening factors such as differential traits of the patients, individual nursing staff, and the physical settings were statistically rather than experimentally controlled by use of multiple linear regression analysis. Measures of the dependent variables—nursing care and subjective responses of the nursing staff—were obtained by work sampling of nursing activity for a three-month period and by questionnaires administered to the nursing personnel during various times in the course of the project.

Trites and his associates (1969a, 1969b) report the results of this research. The initial statistical analysis indicated that the single-corridor unit was the least desirable, both with respect to nursing performance and use of the unit, and that there was no distinct difference between the radial and double-corridor units. But differences between the latter two types of units were found for measures related to location and activity variables, respectively. The researchers felt that such differences might be partially due to including travel necessary for such activities in each activity measurement. Recalculations of the measurements to eliminate travel yielded results which favored the radial unit. Another statistical analysis between the three daily shifts of the nursing staff indicated that the circular unit was superior to the single-corridor design 85 percent of the time, and to the double-corridor unit 60 percent of the time, while the double-corridor design surpassed the single-corridor unit 65 percent of the time. The investigators concluded that the radial design was best, followed by the double- and then the single-corridor designs, in terms of nursing activities and the location in the units where such activities occurred.

Initial results for different subjective feelings of the nursing staff on the three units were somewhat ambiguous and inconclusive. One finding concerning the day shift of the nursing staff indicated that personnel on the circular and single-corridor units felt their workload was heavier than those on the double-corridor units. Other findings for the evening shift suggested that personnel on the single-corridor units had less work satisfaction and that those working on radial and single-corridor units felt less efficient. On the night shift, nurses in the single-corridor units reported "unwinding" and going to sleep faster after their previous workshift, while those in the circular units reported more fatigue before starting the shift. After serving on a night shift those on single-corridor units reported feelings of more efficiency in their work. [2]

Because of these inconclusive findings, the researchers used two indirect measures of the nurses' feelings, by measuring staff absenteeism and accidents to staff members on the differently designed units. The radial units exhibited the least staff absences, the next fewest were on the double-corridor units, and the most on the single-corridor units. Relatively more staff accidents occurred on the single-corridor unit compared to the radial and double-corridor units. The investigators could not control for extraneous factors for these two variables and thus regard these latter results as tentative.

The effects of electronic modifiers were also studied, by introducing auditory contact between nursing staff and patient rooms via an intercom communications system. Their observations led the investigators to conclude that such systems did not reduce the number of trips into patient rooms by the nursing staff. Despite such findings, the opinions of the nursing staff were highly favorable toward such communication systems. Nursing staff members felt that these systems were important in patient care, improved their work, were often used, and saved the staff trips into patient rooms. Thus, contrary to observations of the nursing staff's actual behavior, the nursing personnel indicated they liked the intercom systems in their units.

The overall results of these studies indicate that nursing personnel on the radial unit spent significantly more time with their patients and less time in travel than did the nurses on the single- and double-corridor units. The researchers further state that, despite these more favorable factors for the radial design, nursing staff on the radial units also were observed more often in the nurses' station and to have more nonproductive time on the day and evening shifts, in contrast to nurses on the other two designs.

Attempting, finally, to convert their findings into cost-analysis, the investigators indicated that in both the double- and single-corridor units the extra travel required cost about $77 more per bed per year than on the radial units. In terms of time spent with patients, it was calculated that the additional time nurses spent with their patients on the radial units was worth $67 more per bed per year when compared to the double corridor units, and worth $97 more per bed per year when compared to the single-corridor units. It was further suggested that these time and dollar savings, when linked to lower absenteeism, fewer accidents, and a high preference among the nursing personnel for the radial design, all "argue conclusively for the superiority of

---

2. Other findings were that the nursing personnel, with some interesting variations, tended overwhelmingly to prefer working on the radial unit. However, this preference for the circular unit declined with decreasing status of the nursing staff, most preferences being held by the registered nurses (87 percent), followed by the licensed practical nurses (81 percent), and nurse aides and ward clerks (65 percent). The RNs also differed from the LPNs and NAs in preference for the double-corridor and single-corridor units, with the RNs preferring next to the radial units the double-corridor design (7 percent) over the single-corridor unit (6 percent), while the LPNs (12 percent) and NAs and WCs (19 percent) chose the single-corridor over the double-corridor design (7 percent, 16 percent).

the radial design." Related preferences for the radial design by physicians and patients further supported their conclusion, the investigators stated. Of course, they limited their conclusions to the sizes and types of nursing units studied.

A Social-Psychological Investigation

Between the first Rochester study by Sturdavant and the later studies by Trites and associates, another research endeavor of a similar nature was conducted by Jaco (1970) and his associates in St. Paul, Minnesota, between 1963 and 1967. The major purpose was to evaluate the effectiveness of the radial unit compared to the traditional single-corridor angular unit for intermediate as well as for intensive and minimal levels of patient care in terms of: type, level, and amount of nursing care; nurses' utilization of the unit; patient welfare; satisfaction and reactions to the units by patients, nurses, and physicians; length of patient stay; and care costs for general medical and surgical patients. A second purpose was to appraise the potential intervening influences of such factors as nurse staffing patterns and occupancy levels, and a third was to replicate, as much as feasible and appropriate, Sturdavant's study, and to examine other variables potentially involved with and related to patient care of divergent levels in the radial type of physical design.

Research Design

For intermediate (nonintensive) general medical and surgical patients hospitalized in the same unit, twelve "study situations" were carried out on reasonably comparable radial and angular nursing units in which occupancy level and nurse staffing patterns were deliberately altered. Occupancy levels were altered from high (90 percent filled or more) to low (50 percent filled or less), and the nursing personnel was varied quantitatively at high, average, and low levels, and qualitatively by the ratios of registered nurses, licensed practical nurses, and nurse aides to total staff. Each of the study units contained twenty-two beds composed of two private, six semiprivate (double bedrooms), and two four-bed wards.

Each study situation was maintained for four consecutive weeks. Observations of the nursing staff and patients were made by trained observers using work-sampling methods for a five-day week, twenty-four hours per day (all three shifts). A one-week "resettling period" was held between each study situation to blur any potential "halo" effects. An effort was made to control for differences that might occur in the patient populations admitted to the units during the project by randomizing the assignment of patients to these units by the hospital admitting office. Similarly, an effort was made to use identical nursing personnel in both types of units during the study so that each nurse would be her own control for individual differences among the nursing staff, although this was not always feasible due to turnover of staff.

Nursing staff were interviewed privately at the end of each study situation, and physicians who had admitted patients to the study units were interviewed privately at the midpoint and end of the study. Nursing staff completed certain research forms daily in the unit. Patients were privately interviewed just prior to their discharge. A recording clerk, located in the nurses' station on the radial unit, recorded trips by nurses to the patient rooms and other areas to supplement the observations of the observing staff. Observations were made about five times per hour of every member of the nursing staff in ten randomly assigned sampling areas in the units. Appropriate probability statistical tests were computed for significant differences in the variables between the two physical designs.

Intensive level of care was studied only in the radial shaped unit, due to the many obstacles and potential hazards involved in trying to convert the angular unit into such a service. The existing minimal care (self-care) unit in the study hospital was a single-corridor unit which was observed for a one-month period, after which the nursing staff was transferred to a radial unit similarly arranged in accommodations to provide a comparative study of minimal care on both designs. Since three major levels of patient care—intensive, intermediate, and minimal—were studied on circular units, and the later two levels also on angular-shaped designs, the unusual opportunity arose to examine some of the different factors involved in progressive patient care for both physical designs.

Patient Care in Radial and Angular Shaped Units

The results for intermediate-level care were mixed and often surprising. The type of nursing care differed significantly between the radial and angular designs. From more than 200,000 observations over a two-year period, approximately the same nursing staff gave on the radial unit *more* indirect care and general assistance and took more time out, but gave *less* direct bedside care, showed less standby, and traveled less than when on the angular shaped unit. This paralleled somewhat the results of Sturdavant, who also found less direct care on the radial than the rectangular unit for a more severely ill patient population. However, the ratio of patient-involved care (direct care combined with indirect care and general assistance) to nonpatient-involved activity (standby and time out) was somewhat higher on the circular than on the angular unit. More physical and less social types of direct care were given on the radial than on the angular unit, and no difference in direct medical care between the two designs was found.

The head and charge nurses on the circular unit provided more indirect care and general assistance, and took more time out with less standby and travel, than when on the angular unit. They gave about the same amount of direct care on both units. The registered nurses showed a somewhat different pattern than the head nurses, giving on the circle *more* indirect care and general assistance and *less* direct care than on the single corridor unit. They also traveled less, and there was no difference in standby and time out. The licensed practical nurses differed from the RNs in providing on the circular unit *more* direct and indirect care and general assistance; they also took more time out than on the angular unit, while standby and travel were the same on both units. The nurse aides also diverged in their pattern of activity, giving *more* indirect and *less* direct care on the radial than on the angular unit; they showed more time out and travel, and no difference in general assistance and standby.

From these findings it can be seen that the different nursing personnel performed different functions and activities on the two units. On the premise that care provided by the more professionally trained nursing staff, such as head nurses and RNs, is of a higher level than that provided by LPNs and NAs, the ratio of care provided by the former compared to the latter types of personnel should be an indicator of higher level of patient care. It was found that a slightly higher level of care was provided on the radial than on the angular unit, particularly when the measure included indirect care and general assistance.

The amount of nursing care was measured by the number of staff trips to the patient rooms, classified as nurse-initiated or patient-initiated trips. Trips made in the patient's absence, as well as those involving patients, and staff-to-staff room visits were considered. The results were somewhat surprising in that the nursing staff on the radial unit made far *more* nurse-initiated trips and *fewer* visits when the patients were absent from the room, but about the same patient-initiated and staff-to-staff trips, on the two units. The nursing staff on the circle also exhibited a higher ratio of nurse-initiated to patient-initiated trips, and a somewhat higher ratio of nurse-initiated trips to trips when the patient was out of the room. These ratios suggest that patients on the circular unit received a higher amount of nursing care than those on the angular unit during this study.

A more direct index of impact of the physical design involved those factors indicating the nursing staff's utilization of various areas within the units during their activities. An efficiency index comprised of three measures was developed: a ratio of times nursing staff was observed in patient rooms when the patient was present to times when the patient was absent; a ratio of times observed in the corridors of the unit to other areas within the unit; and a ratio of times the staff was observed performing professional services in patient rooms to those times they were using unoccupied patient rooms for personal reasons. Other indicators were the proportions of time nursing staff was observed in patient rooms compared to other areas of the unit, and the proportion of times staff was in the unit but out of patient rooms.

The results suggest that the nursing staff on the radial unit spent slightly less time in the corridors than on the angular unit, but there was no difference in ratios of time spent in patient rooms when the patient was present or absent. More striking was the finding that the radial-unit staff used unoccupied patient rooms for personal rather than professional reasons more than on the angular unit during periods of low unit occupancy. Also the staff on the circular unit spent a greater proportion of their time off the unit entirely than when on the angular unit, indicating that nursing usage of areas and facilities off the unit itself does play a part in the utilization of nursing time which is independent of the shape or design of the nursing unit itself. Thus while the radial unit was only slightly more efficient in use of corridor space than was the angular unit, this did not result in bringing staff into the patient rooms any more, or in preventing fewer unnecessary trips to the patient rooms when the patients were absent.

Patient welfare was measured with three scales developed by Aydelotte and her associates (1960)—mental attitude, physical independence, and mobility—based on daily ratings of patient status by the nursing staff in their charge. The results showed no difference for any of the three scales for patients hospitalized during the study in the two units. The average length of stay of patients also did not differ significantly between the two units during the project.

Patient reactions. An attempt was made to replicate certain types of questions asked of hospitalized patients prior to their discharge that were also used in Sturdavant's Rochester study. Other questions were added to the interview schedule to examine factors that might reveal how the patients felt about the nursing service and the various physical and nonphysical features of the units and their rooms. One of the more significant questions asked of patients was if there were anything about the unit that they particularly liked. Most of the items spontaneously mentioned by the patients were items in their *rooms* rather than in the *unit*, such as their electric beds, handy bathroom, lavatory, air conditioning, television, telephone, call button, windows, lighting, furnishings, and the like. Responses to this question revealed that patients on the circular unit reported more features of their rooms *and* unit than patients on the angular type, the former averaging two items per patient and the latter 1.7 items per patient. This difference occurred despite the fact that both units and rooms in the two units were quite similar in decor, newness, air conditioning, etc.

This question was further analyzed by measuring the ratio of items mentioned that pertained strictly to the patients' rooms and those related to aspects outside their rooms, such as the windows, the sundeck, and lounge. The results showed that patients on the circular unit reported twice as many "particularly liked" items related to the *external* environment out of their rooms than did patients on the angular unit. It seems obvious that the high visual contact in the radial unit plus the large picture windows on the external wall in this unit may have affected the patients' reactions to their external milieu more on the circular than on the angular unit where such visibility was much lower.

This is further supported by the patients' responses to a question asking them how they compared their unit with others in which they had been previously hospitalized. The results were as follows:

Patients on Circular Unit		*Patients on Angular Unit*	
Positive toward the Circle	37%	Positive toward Angle	14%
Negative toward the Circle	2%	Negative toward Angle	9%
Neutral	61%	Neutral	77%
(Based on 401 patient interviews)		(Based on 395 patient interviews)	

When the patients were requested to rate the nursing service in terms of poor, fair, good, very good, and excellent, the results were surprising in view of the reported preference for the circular unit. A small but somewhat higher percentage of patients gave a "poor" rating to the nursing service they received on the circular unit contrasted to that on the angular unit, although a higher overall percentage gave a positive rating to their nursing service on the circular unit. A much higher percentage of patients on the angular unit, however, either refused to comment or said they "didn't know" in responding to this question, and this could imply that at least a certain portion of this group had negative feelings they did not want to express. Also the negative comments on the circle were confined to only a few study situations. Certainly, visual contact on the radial unit permits far greater observation than on the traditional angular unit, and perhaps it is easier for patients to be critical of what is often observed. Nevertheless, a higher percentage on the radial unit than on the angular one also expressed positive ratings about their nursing service, but the percentage from the angular unit could easily change if the interviewer had persisted in obtaining an evaluation from a higher proportion of patients. This renders interpretation of the responses to this question somewhat ambiguous and uncertain.

When asked if they were bothered by activity outside their room, significantly more patients on the angular unit reported being bothered by outside activity than those on the circle. Only 3 percent of the patients interviewed on the circular unit reported being bothered, while 14 percent did report this on the angular unit. Thus visual contact on the circular unit apparently was not a cause of concern to the patients. When asked about the amount of privacy on their units, however, significantly more patients indicated dissatisfaction with the amount of privacy on the circular than angular unit. Dissatisfaction with privacy was reported by 11 percent on the circle while only 5 percent did the same on the angular unit. This was not entirely surprising since lack of privacy on the radial unit was a frequent complaint by patients in the series of interviews conducted.

The patients were also asked to rate their satisfaction or dissatisfaction with eleven specific items: cleanliness, view from the window, room size, toilet facilities, privacy, bath and shower, room type, amount of noise, air freshness, storage space, and window space. Their responses were scored, and a total satisfaction score was computed for each patient and compared for the two units. Results showed only a slightly higher average score for the circular unit than the angular unit, indicating that *total satisfaction* with the two units was quite similar, and quite good, for the patients in them. Similarly, no difference was found in effect of the two units on the morale of patients, although a slightly higher percentage of patients on the circular unit felt that the unit had improved their morale (80 percent) compared to those on the angular unit (78 percent).

When asked to evaluate the charges for their rooms (which were identical for both units), no significant differences were found, although a slightly higher percentage of patients on the circular unit felt their room rates were too high than those on the angular unit (38 percent on the circle, 33 percent on the angle). Again, however, there was a higher percentage of "don't know" responses on the angular than the circular unit that could alter the total results if complete responses had been elicited in the interviews. These differences could have been due to chance alone.

In summary, the results concerning patient satisfaction indicate mixed reactions to both types of units. More positive features of the room and the unit were reported by the patients on the circular units. These patients had a more positive awareness of their environment, were less bothered by activity outside their rooms, gave more positive but also more negative evaluations of their nursing service, and mentioned more complaints about lack of privacy and about room charges. But generally, there was not much difference in overall satisfaction between the two units. The patients from the circular unit were somewhat more free to express their negative as well as positive reactions than were those on the angular unit, a factor which may have been influenced by having been on that kind of unit in itself. Thus we find some mixed reactions to the circular unit among the patients interviewed, although in general this unit was more positively favored for its physical features, especially features outside the rooms, than the angular unit, despite the fact that the two settings were quite similar in newness, decor, and related aspects.

Nursing staff attitudes. Private interviews were also conducted with the nursing staff. The interviews were held prior to initiating the study and periodically after each study situation during the course of the investigation on both units, to determine any possible shifts in opinions about the units by the staff. The more salient responses to the questions are reported here.

At the onset of the project, the participating nursing staff overwhelmingly favored the radial over the angular unit. Of the nursing personnel initially interviewed, 75 percent preferred the circular to the angular unit, 11 percent the angular to the circular, and 14 percent did not favor one over the other. It is of interest to note, however, that preference for the circular unit was related to status position within the nursing personnel. Specifically, at the time of their first interview, 100 percent of the head nurses, 74 percent of the RNs, 67 percent of the LPNs, 77 percent of the NAs, and 100 percent of the ward clerks favored the circular unit, reflecting a relationship between nursing staff status and unit preference.

During the two and a half year course of this project, only 5 percent of the nurses revealed that their preference had been altered, and in divergent ways. Of the five reporting a change of opinion, two were RNs, two LPNs, and one an NA. One of the RNs would not reveal in which direction her preference had shifted, while the other RN first changed her preference from negative to positive toward the angular unit, then later from positive to negative. The two LPNs and one NA changed from negative to positive regarding the angular type of unit. The lower staff levels thus still continued to show proportionately more positive feelings toward the angular type of unit than the higher level RNs. The total nursing personnel nevertheless largely and persistently favored the circular over the angular unit.

When asked what specific features they liked about the circular unit, by far the majority of the nursing staff mentioned attributes more related to their own convenience in performing their work than attributes favoring the care of patients. Features related to convenience of the nursing staff alone were mentioned by 41 percent while only 3 percent mentioned features involving direct benefit to patients alone. When asked to compare specifically the radial to the angular type of unit, the nursing staff similarly gave a more favorable evaluation to the circular unit, in varying degrees, as follows:

1. *Efficiency of the unit:* 86 percent of the total nursing staff preferred the circular to the angular type of unit, 1 percent the angular unit, and 13 percent felt no real difference.
2. *Convenience of the unit:* 82 percent favored the circular type, 2 percent the angular type, and 16 percent neither.
3. *Patient care:* 73 percent preferred the circular type of unit, 2 percent the angular, and 24 percent felt there was no difference.
4. *Relations to fellow nursing staff:* 34 percent favored the circular type of unit, 2 percent the angular type, and 63 percent felt there was no difference.
5. *Relations to patients:* 53 percent preferred the circular type of unit, 2 percent the angular type, and 44 percent felt there was no real difference for this factor.

Thus, according to these responses regarding specific attributes of the two units, the percentage favoring the circular to the angular unit was highest when efficiency and convenience for staff were concerned, but declining and shifting toward no difference as the factors of interpresonal relationships and patient care were involved. Nevertheless, the total nursing personnel working on these two types of units during the course of the project generally preferred the radial to the angular unit when a choice was involved.

Physician attitudes. A sample of physicians who had attended patients on both types of units was interviewed during the time periods when the project staff was conducting their observations. All physicians were privately interviewed and their responses recorded by the same interviewer who interviewed the patients and the nursing staff. In general the physicians tended to prefer the radial unit for the majority of their patients, although some interesting mixed reactions and preferences also occurred.

Asked if patient care was better on the circular or the angular unit, 48 percent of physicians having patients on the circle reported better care on the circular unit while 52 percent felt there was no difference; none reported that care was worse on the circle. Of the physicians having patients on the angular unit during this part of the study, 66 percent reported that the circular unit gave better care than did the angular unit. In both instances there was no difference between the general practitioners and the specialists among the physicians interviewed. When asked for specific reasons why they believed their patients obtained better care on the radial than the angular, the doctors most frequently mentioned such factors as closer observation of patients, efficiency, and convenience for both nursing and medical staff.

When specifically queried about particular attributes of the two units, the physicians reported as follows:

1. *Patient progress:* The radial unit was favored over the angular for this factor, but not to the same extent as for the other factors explored. The general practitioners tended to favor the circular unit somewhat more than the specialists for this factor.
2. *Patient attitude or morale:* The specialists favored the circular unit more than did the general pactitioners for this factor, but both tended to heavily favor the circle.
3. *Nursing care:* Both specialists and general practitioners favored the circle for this factor, with the former being somewhat more favorable in their responses.
4. *Convenience of the medical staff:* The physicians generally were overwhelmingly in favor of the circular unit for this factor, with the general practitioners somewhat more so than the specialists.

Although preference for the circular unit varied for the above factors, the preference was quite consistent for all for the radial over the angular unit. When asked if the circular unit had any specific drawbacks, the physicians mentioned lack of privacy together with lack of private rooms, which existed in these units at the time this study was initiated, as the major disadvantages of the present radial unit. Distance from nurses' station to patient rooms and lack of visibility were mentioned as drawbacks for the angular unit. Consequently, similar physical features were criticized for their presence or absence in both types of units by different physicians. Also of interest was the finding that the circular unit was reported as having "no drawbacks at all" by more physicians than was the angular unit.

This factor was perhaps related to the next question which inquired if the physicians had had any patients they would prefer not to admit to the circular unit. They were unanimous in having had patients they would not admit to the circle, with the general practitioners reporting this more than the specialists. Reasons mentioned for not admitting patients to the circular unit were: patient *wanted* a private room; patient *needed* a private room; patient was emotionally disturbed or under psychiatric care; patient was senile or disoriented; patient was an intolerant complainer; and patient was terminal. Moreover, all the physicians reported having patients who did not want to be admitted to the radial unit. The wish for privacy and for a private room were the major reasons given.

All of the doctors reported having had patients requesting transfer from the circular to the angular unit, and vice versa. The general practitioners had more patients wanting to transfer from the angular to the circular, while the specialists had the same percentage (60 percent) wanting to transfer to and from both units. By far the most frequent reason for wanting such a transfer from the circular unit was to obtain a private room. Whether such a wish for a private room included the desire for privacy off the circle was not clarified in their responses. When asked if they had a preference in admitting a patient to the two types of units, eight out of ten preferred the circular to the angular unit, one of ten preferred the angular unit, and one of ten had no real preference. Convenience of the nurses and physicians and high visibility were the reasons the physicians gave for preferring the circular unit, despite the previous reporting of lack of privacy as the major drawback of this type of unit.

In summary, the physicians by and large preferred the radial unit to the angular, recognized its virtues as well as drawbacks, indicated that they had patients not liking the circle and wanting to be transferred out of the circle, and even indicated some patients they treated would not be admitted to this kind of nursing unit under their care. Thus, as in the case of the nursing staff, there were some mixed reactions to the radial unit by the physicians interviewed, indicating that this type of unit, while more popular with the doctors than the angular unit, still is not universally or categorically preferred by the entire medical staff of the study hospital. It is thus very likely that if the hospital had only circular nursing units, even with private rooms, there would still be a loss of some patients who would prefer, or perhaps even need, the more traditional angular unit.

Costs. During the four-month period from October 1, 1966, through January 31, 1967, hospital operating costs for the two study units were measured after both units had returned to normal operation following completion of their phases of the overall study. The results of the cost analysis of the radial and angular units, under normal operating conditions for this period, were as follows:

Direct Costs	Circular Unit	Angular Unit
Salaries	$26,096	$37,431
Supplies	498	850
Payroll Fringe Benefits	1,577	1,706
Total:	$28,171	$39,987
Indirect Costs	Circular Unit	Angular Unit
Laundry (allocated by pound)	$527	$1,769
Housekeeping (allocated by salary)	442	662
Maintenance	559	839
Total:	$ 1,528	$ 3,270
Grand Total:	$29,699	$43,257
Number of Beds:	20	26
Total Costs per Bed		
Direct Costs	$1,408	$1,538
Indirect Costs	76	126
Total Costs:	$1,484	$1,664

The above typical cost-accounting system of general hospitals, which traditionally allocates indirect costs by beds in each hospital unit, indicates that the lower operating costs of the circular unit per bed are due to lower *direct* costs, particularly for salaries of nursing personnel on the unit. Thus the radial unit in the study hospital was operated at lower per bed cost than the angular unit, essentially by having a smaller nursing staff to provide for the bed patients in its care, a saving of slightly less than 10 percent per bed.

For average per diem costs per patient during this same four-month period for the two types of nursing units, we find a somewhat opposite occurrence.

Range of Average per Diem Charges to Patients

| | | Range | | |
		Low	High	Total
Radial Unit Patients:	Medical	$16.47	$176.15	$159.68
	Surgical	$36.01	190.95	$154.94
Angular Unit Patients:	Medical	$32.97	$116.25	$ 83.28
	Surgical	$33.98	$158.80	$124.82

Average Patient Charges per Day of Stay

	Circular	Angular
Medical Patients	$57.55	$57.73
Surgical Patients	$74.03	$70.96
Total Patients	$65.10	$63.05

Thus the average per diem costs for hospital care were about 3 percent higher per day, for medical and surgical patients combined, on the circular unit. This difference was due entirely to differential billing of surgical patients, since the average per diem patient charges were approximately identical for medical patients on the circular and angular units, while surgical patients averaged 5 percent higher per diem charges on the radial unit during this period. Since charges to patients for care received while in the hospital· understandably tend to be more variable for surgical than medical patients, and are charged in part for services (such as operating room charges, intensive care unit charges at times, dressings, packs and related supplies, and other treatments) whose costs are not related to utilization of the nursing unit, it is likely that per diem charges for care to patients as typically reflected in their billings by the hospital are not related to care received only in such nursing units. In terms of the measures of cost used, we can say that per bed costs to the hospital did vary between the radial and angular units in favor of the radial type, but that such cost differentials were not found to be reflected in the average per diem charges to patients occupying these two types of units during the same period.

Summary. The results concerning intermediate care of general medical and surgical patients without regard to occupancy levels and nurse staffing patterns show that differences were found between the radial and angular units for type of nursing care; level of nursing care; amount of nursing care; utilization of the unit by the nursing staff; patient satisfaction with the unit; nursing staff satisfactions with the unit; physician satisfactions with the unit; and per bed per diem costs to the study hospital for a four-month period. No significant differences were found between the two types of units for patient welfare and average length of stay of patients as measured herein. In all but one of the factors found to differ between the two types of nursing units, such differences tended to favor the radial over the angular unit, the sole exception being utilization of nursing time on the unit, which slightly favored the angular unit. In many instances these results are similar to some of those found by the Rochester studies, but in other instances our results differ. We can thus conclude that the physical shape of the unit was related to the differences in the factors studied and that generally, with some notable exceptions, the radial type of unit was favored over the angular type of unit for this category of acute patients and level of patient care.

When twelve "study situations" were examined for the same intermediate level of care for general medical and surgical patients with occupancy levels and staffing patterns varied, the results provided some surprises. In general, the efficiency of the circular nursing unit was demonstrated in only a few of the twelve study situations. This occurred most significantly when the nursing staff was cut to a minimum and the unit was highly occupied. Under such pressing patient care conditions, the amount of direct bedside care was significantly greater on the radial unit than on the angular, and the level, amount, and patient-involved care were the highest of any of the study situations, when contrasted to the angular unit, under similar stressful conditions for the nursing staff. Indeed, when the nursing staff, comprising the customary components of RNs, LPNs, and NAs, was reduced in quantity for all of these components while conditions of high occupancy prevailed, the circular unit was at its best for intermediate medical and surgical patients.

But when the staff was drastically altered qualitatively, as in the situations of high LPN and high NA, and when the occupancy of the unit was drastically reduced, the features of the circular unit that contributed to high-level patient care in the foregoing situations now became disadvantageous to the nursing staff, and particularly to the head and charge nurses. In contrast to the angular unit having little visual contact between the patients in their rooms and the nursing staff going about their functions around the nurses' station, we found even "misuse" of certain areas of the circular unit, especially by the lesser trained staff such as NAs, particularly for personal activities in the empty patient rooms. The smaller corridor space and visibility of the nursing staff by the patients from their rooms are particular features that disturb the more professionally trained nursing personnel when they become extremely sensitive to patients witnessing anything bordering on substandard nursing performance. In the angular unit, where these features of visibility especially are lacking, the professionally trained nursing staff permit the lesser trained staff to perform many more functions, or are less critical of the performance of such staff, and the entire nursing operation seems to function more harmoniously for all concerned than when on a radial unit.

The major activities observed on the radial unit, contrasted to the angular unit, during these twelve study situations were as follows:

more indirect care than direct care;

more patient-involved than nonpatient-involved care;

more time out and off the unit;

higher level of nursing care, provided by higher trained staff;

usually but not always more efficient use of the unit;

more general assistance;

less direct patient care;

less verbal communication with patients (social direct care);

less use of corridors;

more personal use of unoccupied patient rooms, especially at times of low unit occupancy;

less use of the nurses' conference room;

usually but not always less nonpatient-involved travel;

less use of lesser trained nursing personnel, such as LPNs and NAs, at varying time periods, occupancy conditions, and other conditions in the unit;

perhaps more appropriate performance of nursing care functions, meeting patient needs when necessary and engaging in other activities when patient care is less needed;

perhaps more flexibility in adapting to changing demands of the patient populations in the unit.

While there are possibly other features related to the radial unit than those delineated by this study, the above seem to be the most obvious.

Results Concerning Different Levels of Care

Since the study hospital maintained a progressive patient care program with intensive, intermediate, and minimal or self-care levels provided, it was feasible to study these levels of care in relation to the physical design of the radial and angular shapes. All three of these levels of progressive care were studied in the radial unit; the intermediate and minimal levels were observed in the single-corridor angular units. A summary of the main results is presented below.

On the radial unit the amount of indirect patient care increased as level of care decreased, i.e. going from intensive to minimal levels of care. An inverse relationship also was found for general assistance, which increased as level of care declined in intensity. Standby was positively related to level of care, decreasing as level of care decreased. The categories of direct care, time out, and travel were not found to be related to level of care on the circular unit. Travel and standby were inversely related to intensive and intermediate care, but positively associated with minimal level of care. The intensive care level was associated with more standby and less indirect care, general assistance, and travel than were the lesser care levels. The intermediate level involved more direct care, general assistance, and travel, and less standby, than the other levels of nursing care. The minimal or self-care level was associated with more indirect care and general assistance, less direct care, and also less standby, time out, and travel for nursing staff giving services on these three radially shaped nursing units in the study hospital.

Thus nursing care tended to vary considerably in terms of levels of progressive patient care for the same physical design, supporting the idea that these levels of patient care definitely comprise distinct and separate universes of hosptial patient care. Utilization of the same circular nursing unit by the nursing personnel for these three levels of progressive patient care also was remarkably divergent, despite the fact that nursing care was provided in similar physically designed units, as follows:

Intensive care: When compared to the other two levels of care, the nursing staff was observed *more* in patient rooms with the patient present, utility room, nurses' conference room, miscellaneous areas, and in unassigned patient rooms (professional activity); *less* in the nurses' station, medication area, corridors, tub and shower room, and in unassigned patient rooms (personal activity); and neither more nor less in patient rooms with the patient absent and off the unit.

Intermediate care: When contrasted to the other two levels of care, nurses were found *more* in the medication area, corridors, tub and shower rooms, nurses' conference room, and off the unit; *less* in the nurses' station, utility room, miscellaneous areas, and in unassigned patient rooms (professional activity); and the *same* in patient rooms with the patient present, and absent, and in unassigned patient rooms (personal activity).

Self-care: When contrasted to the other two levels of care, nurses were found to be *more* in the nurses' station, medication area, corridors, patient rooms with patient absent, and in unassigned patient rooms (both personal and professional activity); *less* in patient rooms with patient present, utility room, conference room, miscellaneous areas, and out of the unit; and neither more nor less in the tub and shower room.

When self-care and intermediate care were analyzed for the angular units, some interesting differences were found, contrasted to the radial units. Significantly *more* direct care, standby, and time out occurred for the intermediate care angular unit, under similar staffing and occupancy conditions, and *less* indirect care, general assistance, and travel, while just the directly opposite occurred for the self-care patients on the angular unit. That is, that type of care which was given less for intermediate care patients was given more to self-care patients on the angular unit. The results also show that indirect care increased as level of care decreased, general assistance increased as level of care decreased as level of care decreased. Direct care, time out, and travel, however, differed between radial and angular units. Thus surprisingly, the shape of the unit affects major aspects of nursing care to some extent at all levels of progressive patient care.

The physicians who attended patients during the course of the entire project tended to favor the radial unit increasingly as the need for intensive care correspondingly increased. But radial units came into disfavor as the level of care decreased from intensive to self-care, even to the point where some of the physicians had negative opinions about the radial self-care unit. This could indicate either that the physicians were genuinely accepting the radial unit more for intensive or seriously ill patients than self-care patients, or that they were not sufficiently familiar with the nursing activity observed by the research staff on the circular self-care unit (which indicated more direct care by the NAs on the radial than on the angular self-care units). Another possibility is that the doctors preferred that their patients be provided care by the more professionally trained nursing personnel, especially direct bedside care, rather than by the lesser trained personnel, even then their patients needed only a minimal level of care.

Conclusions and Interpretation

The major conclusions of this study may be stated as follows:

1. Radial types of nursing units have distinctive advantages and also disadvantages for overall patient care in terms of prevailing utilization and traditional nurse staffing patterns.

2. At times when demand for patient care on a hospital is heavy, and when nursing staff is scarce, the radial unit has many advantages in the provision of total patient care over the more traditional angular unit.

3. Although perhaps more inflexible from an architectural standpoint than other shaped units, the radial unit shows promise for much functional flexibility in the provision of various types and levels of nursing and patient care.

4. Provision of patient care is by *people*, and nursing care provided in a radial unit places different demands on the nursing staff, and to some extent on patients, from those in angular units.

5. The radial unit is designed more for nursing and medical staff convenience than for patient convenience, with the patients assumed also to benefit in turn if the nursing and medical staff are benefited. This is a questionable assumption, since reducing the demands of patient care on the nursing staff in the radial unit was detrimental to the morale of the nursing staff contrasted to those on the angular unit.

6. Less professionally trained nursing personnel, such as LPNs and NAs, are less favorable toward the circular unit than are the professionally trained RNs, because they feel less able or permitted to perform higher level nursing functions on the circle due the high visibility of patients and more supervision of their activities by the professional nurses.

7. Some types of patients are not suited to the radial unit, but no such "contraindications" were found for the angular unit. A general hospital having only circular units may thus lose a segment of the patient population to other hospitals in the area having more traditional angular units.

8. Occupancy levels affect the efficient utilization of the radial and angular units in opposite ways. Low occupancy level disrupts the efficient operation of the circular unit at typical nurse staffing patterns, while it improves the operation of the angular unit. High occupancy, with similar nursing staff, improves the efficiency of the radial unit but not always the efficiency of the angular unit when nursing staff are held equal.

9. Nurse staffing patterns affect the efficient use of the radial unit as much, if not more, as the use of the angular type of unit, especially for the lesser trained nursing personnel, such as LPNs and NAs.

10. The radial type of unit has unexplored possibilities for self-care utilization in the acute hospital. To regard the circle as primarily suitable for intensive care patients is contradicted by the results of this study, as all levels of care were benefited.

11. If the circular type of unit is expected to improve inevitably the quality of patient care and upgrade the efficiency of nursing service, then such expectations are unrealistic and disputed consistently by the findings of this study. Many intervening factors prevent the *automatic* improvement of nursing and patient care by physical design and related physical features. Rather, *how* those physical features and design are mobilized, utilized, and managed may enhance or diminish the potential effects of the shape and physical features of a nursing unit.

12. Hospital costs are less in the operation of a circular unit of the size studied than for an angular unit. It is likely that larger sized nursing units (i.e. more bed capacity) of an angular shape could be operated as cheaply as the radial unit by expanding the capacity of beds per nursing staff member, but the effects on quality of nursing care would need to be investigated before the cost-advantages would supersede quality of patient care. Certainly for the 22-bed units studied, the quality of patient care in the circle generally equaled, if not surpassed, that in the angular unit, at less cost per bed under normal operating conditions.

Thus our study replicated many of the findings of the Rochester studies, but qualification of other results was also indicated. Freeing nurses from the demands of other duties does not necessarily lead to more time spent with patients. On the other hand, caring for patients in units of different designs raises some questions about what is regarded as "care." We noticed considerable "nonverbal" communication between patients and nurses in the radial unit, such as waving, smiling at each other from the nurses' station and the patient rooms, which may be regarded as "care" in a different sense from that of conversing with patients at the bedside by the nursing staff.

We also observed that a strong bond quickly developed between patients and nurses, more so in the radial than in the angular unit, since the patients could readily observe when nurses were busy, concerned, fatigued, or relaxed, and could better appreciate the work of nurses than when unable to see such activity in the angular unit. Patients in the circular unit could identify the different status symbols of the nursing staff, such as the caps and uniforms of RNs, LPNs, and NAs, which were related to their activities on the unit, but which could not be done by patients on the angular unit.

It should be also noted that high visual contact seemed more significant in staff-patient relations, and in the care of patients, on the radial unit than any increased physical efficiency from reduced travel time for the nursing staff giving such care. Such visibility provided by the radial unit's shape allowed the nursing staff more options in attending patients than when such visibility was lacking in the angular unit. In the circular units we found less verbal communication with patients by nursing staff (who can easily observe patients from the nurses' station) and more time in standby. This permits the staff more choices in the performance of their roles on the unit, if the nurse so chooses to utilize her time in a particular way.[3]

In short, our study confirmed a connection between physical design and patient care, and between unit design and the activities and responses of nursing staff, medical staff, and patients. But the results also indicated that the relationship was not of a mechanical, one-to-one nature vis-à-vis physical setting or shape. Rather, it appears that the physical setting may provide, on the positive side, certain alternatives or flexible options to human behavior, and negatively certain obstacles or hindrances to such activity within certain ranges or limits. We believe, for instance, that the radial unit provides more *potential* flexibility in nurse staffing patterns to care for the same level and number of patients than does the angular shaped unit. The high visual contact in the radial unit allows the nurse to elect many more options in giving patient care than do units whose shape curtails or prevents such visibility.

But high visibility may have certain disadvantages in reducing personal privacy for patients in their rooms, which may eliminate the advantage of vistual contact. And the more sensitive nursing staff member may dislike the "on-stage" effect of being constantly watched by patients from their rooms. Consequently, hospital physical design can affect nursing staff and patient behavior for better or for worse. We do not yet know enough about the connection between hospital settings and staff and patient behavior to predict precisely how and what the effects will be. But we can conclude from our study that hospital design at least partially affects staff behavior and patient conduct, and this seems to depend largely upon how such units, once designed physically, are utilized socially, psychologically, medically, and administratively. Physical design alone is insufficient to account for such outcomes.

Conclusions

We have presented some theoretical considerations of man's use of physical space, and dealt with the problem of the effects of different work settings on his behavior and responses. Several studies of the effects of physical design or ecology of the hospital upon staff and patients were reported. These suggest that the hospital spatial environment has some impact upon staff behavior and attitudes and patient care. Despite the elaborate studies described, however, it is our assessment that only a small beginning has been made toward the development of secure knowledge about the intricate and complex relationships between physical design and hospital care. The need to conduct a vast array of research on this topic is still very great.

The following are some suggested areas in need of research attention:
   1. It seems important that we introduce more theoretical and conceptu-

---

3. It should be pointed out also that high visual contact between patients and staff can be provided by physical designs other than radial. A square unit, or one octagonal, spherical, and so on, can also provide high visibility so long as the nurses' station and the patient rooms are visible to each other in the unit layout.

al aspects of human ecology, "ecological psychology," and "proxemics" into research on hospital physical design, so that more systematic and fruitful approaches may be developed and help guide such research. Osmond's concepts of "sociopetal" and "sociofugal" arrangements of the physical environment, for example, hold much promise in further conceptualizing spatial arrangements which pull people together or keep them apart. The radial-designed nursing unit would be an example of the "sociopetal" arrangement while the single-corridor angular shaped unit would exemplify the "sociofugal" arrangement, the former tending to bring individuals more together and the latter separating them. The concepts of "personal space" and "territory" also have much potential for use in future studies.

2. The factor of arrangement of spaces and furnishings may be of equal, or even greater, significance to the activities and organizational relationships of persons using such items as the physical layout or shape of patient units. For instance, arranging hospital beds so that patients can face each other might enhance interaction and communication between patients in double rooms and wards should this be desired. Locating such functional areas as the utility room, supply and storage area, and nurses' conference room adjacent to the patient bedrooms could well affect staff use of the unit differently than when these are placed off the unit or in areas away from patient rooms. Location of the nurses' station within the unit is a critical matter in traditional hospital physical design, although there is some question about the universal utility, or even need, for such a space in tomorrow's hospital. The arrangement of different room accommodations within the unit may also affect how such rooms are utilized by patients and staff.

3. Progressive patient care programs whereby different physical spaces in the hospital are set up for different levels of patient care, ranging from intensive to minimal levels, need to be more thoroughly examined for corresponding variances in spatial design as well as unit arrangement. The unexpected finding that the radial unit in our study provided more positive aspects of patient care than the single-corridor angular unit for minimal or self-care patients suggests that the physical setting is as important for this level of care as for the more seriously ill categories.

4. As the more modern and larger short-term hospitals develop more segregated spaces for specialized categories of patient care, the need to study optimum kinds of spatial arrangements and settings for these services becomes increasingly important. Our study hospital also had radial units for obstetrical patients and an adjacent nursery for the newborn infants which permitted considerable visual contact between mothers and their babies while occupying these separate spaces. Our impression is that this helped to sustain a high morale for the new mothers who could observe their babies in their cribs while lying in their own beds. Possibly other spatial arrangements are indicated for other categories of patients, such as pediatric, orthopedic, cardiac, and psychiatric.

Other functional uses of hospital space may also need reexamination for such functions as those related to pathology, the laboratories, radiologic services, postoperative and recovery rooms, surgical suites, and examining rooms. In particular, the emergency room and out-patient department of short-term hospitals require reevaluation of their spatial arrangments and settings. Similarly, spaces for the service functions, such as hospital laundry, kitchen, power plant, maintenance and repair, and storage can stand hard scrutiny as to efficient layout, arrangement, and location within the total hospital environment. Even the physical layout and location of administrative offices, physician lounges, meeting rooms, and visitor lounges may need examination. Any physical space utilized by people needs study as to its optimum provisions for human use.

5. People tend to develop an identification with various components of space and the physical environment in which they work, live, and play. Anyone familiar with hospital life is aware of the strong identification that nursing staff members, for example, soon acquire for their stations, regarding their units as "homes," as we have heard it expressed by nursing personnel. How this identification develops and what elements enter into the acquisition of such "territory" by hospital staff needs further study. Such identification is perhaps a major reason why nurses dislike "floating" between different nursing units or dislike shifting their assigned areas within units, even though such resistance may be rationalized, e.g. by claims that floating prevents continuity of patient care by the nurses.

6. While our discussion has focused almost entirely on short-term or acute care facilities, there is an even greater need to study spatial design and arrangements appropriate to extended care facilities and services for the chronically ill and convalescing categories of patients. When patients are hospitalized for long periods of time in the same facility or the unit, the physical environment becomes even more important to their overall care than it is for the patient hospitalized for the typical eight or nine days in today's acute general hosptial. The need to cope with "hospitalitis" and other pathologic effects of institutionalization is well known, but the specific effects of physical design, arrangement, and furnishings are still largely unknown for the long-term patient populations. What may be an appropriate or optimum environment for the acutely ill short-term patient, of course, may not be optimal for the chronically ill long-term patient.

There is no longer any need to inquire "if" there is any relationship between the hospital physical environment and the activities and functioning of personnel and patients. Rather, the question is *how specifically* certain aspects of the physical setting, its composition, geometry, arrangement, layout, furnishings, and decor affect behavior and the responses of individuals interacting in such spaces. Furthermore, the impact of the physical environment on groups, organizational behavior, and social structures of the health care facility is perhaps an even greater area for significant research than is the impact on individual behavior.

The need to improve the methodology of future ecological studies of hospitals is definitely indicated. Many previous studies have relied heavily on impressions, observations, and logical inferences. Others, particularly "efficiency" studies, have used highly quantitative data and mathematical models but have lacked comprehension of the "human" element. Some have used work-sampling methods, which usually generate more gross kinds of measurements that lack a desired degree of precision. There is also a question about the reliability and validity of such measures of the true parameters of staff and patient behavior in the hospital. To some extent, these shortcomings are related to the overall embryonic scientific development of the ecological and social sciences. Nevertheless, the need for so-called pure or basic methodological studies to devise more and better measurements and research instruments is evident, and should stimulate important research activity in this area.

Finally, we do not wish to exaggerate the relative importance of the physical environment in hospital organizational research. While the physical setting and its arrangements are indeed significant, and have been a neglected realm of hospital research, they are only one among many aspects and dimensions of health care facilities and systems related to the organization, structure, role, and functioning of such facilities and services. When our knowledge of the full effects of the physical environment on hospital care becomes better and more explicitly developed, then we shall be in a strategic position to evaluate how significant and important the physical setting is in relation to other factors involving hospital organization and functioning. It is likely that physical space and its arrangements may have more impact on some aspects of hospital care than on others, in a manner and degree similar to other factors of hospital organization and behavior. The need to conduct research into every phase of hospital operation is immense. We strongly suggest that the phase of physical design and ecology should be included in any sophisticated research program of hospitals and related health care facilities and services.

References

Aydelotte, M. K., *et al. An investigation of the relation between nursing activity and patient welfare.* Iowa City: State University of Iowa, 1960.

Barker, R. G. *Ecological psychology concepts and methods for studying the environment of human behavior.* Stanford: Stanford University Press, 1968.

Brunswik, E. The conceptual framework of psychology. *International Encyclopedia of Unified Science* (Vol. 1, Pt. 2, 656, 750). Chicago: University of Chicago Press.

Coser, R. L. Authority and decision-making in a hospital. *American Sociological Review*, 1958, *23*, 56-63.

Duncan, O. D., and Schnore, L. Cultural behavioral, and ecological perspectives in the study of social organization. *American Journal of Sociology*, 1959, *65*, 132-146.

Freeman, J. R. Quantitative criteria for hospital inpatient unit design. Doctoral dissertation, School of Industrial Engineering. Georgia Institute of Technology, 1967.

Freidson, E. Client control and medical practice. *American Journal of Sociology*, 1960, *65*, 364-382.

Hall, E. T. Proxemics. *Current Anthropology*, 1968, *9*, 83-108.

Hall, E. T. Proxemics: the study of man's spatial relations. In I. Galdston (Ed.) *Man's image in medicine and anthropology.* New York: International Universities Press, 1963 (a).

Hall, E. T. Quality in architecture: an anthropological view. *Journal of the American Institute of Architects*, 1963 (b), *40*, 44-48.

Hawley, A. H. *Human Ecology.* New York: Ronald, 1950.

Jaco, E. G. *Hospital design and patient care.* Syracuse: Systems Educators, 1970.

Jaco, E. G. Final report on research project titled: Evaluation of nursing and patient care in a circular and rectangular hospital unit (dittoed, available from author).

Lewin, K. *Field theory in social science.* New York: Harper, 1951.

Lippert, S. Travel as a function of nursing unit layout. Tufts University, Human Engineering Information and Analysis Service Report No. 113, and Tufts-New England Medical Center Planning Office Report No. 1, March 12, 1969.

McLaughlin, H. P. Are circular units overrated? *Modern Hospital,* 1961, *96,* 81-87.

McLaughlin, H. P. What shape is best for nursing units? *Modern Hospital,* 1964, *103,* 84-89.

Mintz, N. L. Effects of esthetic surroundings, part II: Prolonged and repeated experience in a "beautiful" and an "ugly" room. *Journal of Psychology,* 1956, *41,* 459-466.

Osmond, H. Function as the basis of psychiatric ward design. *Mental Hospitals,* 1957, *8,* No. 4, 23-29.

Osmond, H. The historical and sociological: The relationship between architect and psychiatrist, and Development of mental hospitals. In C. Goshen (Ed.) *Psychiatric architecture.* Washington: American Psychiatric Association, 1959.

Pace, R. E. Situational therapy. *Journal of Personality,* 1957, *25,* 578-588.

Pelletier, R. J., and Thompson, J. D. Yale index measures design efficiency. *Modern Hospital,* 1960, *95,* 73-77.

Quinn, J. A. *Human ecology.* Englewood Cliffs, N.J.: Prentice-Hall, 1950.

Robinson, W. S. Ecological correlations and the behavior of individuals. *American Sociological Review,* 1950, *15,* 351-357.

Rosengren, W. R., and DeVault, S. The sociology of time and space in an obstetrical hospital. In E. Freidson (Ed.) *The hospital in modern society.* New York: The Free Press, 1963.

Simmel, G. Social interaction as the definition of the group in time and space (translated from Georg Simmel, *Soziologie,* by Albion W. Small). In R. E. Park and E. W. Burgess (Eds.) *Introduction to the science of sociology.* Chicago: University of Chicago Press, 1921.

Sommer, R. Studies in personal space. *Sociometry,* 1959, *22,* 247-260.

Sommer, R. Man's proximate environment. *Journal of Social Issues,* 1966, *22,* 59-70.

Sommer, R. Classroom ecology. *Journal of Applied Behavioral Science,* 1967 (a), *3,* 489-503.

Sommer, R. Sociofugal space. *American Journal of Sociology,* 1967 (b), *72,* 654-660.

Sommer, R., and Dewar, R. The physical environment of the ward. In E. Freidson (Ed.) *The hospital in modern society.* New York: Free Press, 1963.

Sommer, R., and Ross, H. Social interaction on a geriatric ward. *International Journal of Social Psychiatry,* 1958, *4,* 128-133.

Sorokin, P. A. *Sociocultural causality, space, time.* Durham: Duke University Press, 1943.

Sturdavant, M. Intensive nursing service in circular and rectangular units compared. *Hospitals,* 1960, *34,* No. 14, 46-48.

Sturdavant, M., et al. *Comparisons of intensive nursing service in a ciruclar and a rectangular unit.* Chicago: American Hospital Association, Hospital Monograph Series No. 8, 1960.

Thompson, J. D. Patients like these four-bed wards. *Modern Hospital,* 1955, *85,* 84-86.

Trites, D. K., Galbraith, F. D., Jr., Sturdavant, M., and Leckwart, J. F. Final report of research project titled: *Influence of nursing unit design on the activities and subjective feelings of nursing personnel.* Rochester, Minnesota, Research Office, Rochester Methodist Hospital, 1969 (a).

Trites, D. K., Galbraith, F. D., Jr., Sturdavant, M., and Leckward, J. F. Radial nursing units prove best in controlled study. *Modern Hospital,* 1969 (b), *109,* 94-99.

Wheeler, E. T. *Hospital design and function.* New York: McGraw-Hill, 1964.

Wilson, R. N. Teamwork in the operating room. *Human Organization,* 1954, *12,* 9-14.

11

ISSUES AND DISCUSSION OF PART FOUR

Hospital Organization and Patient-Centered Goals

Presentation Highlights: R. Straus

In this paper I have tried to present a kind of synthesis of personal thinking, and of the thinking of others, over a long period of time. I suppose I could identify some of the influences. These would include my being trained in a department of sociology which insisted that its majors have some work in biology, and also the chance and good fortune of exposure to B. Malinowski in the last year of his life, when I was an undergraduate. As I try to analyze the way I think, I believe this was indirectly a considerable influence.

I also have tried to look at the whole issue of studying hospital organization from the point of view of the broader problem of the gap today between the potentialities of medical science and our capacity for delivering medical care, seeing the hospital as playing one part in this total open system. I think there are some consistencies here with some of the other papers. The question of goals, for example, is particularly germane for transition into this paper because I am, in essence, pleading a case for looking at the hospital in terms of what we call patient-centered goals. I am suggesting at least that in the more rigorous research that has gone on involving hospitals, we have not really looked at this as much as we need to.

If we focus on the patient it is worth realizing that there is this historical thread of incarceration associated with the hospitalization of patients. The role that many kinds of hospitals have played in the history of mankind, that of protecting society from people who were in hospitals, has had a significant carryover to the modern scene, where we are, indeed, trying to do something for patients in addition to protecting society from them. The role into which hospital patients are forced, involving institutional dependency and a whole variety of other social experiences which have been commented on liberally in the literature, has significance in terms of these historical threads. I do not think that the concept of confinement is irrelevant. The fact that many kinds of hospitals until recently were constructed outside of communities rather than inside of communities is not insignificant. In other words, patients historically were prisoners and I think that patients today still have to assume a certain aspect of this role.

Another factor that I think is terribly important in looking at the hospital, and this ties in with the concept of sanctions that has already been mentioned, is the very weak position of the patient as a sanctioning agent. This is partly due to the role that I have mentioned and partly to the patient's transiency in a general hospital. The patient has very little purse around which to localize sanction. The individual doctor's position, if he looks to his position as a primary advocate for the patient, is also somewhat of a tangent in many of our hospitals. Depending on his place in the parastructure of the hospital, the physician may have very little force as an advocate for his patient. He himelf is in and out of the hospital a great deal.

Now, I chose to make a comparison between a hospital and a factory, in part to emphasize certain points. I think that it is important to realize that factories have certain forces that enforce efficiency and the necessity to show a profit which over time have made them responsive to change in ways which hospitals have not experienced. I chose to use an example in the paper of some experiments in a particular factory which tried to enable its workers to identify with the end product. I think there is a good deal of material in organizational research on factories around the relationship between the degree to which a worker can identify with the product and certain aspects of his productivity. (*Question:* Do you mean job enlargement? *Answer:* Yes.)

In this particular instance I think it is interesting that they experimented with a whole range of alternatives, including one man producing one typewriter, which incidently showed up extraordinarily favorably in terms of quality and quantity in production. But they had to throw this pattern out, largely on engineering grounds. Simply, they could not find a way to deliver all the components to the worker. Eventually, they did adopt a pattern in which workers produce identifiable products and they have tied this, with their computers, to immediate feedback on quality evaluation, so that not only does the worker produce something that he can identify, but within minutes he has a report back on how good it was. They have also tied the sanction and reward system to the worker's ability to do well at a particular level of complexity of the unit that he is producing, and to promotion to something a little more complex. But in doing this they have found it effective to eliminate most of the usual controls of the behavior of the individual. For example, a worker can stop at any time he wants to and have coffee, have a smoke, visit with other people. There is almost no policing of people in the factory.

It is ironic that in industry there is this movement to humanize the product and, even on production lines, to vary workers' activity a little bit in order to try and get some identification. At the same time, it seems to me, the trend in hospitals over a long period of time has been to dehumanize and subvert the individuality of the patient. Instead, the hospitals have tried to maximize the ability of the worker to treat the patient as a diseased entity rather than as a unique human being.

The second major point that I have discussed in the paper is the importance to understanding human behavior of a concept, or an approach, that assumes and incorporates the recognition of a fundamental relationship among the different characteristics of the organism—its structure, function, chemistry, genetic characteristics, etc. An approach is needed to integrate the patient's personality, physical environment, social elements (meaning essentially man's roles in various social systems), normative behavior and material aspects of his culture, and what I call the temproal element. As we look at this in relation to the hospital, I think we have to recognize that most patients are suffering from some disbalance in some of their basic body systems. We tend to recognize this almost excluseively, however, without keeping in mind the impact of this disbalance on the various other systems and experiences of the patient or on the process of trying to achieve a rebalance.

Under relevant psychological components, for example, we can identify a large number of aspects of the experience of being a patient which inflict psychological stress, which are deleterious to the patient's well-being, and which can very clearly negate certain benefits of his organic treatment. These are particularly evident in many of the diseases for which physical rest is deemed important, and they are measurable. Despite our clear evidence of the relationship between anxiety, or psychological stress, and the ability to actually experience physical stress, however, we put emphasis on the body and on resting the body, even to imposing rest which induces isolation from social activity—a condition which, for many patients, can lead to anxiety.

Concerning the environment which Dr. Jaco's paper deals with in considerable length, we have only begun to scratch the surface. Recognizing the enormous number of factors associated both with the external milieu in which the hospital is set and the internal design (lighting, ventilation, furnishing, colos, sounds, smells), and all those things that impose on the basic senses of the human beings, there is much research that can be done in this area and measured in terms of the physiological and psychological responses of individuals. Such simple frustrations as the inability of individuals to control the temperature of their room, the irregularity of noises imposed upon the patient, the inability of the patient to have any control over the door and who comes in and when, and generally the inability of the patient to control the social environment are all factors which can have an enormous bearing on the patient's ability to maximize medical benefits, including treatment of the organic problem.

In the area of the social components of behavior, and here there is quite a bit of literature, again the hospital does not really give a great deal of attention to such things as sex. They may give attention to sex in terms of separation of sexes but not in terms of other considerations that may be very important to people who spend any considerable time in hospitals. For example, normal heterosexual activity when not medically contraindicated is not considered. This, again, is part of the prison concept that carries over to hospitals. The same may be said about age. Beyond pediatrics and adult care, we give very little attention to groupings of patients, or social intercourse, according to age.

In the area of biological and intellectual attributes, again there are problems. We look at biological attributes primarily in terms of the system involved, not in terms of such things as the biological timetable of the human being and what we do to this biological timetable when we impose, for example, three meals a day concentrated within an eight-hour shift. Similarly, the biological intrusions on elimination systems and a whole number of other factors are not taken into account. We are afraid really, in hospitals, of recognizing who this individual is in terms of the roles that he plays in the outside society. We try to reduce him to some common denominator. This phenomenon of stripping, which Parsons may have been one of the early people to discuss and which others have described, is really a stripping of roles, of social identity. We do not take into account the social roles that an individual must be prepared to reassume when he leaves hospitalization. We have very little in patients' hospital experience preparing them for a transition back into their family, job and community roles.

I am also concerned with cultural norms and the concept of culture shock. The capacity of any individual to experience culture shock is going to be less when he is seriously sick or injured, in pain, or in great anxiety. At the same time that a patient is experiencing this shock he is deprived of the support of relatives or friends and thrust into a total alien social setting. We expect people to make this adaptation at the same time that they are weak or in pain.

With respect to temporal factors, I mentioned basic body functions in relation to the biological timetables of people. We also have to consider, and do not in medicine, the general time orientation that people have with respect to the meaning of time in relation to medications—something that is totally overlooked in hospitals. We give people instructions and medications according to time, but without finding out what this means to them. In the whole area of preventive medicine, we do not try to find whether future orientation means anything, if we are thinking in terms of the future at all. The past, present, and future orientation of patients can have an enormous impact on how they experience hospitalization and how the activities of the hospital impinge upon them.

In the section on the experience of being a patient, I am suggesting that good medical care from the narrow point of view is not always good patient care, if I could use this kind of dichotomy. Many of the requirements of the hospital, and of its medical, nursing, and administrative subsystems, pose demands on the patient which are contraindicated by the requirements of his care or are in conflict with his total health and well being. We need to look at the patient as a human being with a life style, with entrenched habits, with prior experiences, and with certain expectations which he brings to the hospital. We do not ask patients what they expect when they come in.

We must also look at the illness of the patient. Illness itself is a factor which is associated with a good deal of human discrimination. Responses of others to the patient, for example, vary widely depending on whether his illness is perceived as life-threatening, painful, severe, disfiguring, disabling, or whether it is seen as transitory, mild, and subject to total cure. We need to do a great deal of research in this area of the responses of human beings to pain and suffering or crises in other people. There are some beginnings now in the social-psychological literature at the laboratory level of how people respond to pain and suffering of others. In part, I think, the nature of the response depends upon whether people perceive patients as innocent victims or as contributing to their disease, and whether they consider them as nonthreatening to others or as a threat to the well-being of others. These things need to be studied, and the product of this research should become part of the in-service training and education of hospital personnel.

The external culture of the hospital—the characteristics of the environment in which it lives and the society in which it serves—can greatly affect the impact of the hospital on a patient. Who are the employees, where do they come from, and what are their values and attitudes? In a little project, for example, we found a great deal of discrimination going on in a hospital on the part of the nonskilled employees toward patients whom they perceived to be "uppity." These patients were innocent victims. I think they were perceived to be uppity not on the basis of their behavior, but on the basis of a few labels that happened to slip in with them. There are also a few references to discrimination on the part of hospital people toward patients who are perceived to be of a lower class. There are a lot of other kinds of biases and prejudices operating within a hospital. This is part of the internal culture of the hospital.

There are two or three other items that I want to mention. One is the communication process. This is both understudied and underrecognized in hospitals, and I am not just talking about communication with and about patients, but communication between members of the medical team as well. The traditional medical chart has become almost completely, I think, obsolete in its ability to deal with the kinds of information that are germane to modern medical care. One of the great problems that we have in hospitals today is the fact that patients come in and are expected to behave appropriately with very little communication as to how they should behave. They are classified and responded to in terms of how they have been able to anticipate what the staff may consider as appropriate behavior—depending, in other words, on whether they are seen as "good" or "bad" patients. The majority of the patients coming into the hospital have no idea what to expect from their hospitalization, and some have perceptions of their own problems which are quite different from those of the hospital staff—and whichever is right does not really matter. The important thing is that such a situation suggests severe problems in communication and misinterpretation of the patient's behavior.

We also need to study the imposition of hospital routine on patients, again in terms of the conflict between the goals of medical care and the goals of patient care or of nursing care or of administration. For example, I referred to the matter of rest. Hospitals are very difficult places for people to relax and really get rest, short of sedation. Patients must try to sleep in close proximity with other people whose personal habits and periods of wakefulness and sleep, desires for entertainment, requirements for medical attention, etc., vary from their own. Patients report great difficulty in getting uninterrupted sleep, for a variety of reasons such as these.

Patients become lost in the organization of the hospital, in which, more and more, we tend to fragment attention to the patient. When you try to identify the people whom patients remember, this usually comes down to rather extraordinary anecdotal type of situations. A related issue is that of the dependency status which is imposed on patients, and which often forces them to become needlessly dependent upon the institution. And here I think we must recognize different points of view. There certainly is a strong argument from some medical sources that in order to make the patient receptive to appropriate medical intervention, a kind of dependency imposition is therapeutically necessary. To a certain extent perhaps this is true. For convenience and for historical reasons, however, we continue to impose on patients all sorts of unnecessary dependency criteria in the areas of food, clothing, expression of initiative, and ability to engage in discussion on their own problems. This whole idea that patients have no business knowing anything about their medication, for example, is not only a carryover from the prisoner ideology, but it is also a cause of poor communication. We are beginning to get some idea about the enormous gaps which exist, say, between what a physician is telling a patient, what he may actually convey, what a patient may hear, what he can repeat five minutes or an hour later, and what he does to realize that this is an area where communication is extraordinarily important.

I conclude the paper with some comments on inquiry and experimentation. I first cite that hospitals are quite reluctant to be studied, particularly in this area of the impact of the hospital process on patients. One of the rationales I have heard frequently in this regard is that we must not do anything that will impose on the patient's privacy, dignity, or medical care. I think this is interesting, and I have good friends who represent quite the opposite of this philosophy. But they too will recognize that we have mutual colleagues who were successful over long periods of time in imposing barriers to effective research and to the development of effective research strategy with regard to patient care. It would be very helpful in this regard, going back to Malinowski and the very simple concept of functions, to identify clearly the various needs and expectations of people, or the purposes of the behavior of the participants. We should try to identify the behavior of all involved in terms of the interaction of people in their varied roles in the hospital, and see how these relate to the end result of the system.

I also believe that in our research we must go beyond the area of careful, insightful, but rather idiosyncratic observation, such as represented by Taylor or Lucille Brown for example. Through rigorous observation and measurement of the detailed experience of being a patient, one could come up with extremely useful insights. This could be approached in two ways: through the active participation of patients, and through maintaining careful records. I do not think this is necessarily therapeutically contraindicated, and in fact for many patients it could be quite useful therapeutically. I think we can, without violating patient rights, introduce both human observers who are physically present and devices such as electronic monitoring devices. We are doing this in relation to specific diseases now, for example monitoring patients' heart function and other kinds of physiological fundtions. This can be done in such ways that patients will accept and be relaxed with (the most useful device we have for letting patients be comfortable is to create enough consciousness of the situation so that they put us at ease). The principle here is that this kind of research does not necessarily involve imposition on patient rights, it is not necessarily therapeutically contraindicated, and it is the kind of research we really need to begin to develop if we are going to study patient care.

Second, we need some strategies of experimental design. Here again it is ironic that although we have long used experimental design in studies of drug efficacy, we have structured it so narrowly that we often do not really know what the patients are taking, how they are taking it, or whether they are taking it with other drugs, but at least we do introduce a concept of experimental design. I think we can introduce experimental design in hospital research now, and I particularly would like to see it introduced in the area of the structure of patient care. I would like to see us experiment, just as they did in the factory I mention, with various kinds of alternatives. I would like to see us take a unit of work and experiment with how a few people can do more things for a smaller number of patients, and introduce some hypotheses to be tested with measurements of the physiological, psychological, and social experiences of patients, and even measurements in terms of the patient's ability to readapt to society after leaving the hospital. We can also measure patient care in terms of the impact on the people who are performing care functions themselves.

Finally, another point I would like to introduce concerns the concept of patient advocate as something that can be studied in experimental design. I have become convinced that this patient advocate role exists in hospitals all the time. In almost any hospital there are some physicians who have found that the way to take good care of their patients is to find somebody—maybe a nurse, maybe a social worker, it may be a secretary—to see that the needs of their patients are implemented through the system. And I know of one group of physicians, a large group with a very influential clientele, who have really put this on a very formal basis in the hospital. I am suggesting, perhaps, that we need to structure the experience of the patient around a person. This can be a person, perhaps without a great deal of technical training, whose main job would be to prepare and help the patient for entering the hospital and receiving good care while there. In other words, I see this role picking up not when the patient reports but before, and following the patient out of the hospital. This would be the person who looks to communication (this person would not necessarily do all the interpretation) and makes sure that necessary things are interpreted to the patients. This person would find out where the stress was being experienced by the patient and do something about it. I am thinking here of such things in the system as the problems of long wait, of anonymity, and of situations in which nobody knows where a particular patient is at a particular time. The patient advocate would know where his or her patient was at any particular time.

Discussion

Comment: Your analogy of factory to hospital is very interesting, at least from the point of view of lack of patient control. I think you implied this when you pointed out that the patient cannot even control the opening and shutting of the door. Incidentally, years ago, Charles Walker and I (Dr. Guest speaking) wrote a book called *Man on the Assembly Line,* and our general conclusion was that assembly-line workers are incarcerated if anybody was incarcerated. But then management came along and started to attempt to humanize the work. One of the things that I tend to regret has to do with "job enlargement"—again Walker and I coined the original phrase in 1947, based upon our observations of what happened when a company tried to have a woman do her own setups, produce, inspect, and so on. The concept caught on, articles went out, and it was popularized. Then we started to get a stream of letters back: this "job-enlargement stuff is for the birds, says management." Why? We went to the workers, and we said: "We are going to enlarge your job, we are going to make it bigger and better." And, of course, the reaction of the workers was, "The hell you are, you are going to pay me more if you are."

The fundamental fault was the notion that "Daddy knows best, and we are going to make you workers happy down there." As we reflect on your very insightful comments on the hospital, we should watch out about the "Daddy knows best for the patients" phenomenon. I think the patient ought to be given more control. I am not an expert in this field, I am more in the factory field, but there is something very central to what you said. All I am saying is that we avoid the errors that have been made in industry when we go the direction you suggest. I think you suggest a sort of ombudsman. But it is more than that; it is more than just reporting problems. Still I believe we can get the patient to initiate change and do things, as well as make sure that we take care of these things.

Comment: I would like to make one comment related to this. Last year we looked at certain management innovations, incentive programs for upgrading productivity among hospital employees, and similar industrial engineering developments. We went to one hospital, a nice rural 500-bed hospital in the Western part of the country, where they were rewarding nurses with a cash bonus. If they could keep the census of their unit up and the costs of supplying and operating it down, they would get something in the neighborhood of a maximum of $50 a month each. And this was not working. It seems to me that the traditional models of input-output, and of productivity, incentive, and rewards, do not apply whatsoever to the hospital world. There are a number of reasons, mostly social-psychological and partly economic. First of all, in the hospital you have professionalism. The professionalism of the nursing staff, the medical staff, and the administrative staff goes counter to cash bonus incentives for performance. The value system of the professional is not compatible with the value system of the production assembly-line worker in private industry. You are dealing with an entirely different world of values in the hospital, those of a nonprofit system. Basically, the hospital is a nonprofit institution; it is not geared up to making a profit. Even proprietary hospitals in California, which are geared to make a profit, just do not make one.

In short, the worlds of factories and hospitals are separate worlds, so that

"What is good for General Motors is not good for General Hospital." The models of performance and the incentive and reward patterns of industry are not transferable to the hospital. It is interesting that this was confirmed, I think, by the fact that bonus systems were effective only in those components of the hospital organization that most resembled the assembly line, e.g. the laundry and the kitchen in the food service area—those unionized components which resembled the industrial work situation. Although we have not yet said much about unionization and hospital organization, this is a very important factor. Unionization of janitors, floor maids, laundry workers, etc., is now coming into the picture, particularly among the nonprofessional staff. But when you get into the patient care spheres of the hospital, the analogy breaks down.

This is why I have never run across some more frustrated industrial engineers in my life than those in hospitals. They were frustrated because they were not doing what they thought they could expect to do, and they could not understand why. Primarily, the reason was that the organization, the values of the participants, and the motivational systems encountered in a service organization are not the same as those encountered in organizations producing a tangible product. Patient care is a complicated service, not a product like a typewriter, an automobile, or a refrigerator.

Question: But you do agree with the basic thesis, do you not, of the necessity of the patient being more involved in his own care and having an influence or more control over his immediate environment, which is parallel to what we find for workers?

Answer: I know some hospitals now, particularly under the influence of planning and funding agencies, which make allowances for the role of the consumer, and which are a little sensitive to thinking that they can learn some things from patients.

Comment: My experience in that regard suggests that this usually is approached very naively. In the first place, patients in hospitals are dependent upon the system, and I think there is pretty clear evidence that we have not yet identified, or used, very sophisticated ways of measuring patient satisfaction. Having Gray Ladies, for example, ask patients whether they like things at the very time that the patient feels terribly constrained, terribly dependent, and quite concerned about offending this system does not provide a solution to the problem. We need more innovative strategies to get at this point, which is rather complex. A study was done in which the same questions were asked of a group of patients while they were still in the hospital, just prior to discharge, and then after discharge, and this satisfaction/dissatisfaction dimension turned something like 30 percent vs. 70 percent upsidedown. Once the patients were free of the system, they were willing to express criticism which they would not express even up to the point of their getting out of that place.

Comment: That is right; I am just oversimplifying it. In our study we used just plain social workers, and our biggest obstacle to overcome was this inhibition to offend, or report complaints, on the part of patients. There is no question about that. But the skilled interviewer can probe into that, and finally get them to speak up. I was being more symbolic. In fact the administration in the hospital we studied was shocked about some things that they did not know were going on until the patients and our research fed it back to them. Patients can be a gold mine of information about what goes on in the whole hospital facility.

Comment: This also has methodological implications. In a study we did, we tried to use different methodologies to get at patient views, and in one case we had an overlapping group where some of the patients were subjected to two methodologies. We used interviewing, and with very extensive two-hour interviews it was possible to penetrate to a real representation what it is like to be a patient. But even the same patient, when given a questionnaire, came through with what we finally called "the good patient role." The normative present, where you have to respond in terms of maintenance of a complete dependency role, which would pose a risk to the respondent, affects the reactions of patients very significantly. Incidentally, in another study in an intensive cardiac care unit we used galvanic skin response measures, much to the dismay of the cardiologist. The highest deviation on the galvanic skin response of patients occurred whenever the physician came onto the unit. The nurse was next, in this respect, followed by a couple of my people who were interviewing, and then was the family. The least deviation occurred with maintenance personnel. This is one kind of research that we need to work on in this area.

Comment: I very much agree with you that we need to move in the direction of greater control by the patient, the consumer of the process. The question of "what is the whole business for" is very important. But I think when we measure satisfaction, or patient participation, we often miss the key points. One of these is whether the patient got from the hospital what he came there to get. I have conducted some of my own studies in this area, and there are a lot of patient expectations of the physician as well as of the hospital. Satisfaction with the food and the like are of some importance, but they are one small segment of what the patient came there for. As I talked to people over a period of years, I found that patient dissatisfaction relates to some of those sacred areas which people say cannot be invaded, but I think they must and can be. Mainly, it relates to such feelings by the patient as "I do not really feel that I got competent care; I do not really feel that they understood me, and no one enabled me to understand."

This goes back to a series of very simple questions that enter the patient's mind when he makes contact with a medical care outpost, whether it is a doctor, a nurse, or whatever: "What is wrong with me? How did I get that way? How serious is it? Is it going to mean disability or my death? Will I have to change my way of life? Can you do something about it? Is it painful to do something about it? What is it going to cost in dollars, time, and so on? Can you prevent it?" These kinds of simple questions go unanswered. Often you hear people say, over and over again, "But I came for a headache and they did everything else except help that." Those who are designing interviews should try to put these questions in terms of patient expectations.

Comment: I might say, to support your point, that if you look over the long list of job satisfaction studies you will find most of them to be pretty superficial. More recently, you do not see many journal articles on job satisfaction.

Comment (Dr. Pellegrino): May I make one very brief point in support of another point made earlier that bears on this point too? The reward system in the hospital is different from that in industry. I attempted to get residents to report adverse drug reactions by paying them five dollars per incident reported. Now when I was a resident that was a lot of money, and it still is pretty good if you can pile them up, you know, because the number of drug incidents and adverse drug reactions on any floor is significant in dollars and in quality of care. And yet nothing happened. When I said to the pharmacy students, "You come in, you come on the floors, into this sacred relationship, and you tell us," it worked well. That was job enrichment for them, you see; it had meaning, and it gave them satisfaction. I think we need to take a different approach if we want to increase the involvement of these people. Much depends on the development of job satisfaction in the sense of having them doing something useful and something a little more sophisticated than they may be doing.

Comment: I have one anecdote which I think highlights an extremely crucial point. In our interviewing of patients we have felt that it is the relative world of the patient and the continuity of his expectations which make the difference for real satisfaction. One of the more dramatic incidents we encountered involved a young woman whom we interviewed and who, after the first few moments, broke into hysterical tears. What came out was that she was hospitalized at that time for a lump in her breast which was found to be benign, but also the root of her dissatisfaction. She was very dissatisfied because, as she was able to conceptualize most beautifully, "Everyone here defines me as lucky because they compare me with all the many cancer patients they know, and I consider I have gone through hell, which nobody understands. I compare myself with the millions of females who do not have to go through that."

Comment: I would like to make one comment on your paper, Dr. Straus. It seems like there is a little bit of sleight of hand in the argument as I understand it. First you compare the patients to typewriters, which is fine, but then you do not talk about the satisfactions of typewriters, you talk about the satisfactions of the workers who perform on the typewriters. Job enlargement has satisfaction for the people who do the work on the typewriters, not necessarily for the typewriter. They may or may not be satisified; it may be just one worker there. I think that there is no question that, for the patient, some of the problems and horrors of being in the hospital that you describe are real and could perhaps be solved in some of the ways you suggest. I am not at all sure that this, in turn, is going to in any sense increase the satisfaction of the people who work on patients. One of the important factors determining the division of labor in hospitals is that people define themselves out of work that they regard as inappropriate, work that they have no control over, or work that they do not want to get involved in. The financial problems of the patient may be another matter altogether, or they may be the social worker's job. But a lot of the dividing of work in the organization goes on for the convenience of the people who make those distinctions, and these are very often distinctions that they are quite happy to make.

Answer (Dr. Straus): I am sorry. I was not trying to emphasize this in terms of job satisfaction, only in terms of quantity and quality of production of typewriters. In other words, in making the analogy what I meant to stress was the end product. The quality and quantity of the end product was the factor I was looking at, just as I am looking at the patient as the end product of the hospital. The reorganization of the workers was not considered in terms of whether they were satisfied or not, but was considered in terms of how many typewriters they turned out and what was the quality rate on the typewriters. This, then, has the analogy to the suggestion of an experiment in which one would reallocate the functions of people who are concerned with patient care to see if there are some other models that are more effective than those in use, somewhere between one nurse or physician who does everything for a patient and sixty people who each do different things. Some model or models in between, depending on the different areas in which we are working, might be more effective in terms of both quality and quantity, and even cost, of the product of patient care.

Comment: My prediction would be that probably you would increase the quality of care but at the cost of, perhaps, lower staff satisfaction.

Answer: This would be something that would have to be measured.

Comment (Dean Christman): I would like to make a comment on this. We have a small grant to develop a model of patient care, on an experimental basis, in which we are attempting to do the very thing you suggest. It has been underway for about a year now. Because of funding limitations, we have only one experimental and one control unit. One of the things we are doing is to have one nurse, one physician, and one general health care worker for a group of patients. Instead of a nurse performing certain tasks and taking care of sixty patients, one nurse is caring for six patients, along with one general health care worker and the same physician. The three are working as a team. Even when the nurses go on the evening shift, they still carry the same patients; they do not change patients. The whole communication process and the whole delivery of care are showing phenomenal differences compared to the rest of the hospital.

Comment: It sounds kind of expensive though, is it not?

Answer: No, it is no more expensive. The staff ratio is pretty good, but it has nothing to do with staff relationships. Staff relations have to do with severity of illness, not with how many there are on a unit. We just happen to have a high severity of illness unit that we are testing this on. But theoretically the model is so built that it has all kinds of sliding scales as to how many patients can be managed by these kinds of arrangements. On a convelescent unit, for example, the ratio of staff to patients would drop substantially, so that if you take the entire hospital into account no more staff would be added. In fact we are predicting that there is a good possibility of eliminating all the nurse's aides entirely.

Comment: This is fascinating to me. To go back to an earlier comment on satisfaction, I think we have one doctoral dissertation which started out with the hope that we could actually measure job satisfaction in controlled situations, but then ran into trouble with controlling the situation. It ended up comparing satisfaction among a number of existing types of service, including the intensive care unit, which fortunately had some of the elements that we had wanted to test. We also used the operating room, and the recovery room versus a general floor. But out of this study, which was focusing strictly on job satisfaction, turnover, absenteeism, and a number of direct and indirect measures of job satisfaction, the man did come out with suggestions, at least, that those areas of the hospital where the nurse has a greater opportunity to identify with patients were the ones associated with higher job satisfaction.

Comment: I think one of the things that you have to control here is the medical interest of the patient. With small numbers of patients, there are a lot of useful things for the nurse to do.

Comment: I would like to support this at another level. A hospital in Minneapolis has experimented on getting the nurse back to nursing. They have a rule that if a nurse is caught in a nurses' station she is fired. She has no business in there. The nurses are doing patient management, they are interviewing all patients, and they are in charge of setting up procedures for the care of the patient. In other words, they are doing what they were trained to do, not what they had to do to make a better wage by moving into administrative functions for which they are not trained. We all know the problem—the nurses do not do nursing. In this hospital they tried to solve this by getting the nurses back to the bedside of the patient. The only place the nurse can sit down in that hospital is either in the patient's room or in the ladies room, but not in the station.

Interestingly, this hospital is the only hospital in the upper Midwest that has a waiting list of nurses. They do not pay the nurses more than other hospitals do, but the satisfaction level among the nurses is fantastic, and they have a waiting list. They have the lowest turnover rate of nursing staff in the whole upper Midwest, since they have installed this system which allows the nurses to do what they want to do and what they were initially motivated to do when they went into nursing.

Comment: This example, however, does not answer the problem of why was this not responded to as it was at the time of the Peter New and Gladys Nite study.

Answer: I can tell you why. It is because Peter New and Gladys Nite built no clinical leadership into the unit; they just added more workers. Adding more workers without changing any other variable amounts to zero output.

Comment: The case described does involve institutional process devices that avoid the problem of nurses saying "This is merely imposed from above without being generically rooted," and this raises a fundamental question which I think is similar to the question that you raised.

Comment (Dean Christman): In our experiment we involved people to some extent in generating the model. But with reference to nurse satisfaction, I think we have an interesting figure. The only turnover we have in our study unit is due either to the husband moving out of town or to pregnancy. We have no other turnover of any kind. So one almost assumes that there is a high degree of professional satisfaction.

Comment: Again, I think this goes back to the earlier issue of what is defined as medically interesting. One of the things which needs to be studied in this connection in the case of the Minneapolis hospital is whether, symbolically at least, this organizational change in locus of sitting down involves or is parallel to changes in the definition of what is interesting. There almost has to be a correlation between the two for the program to be effective.

Comment: I want to raise another point, if I may. It seems to me that the ombudsman, the patient follower, represents a very real alternative to the structural change that is being suggested here. In one case you are saying "fit the structure to what you want it to do." In the other case you say "give up on the structure and superimpose the patient advocate." It seems to me that if you have some real suspicions about whether the structure can change because of technology forces (e.g. the technology requires a great multiplicity of contacts with severely ill patients), then you almost have to have three things: the control, the ombudsman, and the reduction of the number of people.

The next point I wanted to suggest is that the concept of a person not necessarily technically competent following the patient really evokes some of the sounds that come out of nursing schools as to what the truly professional nurse ought to be. As you design an experiment of the kinds mentioned, it seems to me that you have to go back to what is the content of the training of the nurses who are going to be moving into this. You can have high dissonance or you can have high consonance, according to whether the nurses are prepared for the role that is envisioned.

Chairman: These comments take us back to the area of social control. The connection is obvious, particularly since the idea of the ombudsman, which comes from societal pressures, has been proposed in other areas as well, for example, in the academic field. The concept clearly ties to such issues as those of social control, control agents, consumer influence, and environmental constraints—issues that we have been discussing. Perhaps we may want to return to discuss some of these further, but at the moment the alloted time is running out.

Comment: I too would like to make a comment on this ombudsman and social control kind of problem, looking at it from the inside. I do not know whether others would agree with me or not, but if we could change the structure so that the value system in turn would have a structural rein on action, we may not need this additional person injected into the situation that can cause another coordination strain. The thing that gets in the way of monitoring effective patient care, or the follow-through process phenomena, is the submarine and salami kind of thing that was discussed earlier. If the patient care process were structured and viewed in terms of continuity of behavior, instead of as a series of discrete and discontinuous acts, an ombudsman would not be needed.

Comment (Dr. Straus): Actually I have my tongue in my cheek a little bit on this patient advocate thing. What I meant, and perhaps this did not come clear in my paper, is that such a role would be a way of introducing an experimental design for coping with the system as it exists.

Comment: Experience with the ombudsman in other areas of life has not met expectations. Certainly in universities the ombudsman is going through the same problem of running against the structure and exercising no leadership. It is only solving superficial symptoms without getting at the heart of the problems.

Comment: No matter how we change the structure, I think we are going to have some need for an advocacy role somewhere built within the system. No matter how we structure the hospital, we are not going to structure it perfectly, and we need the kind of dither that a role of that kind represents. But I do not think we can depend on it to deal with the problems of structure, the problems of institutional goals, or the problems of the action of physicians.

Question: But could it not be an ombudsman for a professional discipline, working with that professional discipline, rather than for the patient?

Answer: No. I think it must be for the patient. I think that no matter how we structure the situation, the complexities of medical care are going to be such that there is a need for someone who always speaks up and says: "Look, this guy is not getting what he is supposed to get." I think we need both to change the structure and an advocacy role.

Comment (Dr. Scott): I want to add to my share of the concern for the ombudsman approach because it seems to have serious deficiencies from the point of view of the system. The ombudsman approach is very much a "subject-oriented" approach. That is, it is concerned with such things as: what are the outputs that a person gets, and is a person getting what he is entitled to within some kind of a framework. But it never asks fundamental questions about the system itself or about the way in which ther person participates in that system. It also has a peculiar contemporary sense and its roots are in what you might call the adversary philosophy or the adversary perspective on society—adversary between the establishment and the victim. And in this sense it may be a political consequence of current trends, without necessarily being institutionally necessary.

Comment: Yes, you are right, and I would like to add to that point. It seems that we have a number of factors here that are social controls of the hospital, and I wonder about how many degrees of freedom we are going to have as, for example, the unions get stronger, and as the new careers movement develops a headway—something which seems to be very fashionable now and which is pushing for ombudsmen and that type of solution. It seems that the hospital now is being used as an employment opportunity. As a consequence, rather than getting more professionally oriented people it is going to be saddled with a number of people who are not professionals, and this leaves us in a very interesting situation.

Comment (Dr. Jaco): I have been in administration about ten years, and we are losing our options fast. The issue of unions came up in our study. Nurse's aides were being unionized, and they were having a big battle with negotiations right in the middle of my project, messing up all my variables. We worked it around to where we could do the project. But my point is we were looking at the various roles when we manipulated nurse staffing patterns in the different study situations, and I know that I could not replicate that study a year later because so many changes had occurred on the personnel requirements. Job descriptions became locked into particular roles and changed role definitions. RNs no longer could make up a bed, for example, even if there was blood all over it. They had to call a floor maid to do that, because it was within the union's jurisdiction. This kind of thing is happening, and it is quite true that administration is getting squeezed in the process in terms of unionization, in terms of governmental regulations, and in terms of other constraints. The options of administrative decision-making are being narrowed all the time.

Comment: I would like to add a small ancedote that might show the other side of the coin. Some years ago I was asked to be a consultant to a hospital in Detroit in which they had anticipated unionization, and the administration and personnel office had worked out very elaborate and precise job switches with which they were very happy. Then the union bought all of these job descriptions without any controversy, and they thought that they had won the battle. Six months later, however, the hospital was in terrible turmoil because the nurses were not unionized and everything that was not in the job descriptions (the shop stewards enforced the job descriptions) the nurses had to do. They were doing everything from the dregs of the janitor's job, which were not classified, to patient care. The hospital had such an enormous turnover that they could not keep a nurse on their staff.

Chairman: Most of these comments demonstrate the importance of environmental forces, not only as constraints to decision-making but as factors which may change the character of the internal structure of an institution, whether or not the institution responds to them. And that is, in a sense, what we are saying here. Clearly, such things as government regulation agencies, the unions, the opportunity people, and related forces might change the character of the hospital, and perhaps bring it closer to the factory model, particularly if the institution does nothing to alter its traditional structure. The ombudsman idea, perhaps, does not go far enough in this direction. In any case, apart from union, government, and comsumer pressures, urbanization and the other societal trends that we were discussing earlier also are forces which eventually, though perhaps imperceptively, will affect the very structure of the institution. These are not just constraints to decision-making. These are powerful forces in the environment to which the hospital often attempts to adapt in a rather passive way, or only when forced, even though these forces are likely to change its basic structure and character.

Ecology of Work and Patient Care

Presentation Highlights: E. G. Jaco

The area of ecology, space, and temporal aspects of organizational behavior is a very mixed one. It is an area that many people have mixed feelings about, but one that has a certain seductive appeal for people who get involved in research on it. It is easy to go overboard and say "Gee, this is great stuff," and then end up making strong overgeneralized statements on spatial and temporal aspects of social behavior in organizations. This is one reason why we have had uneven cycles of research in this particular area, both in the health care field and in social science. There are a lot of very insightful ideas about the subject but no systematic development of the concepts. There are also some patterns and generalizations upon which we can hopefully build a body of theory and make some predictions.

There has been more emphasis upon what can be called macrospace studies of hospital facilities in contrast to personal space studies focusing on the immediate work surrounding of the individual, whether he be a staff person or a patient. But useful concepts and analytical constructs that might be valuable in conducting useful research of this kind are being developed. To date, however, most of the research on use of space in hospitals has lacked theoretical underpinnings for generating hypotheses to be tested. Studies generally have been on a pragmatic level, revolving around questions of efficiency, such as "Can we get by with fewer nursing staff without jeopardizing the quality of patient care?"

This type of question has been one focus because the cost aspect is certainly an increasingly dominant one in our society. But I am concerned because this focus on efficiency is apparently a motive for the majority of studies on the use of space in the hospital field. This is particularly exemplified by the Yale Traffic Index studies, which look at the unit providing patient care in highly mechanistic, quantitative, statistical terms and completely ignore the humanistic aspect. This is rationalized in many different ways. I still have not forgotten the comment by an architect, for example, that "hospital architects could care a hoot about patient satisfactions when they design a hospital," and they make no bones about it, partly because they do not have enough money to build any so-called luxuries. I do not know whether these are rationalizations, but I know that it is a common statement that you get from architects and administrators who hire them to build these units and then brag about how cheaply they build a unit for so many beds, keep the cost down, and make the trustees happy.

As long as the focus remains on this level, we are going to be limited on what kinds of research are going to be done. Still, there is some insightful work in this area, though most of it is based on anecdotal or observational material. The ecologist Edward Hall has observed, for example, that a physician stands at varying places at the bedside when he makes rounds. If he stands at the foot of the bed, he is probably a surgeon, but if he stands at or near the head of the bed, he is probably an anesthesiologist, the only friend the patient has in the operating room.

Others have come up with some rather clever experiments on the use of space. Particularly interesting are those reported by Sommar. In a mental hospital, for example, chairs were rearranged to increase social interaction. In the morning all chairs were lined up along the halls, and when visiting hours would come, the chairs would be moved in a circle so that relatives and visitors could talk with patients. But the patients would then move the chairs back against the wall. Apparently the patients conformed to a norm that patients are not supposed to disrupt the usual arrangements of the furniture or the setting of the unit.

I do not want to take too long on this because I would like to share with you some of the results of our own studies of radial and angular patient units. Based on the work done to date, however, I would like to suggest that it is no longer fruitful to ask in our research whether space or the physical work environment has an impact on behavior. It is clear to us that it does, and we do not need to study that anymore. The ways in which it affects behavior is what we ought to be studying in the future. The limits, the ranges, and magnitudes of these effects should be the focus, although obviously efficiency and cost also have to be dealt with since they are primary concerns to the architects and most hospital administrators. But the impact of space and physical environment on the patients, doctors, nurses, and other staff working in the patient units should be the principal focus.

It is also important to keep in mind that we are not just talking about the shape of a patient unit per se; we are concerned with the total setting of the immediate physical environment in terms of its arrangement, like the positioning of furniture, distances, convenience, access, etc. The ecologist changing chairs, for example, was creating what Osmond calls a sociopetal arrangement—one that pulls people together. Sociofugal space arrangements, on the other hand, keep people apart and separated. The ideal type of sociofugal space would be a penitentiarry with a long line of cells, down a single corridor, each being a compartment. This would also mean a minimum of communication and social interaction, in contrast to a circular arrangement where everybody is thrown together and must interact. There is an analogy to the hospital here, since Straus suggests the idea that the patient is like a prisoner.

The main point is that the arrangement of the patient facility, including the modern hospital and medical center, segregates its functions into specialized compartments such as operating rooms, recovery rooms, postoperative units, bassinet rooms, nursuries, and obstetrical units. In California there is even a law that all hospitals must segregate physically the obstetrical unit from the rest of the hospital. The administration is left with no choice, and they simply have to shut it down if the occupancy drops too much. Other patients cannot be put in there, for the hospital would lose its license. More generally, the hospital today, the modern general acute hospital, is a composite of specialized functional services that are based on spatial considerations. Under these circumstances the impact of the physical environment on behavior can be both direct and subtle. In terms of impact on communication and action, for example, one study of an obstetrical unit showed that nurses, doctors, and other staff would resolve certain conflicts in the corridors rather than in the particular area where they did most of their work. Obviously, the assumption is that if they were functioning under a different spatial arrangement in that service their behavior and use of space would be different.

In our studies of radial patient units we have an example of a sociopetal space arrangement where staff are thrust together and must interact to some extent. What we were able to do in this particular study of a hospital in St. Paul was to manipulate a number of experimental variables, both independent and intervening, and see to what extent the shape of the patient unit, radial or angular, had an effect on nursing behavior, physician behavior, and patient behavior or reactions.

In the radial unit, the nurses' station was in the center and the patient rooms were arranged along the wall in a circular fashion. Off from the nurses' station were the utility room, the supply room, etc. The distance from the center of the nurses' station to the individual patient's door was eighteen feet. All patient bedroom doors had a glass panel so that a nurse could see the bed from any point in the station and from most parts of the unit. One could lie in a bed and see what the attending physician or the nurse was doing—in fact what most nurses were doing—or look into the other rooms around as well as the nurses' station. The station had a low counter so that the nurse could be sitting down and still see into the rooms and observe the patients. The arrangement of the angular-shaped unit—the more conventional and familiar type of patient unit in hospitals—provided a sharp contrast. These units were both new, a year and a half old. Both were built at the same time, had the same color carpets, corridor area, air conditioning, etc. They had twenty beds each, but before we started the study we changed it to twenty two beds—two private, six semi-private, and two four-bed rooms. Each unit had a total floor space area of about 1000 square feet, and the length of the corridor was identical for both.

We set up twelve study situations by varying the occupancy level and nurse staffing patterns (qualitatively in terms of the ratios of RNs, LPNs, and aides, and quantitatively in terms of numbers of staff). The ratio of staff to patient census was varied from high, to medium, to low. In one situation we had a head nurse and nothing but aides or LPNs (it took a few tranquilizers to get them to do it, but we did), and in another situation we had nothing but RNs. At one point in the low-occupancy condition there was one nurse to one patient, and that is when the circle fell apart; it absolutely collapsed, even though we had a luxurious staffing pattern. In contrast, there was no collapse in the angular unit under the same staffing pattern.

We observed around the clock, five days a week, all three shifts. We used work sampling, but the methodological problems with this still have not been resolved. We collected over 200,000 observations over a period of two years. Essentially, we ran one and the same situation with a varied staffing pattern and occupancy level for four straight weeks. Then a resettling period was allowed to let the unit get back to normal for a couple of weeks, before starting a new study situation. We also had the admitting officer randomize the admission of patients to the units. We interviewed the patients just prior to their discharge, often in a room that we had reserved, using a social worker who was a trained interviewer. In addition, we interviewed, privately, the nurses and also the physicians who had had patients on the study units.

The methodology is one of the things that I certainly think needs examination. Among other techniques, we used traditional work sampling in the study, which is pretty well established in nursing studies. You have someone observing somebody every few minutes on the unit, and then you usually make a summation from which to get distributions of what activities were observed being performed, by whom on the staff, and where on the unit. Personally, I have some serious questions about whether this method of work sampling really gets at a true or accurate measure of the parameters involved in nursing performance. Something as complicated as nursing care, much of which requires continuity of treatment and the like, is probably not well measured with this technique. The best available technique may be work sampling because of reasons of expedience and because it has been in use for a number of years, but it never gets at the quality of nursing care in any direct sense. In other words, when a nurse is observed doing something, say adjusting an I.V. or talking to the patient by the bedside, you do not have a measure of how well she is doing that. Nor do you know whether you are getting biases with this method. Even with closed circuit television, you can scan the performance of nurses but still you do not get a direct measure of the quality of patient care. You only get indirect measures based on assumptions that themselves may be questionable.

Let me give you some of the results. What we found in the circular unit was that within a very short time, perhaps an hour or so, patients knew personally every member of the nursing staff and could distinguish among RNs, aides, LPNs, etc. A definite bond between the patients and the nurses developed very quickly in this unit. These were the same nurses, incidentally, who worked on the different units and study situations on each unit, serving as their own controls. It was the same nursing staff, essentially, performing the same nursing tasks on the two types of units. Yet we did not find the same bond developing quickly on the angular units.

Nearly all RNs preferred the circular over the angular unit, but not the aides. The interviews indicated that aides did not like the circular unit because "nurses keep an eye on me too much." Aides felt that they were on stage and restricted too much. (The dirty word around the hospital was "the fishbowl"—a reference to the circular unit.) If an aide wanted to smoke a cigarette, she had to leave the unit, unlike the case of those working in the angular unit.

These social-psychological differences in staff reactions and behavior were due to the high visual contact that prevailed in the circular unit, which contact in turn was the result of the difference in the shape of the two types of patient units. According to the nurses, the circular unit was ideal for intensive care, because the nurses could take care of the critically ill round-the-clock with a minimum of physical effort or fatigue and, therefore, perhaps also do a better job. But would this hold for less intensive care patients? The results showed that it did not for an intermediate-care situation. We aslo had a minimal self-care service, set up more like a hotel, where patients were ambulatory and could get together or leave and return as they pleased. This service received more positive reactions than either the circular or the angular unit.

While the circular shape of the unit definitely had an impact on patients and staff in many ways, there were also some contrary indications. By and large, among the MDs the specialists preferred this unit. They were very disappointed, however, for certain categories of patients they thought would not do well under this high visibility arrangement. There were also some patients, mostly medical, who demanded to be removed from this unit, often because of severe allergies or migrain which were bothered by all this activity. One patient was disturbed about our observers going around and looking into the rooms, considering this an invasion of privacy.

There was another interesting thing due to the high visibility in the unit that we called the "curtain pulling syndrome." We had a recording clerk sit in the nursing station and record the frequency with which the patient bedside curtain was open, partially closed, or completely closed. Eventually we were able to predict when a patient was ready to go home by how frequently he kept the curtain closed. When they were first admitted, very sick and in an anxious state, they wanted to be observed by the staff and left the curtains open. When they began convelescing, they started closing the curtain more and more. And when they were approaching discharge, they wanted privacy.

The circular unit showed its efficiency particularly when the staff to patient ratio was low. An almost rock bottom staff gave a fantastic amount of bedside care. We did not find this in the angular unit. In the circular unit setting, the social psychology of work was quite different. First, patients could observe each other, as well as the staff. The patients complained of lack of privacy, and the nursing staff complained of being on stage, always being watched by the patients. The head nurse and the charge nurse, in particular, were reluctant, on the circular unit compared to the angular unit, to let an LPN or an aide do certain functions in a patient's room that would be seen by other patients, even when the workload was extremely high. But they had no compunction about sending an aide or LPN to do a lot of things in the single-corridor unit because none of the other patients could observe what was going on. One consequence was that considerable resistance was generated, particularly among LPNs, who resented the fact that they could not do the same bedside functions in one unit that they could do in another.

Further, there was significantly less verbal communication on the radial than on the angular unit, and this raises a question about appropriate care. For example, in one sense the patients felt far more secure in the radial unit than they did on the angular unit. Yet overall they received less bedside care and far less verbal communication from the nursing staff. There was a substitute in the nonverbal area, however: in the circular unit the patients could smile at each other, the nurses would come in and be seen by all patients, and patients and staff would wave at each other. In addition, there were more nurse-initiated trips to the patient rooms on the circular unit, for the simple reason that nurses would see something that had to be done, and they would go do it right away; they spotted it and they could take care of it, without having to wait for a call light. Incidentally, the average time spent per visit to the room by the nurses was very short compared to the angular unit, where things would just pile up.

The question arises about the quality of care or the level of it. We found, for example, that in some situations the RNs gave more care than in others. There was little difference, however, between the two units with respect to the time nurses spent in the nursing station; about a third of their time was spent in the station on both units. But the behavior of the LPNs and the aides varied far more than did the behavior RNs on the two settings.

In any event, the very shape of the unit per se was responsible for the great difference in visual contact that characterized the units. Visual contact, in turn, was the major independent variable accounting for most of the differences in staff behavior. This has many implications for the relationships on the units among the different members of the nursing staff. In some ways, for example, there was more tension on the radial unit, sort of a constant low level tension among all the nurses, that we did not find on the angular unit. And yet one wonders why the reverse should not be the case, since nurses on the former unit could always keep an eye on their patients without any difficulty. Perhaps the architectural inflexibility of the circular unit was the problem. Architecturally the most rigid kind of structure one can have is the circle. If you modify it in any way, immediately vitiate all the advantages of the physical arrangement that it provides.

In summary, no matter how we stacked the cards against the nurses, we found that the seriously ill patients, those requiring intensive care, got the most direct bedside care on the circular unit—much more so than on the angular unit. So in a sense this was more appropriate or better care, and the nursing staff had more options in the ways they provided care. Nurses also could anticipate things better on the circular unit because they had the patients under constant surveillance. This gave the nurse options in performing her services and tasks, at her own discretion, and facilitated decision-making on her part. The virtue of visible contact did not exist on the angular unit. Other findings, however, which are discussed in my paper in detail, show the limitations of radial design for patient care, staff behavior, and patient reactions.

Discussion

Question: A board of trustees, an administrator, and an architect are sitting in a room, and they have hired you. What do you tell them, in terms of your findings Dr. Jaco, when they say, "We have got to be efficient, we can not spend too much money." I would be interested in the process by which this kind of knowledge gets to those who make the building decisions.

Answer: Before I was even able to do the study, I met with the trustees, the administrator, the draftsmen of the project, and others. I asked the trustees individually, as well as some of the others, about the building program, without fully realizing that they had strongly identified with these circular units. This was an old hospital, built in 1867. The structure was practically falling down, and they had to make a decision, like most hospitals do periodically: "Should we remodel or relocate out in the suburbs?" They agreed to stay put, but in looking around got some advice on a new kind of structure that from the outside would change the physical image of the hospital. The circular structure would change the hospital from Old Bailey to something modern, neat, nice and intriguingly different. Without realizing that they had a firm legal involvement, as well as dollar involvement in these circles, I wanted to know their answer to one question before undertaking the research. Specifically, I asked: "Can you accept negative evidence? Can you accept the results, if our study shows that circles are mostly for the birds, and that you have washed all these millions of dollars down the drain?" One trustee, a banker, replied: "Well, if we have made a mistake then we would like every other hospital to know about it so they will not repeat this mistake." Now that is probably unusual.

Comment: I think the question is much broader. Since the different designs are not made in heaven and there are many varieties of spatial arrangements that archietects could design, how does one adopt a schema for decisions not based upon only one or two models? In other words, how do we develop a general concept of space utilization for the medical world? This question is not especially sociological; it is also an architectural question and one of engineering efficiency. As far as I can tell, and you people know better, hospitals are growing up quite haphazardly, by adding a wing here or there when crowded. Somebody says, "Oh, I need another wing," and the outcome is an addition down that corridor, then another wing off at another corridor, and so on. It seems to me the whole process is like a bad dream.

Comment: One of the intriguing and tantalizing things about Dr. Jaco's report is that it is unequivocally ambiguous, and that, I think, is crucial. I apologize for sounding like somebody out of a school of education, but what it really suggests—the data suggest—is that you cannot go further with research in this area unless you consider the articulation of objectives and established hierarchy of priorities among competing objectives. Basically, there are a number of things that are simultaneously in there, and any building is a compromise between various objectives. The fact that we now have hospitals which are built as memorials, you know, or as doctors' laboratories, merely suggests that there are a variety of objectives, and that the architect and those who work with him need to raise the questions that I think are being raised here.

Comment (Dr. Jaco): To get back to the previous question too, as a result of our first study the hospital subsequently added on more circles. And as a result of our study they made several basic changes in the design and the layout, particularly in the nurses' station. This need to achieve a better integration came out in another area of my research. The nurses complained about a lot of things that were in the layout of the station, e.g. the drug cabinet was right in the vortex of the station where a patient could reach right around (although it was locked), grab the key, and help himself to the drugs. They changed that. They also made minor changes to permit more privacy. Originally, there were no private rooms on the circle, and this is certainly why we first started. As a result of our study, however, they were going to have private rooms to permit more privacy for those patients who wanted it.

I think the moral is that no one physical setting is perfect for everybody. I have warned the administration, and I think I have indicated before, that if you completely phase out all your angular units and have nothing but circles you will probably lose 20 percent of your occupancy within a week. There are enough physicians who will not admit patients only to these circles because, for some patients, they consider it medically contraindicated. There are also social-psychological contraindications. Some patients, for example, are chronic complainers, others have paranoid tendencies, and others simply keep hanging around the nursing station interfering with the work of the staff.

This is an area where we need to do more research on the mesh of the patient's needs from a personal, social-psychological view to complement those of a medical, physiological nature within a particular setting—the patient unit. Many of the physicians on the staff told me privately that they wish hospitals would decide for doctors what is the optimum room accommodation for their patients. Doctors do not think they should be the ones to decide but think rather the hospital administration should do that. There certainly is a need to do some studies in this area. If we could get the physician to specify a few major variables, for example, could we predict on a preadmission set-up which of a number of different accommodations would be the optimal one for a patient's medical, psychological, and social needs?

Question: Are you not assuming here that the physician knows a great deal about his patient? Actually, many physicians do not.

Answer: No; the physician is saying that. He does not know what the best accommodation would be but he is stuck with that, and he is the one that gets heat from patients—"How come you put me in that crazy place?" I heard patients complain to their doctors, saying "I do not want to be in this fishbowl," or some other more nasty words. Some demanded to be transfered, and the doctor was the one blamed for it, even though the admitting officer put the patient in there.

Comment: I thought you were suggesting that you would look to the physician for guidance in this assignment.

Answer: No. The physicians told me that they wished the hospital administration and the admitting office had more sophistication about accommodations so they could advise them what would be best for their patients in terms of what they need and in terms of their medical problems. Some needs are obvious. If a patient has a contagious disease, he needs isolation. But in terms of the general patient, or average patient, there is a need for research concerning the matter of optimal accommodation.

Comment: This takes us back to the basic question of "circular floor for what?" For intensive care the circular unit may be appropriate, or even optimal. But for pediatrics or obstetrics the best arrangement may be very different.

Comment: By and large frankly I am giving you a typical episode of acute illness. The patient goes through many stages. The obstetrical service in that hospital was new and beautiful. The unit was a circle, and right off it was the nursery where all new mothers could look right in and see their babies.

Comment: Yes, but some of them get more anxious when they see them and some do not. This raises the question of patient expectations and issues about culture and the patient's mode of living. Can we create a hospital, or a patient unit arrangement, which will minimize the trauma of hospitalization?

Answer: Do we want to? Frankly, I do not think that is always for the good, because you do not want the patients to spend the rest of their lives in the hospital. If you make it too convenient, they will not want to leave.

Question: I do not believe that is our problem; that is another matter. But there is one question I want to ask. In your studies, as I understand, you were looking at this sort of thing. Was there an orientation for the staff regarding the intended objectives of this unit?

Answer: Yes, there was for some of the staff who were going to be assigned to the unit. This continued for a few months after they were ready to accept patients. What we had to do to counteract this was to assign half of the nurses who had no prior experience on a circular unit and half who had. This should equalize any biases on their part or preferences in their performance. But, by and large, if a nurse was going to be assigned to the radial unit, she received some orientation. In some cases they asked a nurse who wanted to be transferred to go to the circular unit, and then they hired a replacement for her. Some of the nurses were brainwashed in the process. Hospital administrators and nursing service personnel sometimes would come and say, "Oh this is the greatest thing in the world," referring to the circle. And I have seen some horrible blunders made because of this.

Question: If you went to the hospital and had a choice between an angular and a circular unit, which one would you choose of the two?

Answer: I do not want anybody poking and invading my personal space, unless he is qualified. Even then, I would like to get it over and done with and get out. Personally I would prefer the angular unit.

Comment: In a small study we took a number of rooms of the hospital, which were the kind of room where here is the washroom, enter here, and then the bed sort of like here. We interviewed about thirty-five patients. They were patients with either gastrointestinal or cardiovascular conditions. Most of the cardiovascular patients were postoperative, and most of the gastrointestinal had ulcers or ulcerative colitis. We asked them about the position of their bed. Almost all of the gastrointestinal patients, and we are not examining other variables here, said "Well, I would not want to be here, but this is fine." In contrast, 80 percent of the cardiovascular patients, all the infarcts, said "Oh, I just do not know; I would much rather be able to see."

Comment: Those were two different populations of patients.

Answer: I know, and that is exactly the point I am making.

Comment: I think this is a psychological factor. If I were critically ill, I would want the round-the-clock observation, but not for intermediate care level.

Comment: I would like to make an observation and raise a question. The observation is that in many hospitals space has become the currency for most managerial decisions. For many decisions, the administrator will say, "Where is the space?" Somebody should study this; it is a very interesting and important area. The question I had is this: With all the hundreds and hundreds of hospitals that have been built in the United States, it amazes me that there has been so little creativity in terms of designing these hospitals, and I wonder—I am not an architect—whether anybody knows of any architectural school which is actually going into this area. I just do not know of any, and it is really shocking to see so little creativity in this area.

Dr. Jaco: I gave these preliminary results to a couple of American Hospital Association institutes on designer instruction. Half of the audience were architects and half were administrators. I was very much impressed with the questioning that is going on now in hospital architecture. Ten years ago, they thought they had all the answers. Also, the VA in Washington, as I understand, has been experimenting with a hospital where they had movable doors and walls. They were going to go into various room sizes and shapes, and different accommodation arrangements. In our study, we interviewed patients who hated those lights above that bed that one of John Thompson's studies said were very good. In a double bedroom, not just wards, if one patient wanted to go to bed a little earlier at night than the other, and the other patient wanted to read, the latter kept his light on and this made it miserable for the other. In part, the problem was that the beds were arranged side by side. We picked up a lot of little tips. In the circular unit you also had to be careful because street lights would shine at night through some drapes that did not quite close, and the lights would bother the patients all night. We also encountered patients who said that the air conditioning made a lot of noise, and "I bet I could fix it if I had a wrench."

You can learn a lot from the patients, particularly about the immediate room. I wish every medical student and every nurse would be a patient in the hospital to see what it is like in that role, or get a little sensitivity training about the role of the patient. A lot of psychological differences are reflected in the nature and frequency of patient complaints, and I am sure we could learn a great deal from the experiences of patients. But there is developing a critical attitude now in hospital architecture that you never found in the past.

Part Five

12

THE ROLE OF THE DOCTOR IN INSTITUTIONAL MANAGEMENT*

Robert H. Guest

The decade of the 1960s brought to a head one of the most difficult issues in the entire arena of human health: the role that medical men play in facilitating the *institutional* functions of American hospitals. This period saw a profound shift away from the traditional role of the doctor as the professional solo practitioner almost completely responsible for care and treatment of patients to one in which he interfaced very directly with almost all functions of hospital management in order to provide what has come to be known as *total* patient care. The means by which the doctor can effectively manage both his professional role and his institutional role may well determine how effectively total patient care is provided in the next decade.

This paper is not a point-by-point review of the literature as such. Rather it is an interpretative summary, beginning with an historical explanation as to why the tradition of the independent solo practice of medicine has made it difficult for doctors to mesh their primary professional tasks with the institutional demands for total patient care in the hospital. It covers what has been observed about the role of the medical staff in policy-making. It does not explicitly deal with the organizational interface of doctors, nurses, and other paramedical groups. The paper concludes with some speculative comments about the future—the future of the doctor's institutional relationships, and the future research challenges with respect to these relationships.

Past Research

In the last decade a considerable volume of literature was generated concerning the doctor's institutional role in the hospital and in the community at large. Much of the published material was written by concerned and responsible observers, including doctors and administrators. The striking fact, however, is that there has been preciously little truly sophisticated research in which hypotheses were posed and rigorously tested under conditions even approaching acceptable standards of behavior research. Most of the literature in this area has been hortatory or observational at best. It could hardly be called *research* in any acceptable sense of the word.

*Paper presented at Conference on Hospital Organization Research, May 22-23, 1970, Institute for Social Research, The University of Michigan, Ann Arbor, Michigan. Robert H. Guest, Ph.D., is Professor of Organizational Behavior, The Amos Tuck School of Business, Dartmouth College. (Some modifications of the original paper have been made by the Editor.)

If one views the spectrum of research in other areas of human activity one cannot fail to see the contrast. Sociologists and psychologists in the 1960s studied intensively the institutional roles of a wide variety of occupations and professions. Important hypotheses have been generated, for example, from the study of the scientist or the engineer and his role relations to the institutions of government and industry. A vast amount of solid research has been produced in the area of management itself, the functional and hierarchical relationships in industry and government, with useful explanations as to the causes of organizational stress. Some of the best survey and experimental research by behavioral scientists has been made in the hopsital itself, but it is usually focused on the nursing profession, on paramedical groups, and on administration per se. The doctor is rarely central to the *research design,* even though it is quite apparent that the doctor's role in the management matrix is crucial to an understanding of how the hospital functions as a purposeful organization.

One can only speculate why we have so little solid research data on the doctor's institutional behavior. This observer can speak only from his own experience. It suggests rather strongly that the basic problem may be one of *entry.* The behavioral science researcher finds it very difficult to convince members of the medical profession that they are proper subjects of "research." Part of the reason is that doctors may feel that a nonmedical researcher would have to delve into behavior that is strictly medical, that any exposure might violate the long-standing ethic of the doctor's confidential relationship with his patient. Some observers have suggested, perhaps irresponsibly, that proposals for research may lead to change, and that this traditionally conservative segment of society, while applauding change in medical science and technology, would resist any possible exposure of their institutional roles. Finally, and the argument is a convincing one, doctors are simply extremely busy people. Time is a valued commodity for one of America's scarcest professional resources.

It is hoped that the present decade will see a change in the pattern of research, and that the medical profession will be willing partners in the effort. The physician's institutional role in hospitals during the past decade was difficult enough for doctors as well as administrators. It will certainly not become less complex when one contemplates the radical changes in medical care and treatment that are bound to come in the next decade. One only has to read Sidney Garfield's article, "The Delivery of Medical Care," in the April 1970 issue of *Scientific American,* to begin to appreciate the enormous changes likely to take place.

The Doctor's Emerging Role in the Hospital: Historical Overview[1]

The role of the doctor, and of the medical staff, as an initiator of and

---

1. Much of the material in this section was derived from "The Role of the Doctor" by the author (Guest, 1966).

responder to policies in hospitals, has deep roots relating to the history of the formation of hospitals themselves of the advances in medicine.

Origin of the Hospital

It is a curious historical fact that the early hospital was not founded for the primary purpose of medical care. The hospital was an outgrowth of the need to found and administer lodging houses by religious organizations assisted by gifts from the wealthy. However,

> in time the hospitals (or lodging houses) began to take in the homeless . . . and give them more permanent lodging . . . . Since many of the homeless unfortunates were physically ill, however, nursing care was necessary, and in time medical consultation was sought. The medicine of the time had really little to offer these patients. Most of them were suffering from chronic or terminal illnesses, and the hospital undertook to make them as comfortable as possible within the resources and knowledge available, until they ended their days . . . . The services of such doctors as did visit the hosptial were often a gift of their time to the unfortunate. They did not see any immediate advantage to themselves in giving their service. Their only reward for succoring the unfortunate lay in their hopes for the life to come. The focus of medical practice at that time was in the home. It was there that the doctor found the resources which he needed for his patients: elatives to provide nursing care, food, and shelter. Even up to the middle of the last century, the hospital provided a wretched substitute for home care. (Burling, Lentz, and Wilson, 1956, p. 4.)

The recognition of Miss Nightingale's role and the relationship between filth and hospital death rates, combined with the scientific explanations by Pasteur among others, set the groundwork for the modern hospital. It was only in the middle part of the nineteenth centrury that the doctor began to play a crucial role in the hospital as an institution. He found that with advances in science and skills, special attention needed to be given to the patient. Hospital attendants were not skilled in the required auxiliary care. The need for more skilled training stimulated the growth of nursing educational facilities. The hospital became the obvious locus for the function of nursing education (Burling, Lentz, and Wilson, 1956).

Thus an institution, both in a physical and organizational sense, already existed for doctors to treat those patients who could not be treated adequately at home. And because medical practice during the 1800s was not advancing at the pace of today's science and technology there were no serious strains on the hospital to meet the doctor's technical requirements. Nor was the relationship between doctor and "management" so complex as to require the medical practitioners to become involved in the kinds of organizational problems which medical staffs face today in hospitals.

Most hospitals were not founded and operated by physicians. Had they been created by the medical profession the entire development of institutional patient care might have been vastly different. Because hospitals were not origingally founded by the medical profession, the doctor was not an integral part of the organization in a strict bureaucratic sense. This was true in spite of the vital relationship between medical practice and the institution. These historical facts help to explain why the doctor, in one sense, was not in control of the institution; he had to perform his work in the kind of relationship that has few parallels in other large-scale organizations. The doctor was and is still officially "a guest" of the open staff hospital. Many of today's most difficult policy questions facing governing boards, administrators, and doctors revolve around this central fact.

Professional Independence of the Doctor and the Shift to Interdependence

In another sense, of course, the doctor and his practicing colleagues were from early times very much in control because of their unquestioned authority in administering to the hospital's most important "product"—the patient.

Not only was the doctor's authority made explicit by the traditions of the profession; he was clothed with an informal authority that was accepted by every segment and function in the institution. His stature stood in marked contrast to the sick, aged, poverty-stricken, and frequently homeless patients he treated. These patients were wholly dependent upon the doctor, yet the doctor was independent of the institution itself. He was responsible to his client, free from formal organizational constraints of the hospital, and he possessed skills of a special intellectual and technical character (Wilson, 1959-60).

Professional independence was reinforced by the fact that for many years the hospital was not the center of the physician's practice. The center of his practice was his home and that of his patient. He "hung up his shingle" and made himself available to all in need in his community. Unlike employees of the growing factory and business organizations he took no orders from agents of any organization. He was responsible only to his patients, and this responsibility was supported by traditions going as far back as Hippocrates. It was assumed that only his independence to care for the welfare of his patients was the overriding consideration. Unheard of was a suggestion that any form of organizational bureaucracy should intervene between himself and his patient (see also Parsons, 1963, p. 26).

As the years passed and the doctor to an increasing extent was practicing in an "institution," he wished to preserve his primary relationship to the patient undisturbed. While utilizing the hospital's new therapeutic facilities, not available in his own office, he jealously guarded his professional rights. In so doing the superintendent (usually a nurse) and all others took a subordinate role to the doctor. This subordination often colored administrative as well as professional matters. By 1900 and, indeed, for the first half of the twentieth century the doctor was fully in command. In most institutions it was the surgeon who gave orders to nurses, students, attendants, orderlies, and many others. As Wilson (1959-60, p 178) points out, "in his absence the organization ran in deference to precedents he had established or in anticipation of those he would establish."

Many institutional forces were coming to bear on the medical practitioner in his *hospital* role. In the first place his own medical education was taking place in increasingly complex medical school organizations. The former individual apprenticeship system had long given way to a training environment which itself was made up of large numbers of people and complex laboratory and clinical facilities.

Upon becoming a member of a hospital staff his "solo" relationship to his patient became more dependent on his being a member of a staff organization, on interacting with colleagues and administrative units. Consultation with other colleagues in the specialties became increasingly important. Laboratory facilities and the relationship to pathologists and others became essential. Patient treatment became more complex. The organization grew in size and complexity. The system of consultation became organized in the form of a medical staff. Rules, regulations, and the routines increased the doctor's dependency on other groups.

The shift from individual practice uninhibited by other external necessities of specialization and professionalization, according to Parsons (1963), meant that "Patient care itself, furthermore, has come increasingly to be carried out not by individual physicians but by teams of service personnel. The consultants on whom a physician in charge of a case becomes dependent constitute one major component of the team. This means that he can function far more effectively as a member of a staff of a hospital or clinic than he can alone or having to make purely private arrangements with his consultants."

Obviously the degree of consultation that was required and the extent of the doctor's relationships to the staff organization differed widely between the more complex metropolitan hospitals and the smaller community general hospitals. Also, in the smaller community hospitals certain doctors continued to play a dominant role in the major policy and administrative matters of the institution.

But even in the smaller institution the move for "professionalization" of hospital and nursing administration was well under way in the post-World War II period. Governing boards, responding to community pressures for expansion and medical pressures for more modern facilities, were taking greater interest in what comprised patient care in the broadest sense. Boards did more than just provide philanthropic financial support. They began asking probing questions about internal operations. In short, hospital trustees and administrators were assuming a larger role in the formulation and implementation of the policies of the institution. All available evidence suggests some lag in the acceptance of these developments by the doctors. Conversely, there was much that nonmedical groups had to learn about the scientific complexities of the modern tools and facilities of medicine.

From the physician's point of view, a view generally shared by the governing board, administration, and the public, his role as medical practitioner was not to be questioned. Also, the authority of the medical staff as a self-governing group was legally delegated by the governing board to the staff; it was manifest in the form of medical staff bylaws. What historically was rarely made explicit was the doctor's responsibility to the institution as distinguished from his responsibility to patients and colleagues. The most critical stresses involving policy matters of the institution can be traced to the confusion arising from the doctor's not clearly defined dual role.

Organizational Constraints on the Doctor

What are some of the changes which, in recent years, find the doctor being subjected increasingly to organizational constraints? Some have already been indicated. Basically, these changes are related to increased specialization of functions and greater professionalization of task performance.

Specialization has resulted from the accelerated innovations of science and the growth of medical technology. The proliferation of new knowledge and techniques not only created new functions in the medical profession; older functions were broken down into a variety of subfunctions. To keep the centrifugal forces from exploding in all directions, hospitals had to develop means and structures for coordinating both the medical and nonmedical specialties. As Wilson (1959-60) points out, coordination had to be formalized with each specialized component having some understanding of its mutual rights and obligations toward others.

Georgopoulos and Mann (1962, pp. 5-6), speaking not of the specialization of the medical profession alone but of the hospital as a whole, make the following observations:

> To do its work the hospital relies upon an extensive division of labor among its members, upon a complex organizational structure which encompasses different departments, staffs, offices, and positions, and upon an elaborate system of coordination of tasks, functions, and social interaction . . . .
>
> Work in the hospital is greatly differentiated and specialized, and of a highly interactional character. It is carried out by a large number of cooperating people whose backgrounds, education, training, skills, and functions are as diverse and heterogeneous as can be found in any of the most complex organizations in existence. And much of the work is not only specialized but also performed by highly trained professionals—the doctors—who require the collaboration, assistance, and services of many other professional and non-professional personnel. In addition to the medical staff, which itself is highly specialized and departmentalized, there is the nursing staff, which includes graduate professional nurses in various supervisory and nonsupervisory position, practical nurses, and untrained nurse's aides. In addition to the nursing staff and the medical staff, which are the two largest groups in the community general hospital, there

are the hospital administrator and a number of administrative-supervisory personnel who head various departments or services (e.g. nursing, dietary, admissions, maintenance, pharmacy, medical records, housekeeping, laundry) and are in charge of the employees in these departments. There are also a number of medical technologists and technicians who work in the laboratory and X-ray departments of the hospital, as well as a number of miscellaneous clerical and secretarial personnel. And apart from all of these staffs and professional-occupational groups, there is a board of trustees which has the overall formal responsibility for the organization, and which consists of a number of prominent people from the outside community. The trustees offer their services to the hosptial without remuneration and are not employees of the organization. In short, professionalization and specialization are two of the hallmarks of the hospital.

The implication of the above as it concerns the doctor's relationship to the total institution can be stated simply: the doctor is no longer either the generalist or the free agent he once was. As Rosen (cf. Wilson, 1959-60, p. 179) puts it, "One may say that the Industrial Revolution has finally caught up with medicine, and that the medical practitioner is being brought into the 'factory' (the hospital and the whole bureaucratic complexity for the provision of medical care) where he is being subjected to the necessary 'labor disciplines.'"

It is in this broader context of the highly specialized and complex organization that one can begin to understand the difficulties faced by the governing board, administrator, and the medical staff in working out policies that simultaneously maintain the integrity of the total organization as well as preserve the professional rights of the doctor himself. It is worth repeating, but from still another observer's point of view, that the installation of administrative controls has substantially altered the human environment within which policies are formulated:

> As the hospital has become more complicated and more critical to all of medical practice, as its uses have multiplied and its patient load has extended rapidly, the administrator has enjoyed an accompanying growth in stature. Rational planning and control, from food management to finances to surgery, have become a hospital necessity. The rationalization of hospital life could not occur without the expansion of old roles, like that of the administrator, and the creation of new ones, like those of personnel director or comptroller. Thus the administrative staff, traditionally seen as the doctor's handmaiden and existing, like the nurse, for his sole convenience, has been transformed into something approaching—although not nearly reaching—the character of executive echelons in corporate or governmental hierarchies (Wilson, 1959-60).

The Doctor's Role in Policy-Making

Underlying all these comments concerning the medical staff-board-administrator relationship is the fact that no one element in the triangle alone "makes" policy for the institution. Although the board, the administrator, and the medical staff are concerned with one basic "service," good patient care, they have special interests in making changes that will improve their own particular functions. Unlike highly decentralized holding companies in industry, a change affecting the total organization can come only through a degree of agreement among all three parties. The special interest of one at the policy level becomes a concern of all. One of the chronic problems found in so many American hospitals stems from the domination of one over the other two or the abrogation of responsibility by one to the other two. In hospitals attached to university medical schools the problems of the doctor's institutional role are somewhat different but not necessarily less complex. In such instances the medical staff must interface with still another complex institution, the university itself. Perhaps an example of the least complex doctor-institutional relationship is found in military and Veterans Administration hospitals.

Policy-Making Agents

The medical activities in the hospital, even on a day-to-day basis, are related to policy considerations which must be considered by the board or by the administrator. What the doctors decide can affect accreditation of the hospital, an agreement with Blue Cross or Blue Shield, the administration of Medicare and Medicaid, or even a fund raising campaign. Such agreements bear on fundamental matters of policy and they cannot be relegated solely to two sectors of the triangle. The board and the administrator can assume primary responsibility for fund-raising, for example, but they quickly find it a crucial necessity to share some of the decisions with the doctors. Policy decisions to establish or enlarge nursing education clearly involve three elements of the basic triangle.

Pointing out that the special character of authority relationships in the triangle cannot be reliably compared with that of other organizations, such as universities, Ray E. Brown (1949) states: "No other formal organization can equal the obstacles to tranquility that are present in the medical staff-administrator-trustee triangle." He then goes on to make the familiar point that doctors are not employees of the institution. They are independent contractors who determine the nature of services to be rendered to the institution's clientele, yet the very nature and quality of the services performed largely determine how well the institution functions. Their livelihood depends less and less on home practice and more and more on the nonmedical staff and facilities of the hospital. Thus they are in the position of having much the same proprietary interest in the success of the organization as scientists have in an industrial enterprise or as teachers in an academic institution. The major difference, at least in open staff community general hospitals, is that they are not paid by the organization. The importance of this difference cannot be underestimated.

Paul Gordon (1962, p. 72) carries this point further by observing that the unique relationship of the doctor in the policy triangle is not something that has evolved out of custom alone. By the very charters of incorporation, no one other than doctors can engage in the practice of medicine. This separation of practice by doctors from "practice" by others who are responsible for other aspects of patient care has been firmly set down in a long series of court interpretations.

Court decisions may have clarified what constitutes medical practice, but they have not solved internal problems of *administrative* authority. The board is held legally responsible for who should be or should not be members of the medical staff, yet, except in medically managed departments, there is no financial contractual relationship between the board and the doctor. The doctor and patient engage in separate financial arrangements. The patient also makes another "contract" with the hospital and is thus subject to two foci or lines of authority. There is a "line" of administrative control from patient to nurse and up through administrator to board. The other line of control is from patient to doctor and to the medical staff. Decisions on diagnosis and orders for treatment are vested in the doctor. Decisions related to providing facilities and personnel to support diagnosis and therapy involve the administrator and board.

In the absence of a single line authority such as one finds in most bureaucratic organizations, certain accommodations are necessary. As previously noted, the board of trustees of the institution has ultimate power to appoint and reappoint doctors. But this power is rarely used as a weapon to coerce the medical staff. To establish some kind of rationale, authority mechanisms evolve with varying degrees of success to clarify the gray area of respective jurisdiction that is between what is clearly medical practice and what is purely and simply administration. Within the medical staff there is a quasi-hierarchical organization made up of officers and the many committees of the staff. The board and the administrator rely on this machinery of self-government by the medical staff organization as the formal link with the hospital organization.

It is through the process of persuasion by means of this linkage system, combined with a high incidence of informal contacts, that rational decisions come to be made to assure accountability for the success of all programs sponsored by the hospital. To bridge the communication gap at the interface, representatives of the medical staff are frequently appointed to program committees set up by the administrator or board. Agreements are reached which spell out what the medical representatives are expected to do over and above simply being medical practitioners. Sometimes such agreements are put in writing while at other times they remain at the verbal level. The success of any hospital-initiated program is dependent upon the doctors' broader commitments to the institution and upon the "climate" of relationships between medical staff and administration.

On many issues accommodation between the parties does not come easily.

Agreements have to be negotiated. Gordon (1962, p. 72) puts it clearly when he says: "The elements . . . stem from the power relationships, the control relationships, and the alternatives available to each group in what can here best be seen as a negotiated relationship and one constantly subject to renegotiation. They stem out of the alternative means of leverage and the amount of power behind that leverage that is available to each party involved in the negotiation . . . . Stated baldy, on a day-to-day basis, the voluntary hospital corporation and its agents have no legal or organizational means of controlling the service that the hospital has been set up to render."

Speaking specifically about the relationship of the administrator to the medical staff, Gordon (1962, p. 72) goes on to say: "The administrator cannot expect to exercise very much 'top-down' executive control over doctors. Legally he cannot control professional practice. Strategically, the doctors can relegate other activities to the sacrosanct area of 'practice' when they want. As with administrators in other lines, the hospital administrator can frequently be most effective in the role of consultation, persuasion, negotiation, integration of diverse interests, and the like.

Gordon as well as other experienced observers point out the fallacies of comparing the hospital administrator with the appointees of heads of other types of organizations. In dealing with the medical staff, the administrator can ill-afford to use autocratic methods in pushing through hospital programs. Likely as not the administrator who resorts to directive leadership over the medical staff will quickly find himself looking for another job. To be effective or to even survive, the administrator must demonstrate unusual skills of interpersonal communication. He must be able to size up the true perceptions of the medical staff. He must know where he can expect support and where he will find resistence. The strategy of his approach to the medical staff is often just as important as the substance of what he is trying to accomplish. Finally, good timing is crucial in his negotiations with the medical staff (Gordon, 1962, p. 72).

Formal Links in the System

Many of the current articles make the plea that the link between doctors, administrators, and policy-makers would be measurably enhanced by explicit representation of the medical staff on the board of trustees of the institution. Indeed, the Joint Commission on Accreditation of Hospitals did, at the end of the last decade, make this a very explicit recommendation for accreditation. In this observer's own research and in observations by others there appear to be strong and varied opinions about the amount and character of medical staff representation on the board. Doctors desiring more representation justify the desire by saying that many decisions are too technical for laymen to make. Lay members of boards express concern that doctors might fail to take a global view of the institution's needs. Also, the danger of greater MD representation could mean that a doctor who was not an official representative of the medical staff might tend to grind a personal axe. He could not speak objectively "wearing two hats," for he might take issue with the official medical representative (the executive committee chairman) and create confusion in his later discussions with colleagues at the hospital.

There is another process of representation often dealt with in the literature, namely, devices for seeing to it that nonmedical groups are more frequently utilized by official bodies of the medical staff itself. Dr. Nelson (1961) put it this way:

> The heads of departments, plus elected members from the medical staff as a whole, should constitute the basic membership of the executive committee of the medical staff or medical board. It is here in this executive committee or medical board that policies and procedures for the medical care of patients should be elaborated. Since this group's function is to set rules for physicians and their work in the hospital with all other groups, it is important that the hospital administrator be present and participate in deliberations. In my judgment, the chief nurse, the chief of radiology, pathology, and other fully organized departments also should be on the board. The executive committee of the medical staff should receive regular reports and participate in discussions on the general operation, including financial operation, of the hospital because the hospital administration needs the help and understanding of the physicians the committee represents.

Greater physician involvement in institutional (managerial) problems is more than merely a plea made by a few isolated or disgruntled administrative types. At least two prestigious national commissions posed the issue in the frankest and strongest terms: The latest official report on the state of our health system's health is that made by the Secretary's Advisory Committee on Hospital Effectiveness, appointed by John W. Gardner, Ph.D., the then Secretary of Health, Education, and Welfare. The committee bluntly recommended that "appropriate members of the medical staff shall be directly involved with the administration in developing the budget and operating plan, and in the achievement of financial and service objectives as budgeted and planned . . . ." The committee was convinced that physician participation in the budget and planning disciplines not only would help the hospital but also would help the physician's own performance—and, of course, the patient! The committee report says: ". . . the physician who has sat through a line-by-line examination of the pharmacy budget may consider that the inventory of tetracyclines could be reduced from five brands to two or three without lasting damage to the cause of medical freedom, for example, and the surgeon who has had to study the nursing department payroll might readily modify some of his demands on nursing department time and temper without lasting damage to either his pride or his patients." Just before the report previously cited came out, anothr study weighted in, this one prepared by the National Advisory Commission on Health Manpower. This commission also found a shocking lack of physician involvement in management process, noting that "although physicians are subordinates in the formal organization of the hospital, they are the leaders in the informal organization that controls most hospital decisions. How to give physicians responsibility commensurate with their authority is a problem. Presently, most physicians feel little responsibility to a hospital because they pay nothing for its use; neither do they suffer any direct consequences when the hospital gets into financial trouble . . . medical and hospital associations should jointly explore means to increase the physician's responsibility for the successful and economical management of hospital operations." (cf. Crosby, 1968, p. 47f.)

Characteristics and Assumptions About Doctor-Hospital Relationships: A Summary

The Relationship Between Doctor and Institution

The observations above serve to highlight some of the central issues concerning the role of the doctor as practitioner and staff member in his relationship to other elements of the hospital institution. Most of the literature appears to confirm what has been said about the basic characteristics of the relationship between the doctor and the institution. These may be summarized as follows:

1. The doctor was and is officially a "guest" of the institution, but his privileges as a "guest" are being limited by increasing pressures to conform to certain organizational constraints of the medical staff, the hospital, and third party agreements.
2. The doctor is the "independent professional," but he is becoming increasingly interdependent in his relationship to his colleagues, other professionals, the administrator, and the governing authority of the institution.
3. The doctor makes his own financial contractual arrangements with his clients but these arrangements are to an increasing extent preestablished in schedules set up under health insurance, Medicare, Medicaid, and other third-party agreements.
4. The doctor has a fundamental right to minister to his client, the patient, but the responsibility for "total patient treatment" appears to be shifting toward greater involvement of other "professionals," including administrators.
5. The knowledge of clinical practice is "owned" by the doctor, but the technical tools of his practice are owned in large degree by the institution which gives him the privilege to practice. Even the doctor's clinical knowledge is being supplemented by specialized knowledge of other, nonmedical, members of the institution.
6. The doctor's role as a member of the hospital organization, as distinguished from his purely professional role, is being made increasingly explicit in bylaws of the medical staff and in written agreements with

administrators, boards, and outside parties of interest.

Medical Staff and the Governing Authority

Both in the literature and in studies by this observer certain basic assumptions about the role of the doctor (and staff) vis-a-vis the governing authority appear to have been accepted, with varying degrees of understanding or commitment, by all persons and groups concerned with setting policy. Generally, it is assumed that:
1. The governing authority (the board) is responsible for the final approval of all major policies pertaining to the hospital;
2. The governing authority has to delegate both responsibility and authority for medical care to the hospital medical staff, and the medical executive committee or its equivalent is the structural instrument for this delegation;
3. The board of trustees has the sole power to appoint all members to the clinical departments as well as the chairman of the executive committee, but only on the recommendation of the medical staff organization;
4. Recommendations for staff membership go to the governing authority and the governing authority must apply certain criteria in determining eligibility for staff appointment; and,
5. Some kind of communication mechanism should be formally established to assure a sustained relationship between the medical staff, the administrator, and the governing authority.

Assumptions about Medical Staff Organization

Another series of frequently made assumptions relevant to prevailing institutional arrangements in hospitals concerns medical staff organization. These assumptions may be articulated as follows:
1. On matters of professional ethics and discipline within the medical staff the responsibility lay with the executive committee or is delegated to the chiefs of the clinical departments with added responsibility vested in the administrator to monitor actions by the medical staff.
2. The approval of credentials (not necessarily the collection of credentials), as well as the evaluation and appraisal of diagnostic and therapeutic activities, is the responsibility of the medical staff executive committee or an equivalent body.
3. The medical executive committee has the authority to organize the departments and the necessary committees for carrying out medical functions.
4. The medical staff, through its executive committee, makes reports to the governing authority or to its representative, the administrator (the amount, the character, and the substance of these reports are are always clearly defined).
5. The medical executive committee should operate in conformity with a set of written bylaws.

6. Bylaws must be approved ultimately by the governing board and, once approved, both governing board and the medical staff are bound by these bylaws.
7. Under no circumstances should any members of the governing board or the administrator attempt to pass judgment on the clinical ability of individual doctors.

An interpretive summary of much of the literature regarding the structural relationships linking board, administration, and medical staff can now be made:

1. The executive committee of the staff is the primary structural unit linking doctor to administrator and the governing board. The relationship of the chairman of the staff executive committee to the board, however, is not precisely that of subordinate to superior. He is a discussant, information-exchanger, and negotiator.
2. Board members and administrators, perhaps somewhat more than doctors, feel the need for more use of existing mechanisms for linking board and medical staff on policy matters.
3. Medical representation on the board is felt to be essential. But where an M.D. board member is not an official representative of the medical staff certain communication difficulties and interpersonal stresses are likely to develop.
4. "Reciprocal representation" is sometimes found to work reasonably effectively. Not only is the administrator present in staff meetings, but officials of the board attend executive committee meetings of the staff. This is wholly accepted and welcomed by the medical representatives in one study conducted by this observer.
5. Major programs developed by administrators as the result of policy decisions are not likely to be implemented if officials of the medical staff are not informed and, indeed, involved.
6. The structure of organization in the medical staff is not viewed as a wholly satisfactory mechanism for either the upward flow of information to the board in making policy decisions or for the flow of information downward. Putting it another way, the incumbents of the positions of formal authority within the medical staff are not ncessarily and at any given given period of time the persons to assure the upward and downward flow of information related to policy matters.
7. Most observers agree that the dynamic links throughout the hospital organization are those forged through informal day to day interactions, not by the periodic "engineering" of structural arrangements.

This last observation is appropriate to underscore as we turn to look at the future. It is in the future, with its increasing complexity, that new imaginative and, perhaps, even revolutionary means must be found to forge "dynamic" links of understanding among all who are concerned about delivering the best posible health service to the American public.

The Challenge of the Future

It appears reasonably certain that as one views the problems and promise of the 1970s it is unlikely that the medical profession can refrain from further involvement in the institutional decision-making process. This is true not only with respect to the hospital but also with respect to other institutions and agencies in the larger community.

This theme was expressed more frequently than any other in the recent literature. The following comment by Crosby (1968) is typical: "We now have to tie the practicing physician, regardless of the type of his practice, into the management of our health care services system. Physicians should be deeply involved in the planning and managing of all aspects of our health services system, inside and outside the hospital."

We have seen and will continue to see the proliferation of hospital insurance plans, expansion and changes in Blue Shield, Blue Cross, and other third-party agreements. Medicare-Medicaid is bound to expand and change. The medical profession's role in these changes will be crucial. Further developments in intensive care and programs for progressive patient care will be stepped up. Group medical practice is likely to grow with changes in state laws. Prepaid comprehensive health schemes could proliferate substantially with basic changes in federal support. New forms of family-centered treatment, home care, links with nursing homes, community health centers (and especially community mental health) are appearing and will continue to expand. The system of nursing education linking hospitals to community colleges should find the medical profession in the center of the decision-making process. Regional planning of facilities involving several hospitals is already appearing as an economic necessity. Service centers in regions are and will provide central laundries, dietary departments, purchasing (including pharmaceuticals), and data processing units to groups of hospitals. The regional medical center concept has been accepted virtually as a matter of national health policy. In such moves the individual hospitals must learn to "give up" some of their cherished independence. Such decisions are more than purely administrative. They involve basic policies with the necessity for the medical profession to have both the knowledge about such decisions and a very direct involvement in them.

Dr. Nelson's (1960, pp. 42-43) observations early in the last decade appear to be valid both today and for tomorrow:

> To meet the growing demand for better and more comprehensive medical care, better organization will be required of physicians on hospital staffs in order to develop patterns for providing a wider range of services in outpatient clinics, rehabilitation units, nursing homes, and related paramedical facilities. The whole concept of the regionalization of hospitals or of creating working affiliations between general hospitals and paramedical institutions can be established administratively with moderate ease, but it could founder and fail unless suitable, workable and agreeable

professional arrangements can be made. The physicians will be apprehensive because of fears of domination and regimentation. They must be reassured that their professional independence will be maintained.

Administrators and doctors, especially deans of medical schools, keep stressing the need for helping medical students to understand better the *organizational* roles they can be expected to play in the professional practice of medicine. As one medical observer (Cadmus, 1965, p. 49) put it: "Should all medical schools ever offer systematized instruction in hospital-physician relations, reenforcement and elaboration during the postgraduate period would still be an asset. Certainly, the understanding of hospital-physician relations can be improved through properly designed education."

Ample warnings are given to the effect that standard and "packaged" programs on management would be useless in the medical school curricula. They must be tailored to the special needs of the profession and not drawn primarily from management programs of industry or the business schools. An observation by a British physician (Anderson, 1967) is quite appropriate to the American picture as well:

A complex and expensive modern hospital can be efficient only when all those who can contribute to this efficiency are prepared, and indeed trained, to exercise the functions which in industry would be described as managerial . . . .

However, the techniques of management as they are defined for industry will probably not be immediately applicable to hospital medicine. It is too easily assumed that analogies can be made between hospitals and industry. Although there is much to be learnt from the expanding experience of business management, many aspects will require fundamental reinterpretation before they can be applied to hospitals. Indeed, it may be sensible to assume that management is not learnt by attendance at an indoctrination course at which some wise men set down a few simple rules. The most that can be done in a management course is to open the minds of the participants to a process of self-examination. The success of any training scheme will be measured by the desire of its participants to conduct a "do-it-yourself" study of some aspect of their own situation and to appreciate the need for expert advice when such studies are planned.

In developing medical school programs and, indeed, in providing the present practitioners with greater understanding of institutional relationships (over and above "patient" relationships), some observers believe the experience of doctors engaged in community and public health programs would be valuable. According to Christman (1965), for example, "Physicians actively engaged in rehabilitation and in community mental health programs appear to be much more sensitive than most physicians in perceiving how patient care is organized as a social process. With the rapidly growing complexity of health care, it seems a foregone conclusion that every member of each discipline will have to be increasingly cognizant of the whole social design of health care."

Some Speculations on Major Trends in Medical Service

We are beginning to see the broad outlines of the so-called whole social design of health care. Some of the parts of the design were alluded to earlier in the mention of comprehensive prepaid schemes linked to group practice. Increased use of paramedicals was also mentioned. The Garfield article (1970) develops the thesis that the traditional fee-for-service treatment is obsolete, that health services will have to be practiced in some form of group practice in a prepayment arrangement. He describes the enormous waste of the MD's time in the way the traditional system of treatment has worked. He suggests that the doctor's major effort should be devoted to sick care and rely more on well-trained paramedical professionals to assume the burden for health-testing service, for health-care service, and for preventive-maintenance service.

According to Garfield's research, "We can save at least 50 percent of our general practitioners', internists', and pediatricians' time." He speculates further about the organizational structure of medical care under the new system as follows: ". . . a central medical center, well staffed and equipped would provide sick care. It could have four or five 'outreach' neighborhood clinics, each providing the three primarily paramedical services: health testing, health care and preventive maintenance. Staffing these services with paramedical personnel should be much less difficult than staffing clinics with doctors."

One may take issue with the details of Garfield's proposal, an idea derived from long experience with the Kaiser-Permanente prepaid comprehensive plan. There is certainly no assurance that the Americal Medical Association will accept the idea readily. There is very serious question that such a major change in the delivery of medical services is possible without massive support from the federal government. But if we can hypothesize that a much larger proportion of the doctor's total professional activity can be carried out by non-MDs we can speculate further on two consequences. First, it could alleviate many of the current stresses we observed as we viewed the doctor's institutional role under the present set-up. As pointed out, these stresses or frictions arose not simply because doctors were poorly trained in dealing with administrative matters; they also emerged from the frustrations which the physicians themselves experienced when they were "pushed" by institutional demands to engage in activities not directly and immediately related to the care of the sick. Second, conversely, the doctors will have to accept new commitments which demand some proportion of their time to new kinds of institutionally related activities. They will have to become directly involved in planning for the training and allocation of the expanded paramedical activities. Further, they must play a major part in organizing outreach clinics whose services revolve around health-testing, health-care, and preventive maintenance.

The application of findings from behavioral science research could be crucial in the solution of future problems. As was suggested in the beginning of this paper, a number of useful contributions have been made by sociologists and psychologists working in many types of institutions, including hospitals. What was lacking in past research was more and better research with doctors on their institutional roles vis-à-vis nonmedical groups. One hopes that the next decade will bring about greater cooperative research effort among those in the medical profession and the behavior disciplines.

References

Anderson, T. The hospital clinician's role from two standpoints. *Lancet,* 1967, *2,* 1246-1248.

Brown, R. E. In the board-administrator relationships hospital tensions threaten tenure. *Modern Hospital,* 1949, *73,* 51-53.

Burling, T., Lentz, E. M., and Wilson, R. N. *The give and take in hospitals.* New York: Putnam, 1956.

Cadmus, R. R. Hospital-physician understanding begins during medical school. *Hospitals,* 1965, *39,* 49.

Christman, L. P. Nurse-physician communications in the hospital. *Journal of the American Medical Association,* 1965, *194,* 539-544.

Crosby, E. L. Physician's place in health care administration. *Hospitals,* 1968, *42,* 47.

Garfield, S. R. The delivery of medical care. *Scientific American,* 1970, *222,* 4, 15-23.

Georgopoulos, B. S., and Mann, F. C. *The community general hospital.* New York: Macmillan, 1962.

Gordon, P. J. The top management triangle in voluntary hospitals, I and II. *Journal of the Academy of Management,* 1961, *4,* 205-214; 1962, *5,* 66-75.

Guest, R. H. The role of the doctor. In A. B. Moss, W. G. Broehl, Jr., R. H. Guest, and J. W. Hennessey, Jr. (Eds) *Hospital policy decisions: process and action.* New York: Putnam, 1966.

Nelson, R. A. Challenge of the sixties: the physician and the hospital. *Hospitals,* 1960, *34,* 42-43.

Nelson, R. A. Physician and the hospital. *Hospitals,* 1961, *35,* 44-47.

Parsons, T. Social change and medical organization in the United States: a sociological perspective. *Annals of the American Academy of Political and Social Science,* 1963, *346,* 21-23.

Rosen, G. Notes on some aspects of the sociology of medicine with particular reference to prepaid group practice. Unpublished manuscript quoted by Robert W. Wilson (1959-60) in "The Physician's changing hospital role."

Wilson, R. N. The physician's changing hospital role. *Human Organization,* 1959-60, *18,* 177-183.

13

THE CHANGING MATRIX OF CLINICAL DECISION-MAKING IN THE HOSPITAL*

Edmund D. Pellegrino

The process of making clinical decisions is the balance wheel of hospital operation. It is central to all the patient-oriented functions of the hospital, and it has remote effects on all major elements of hospital organization—the patient, the health care professionals, administrators, trustees, and the community. It is also the process least accessible to organizational control, the most in need of freedom and yet the most potent of hospital processes for good and evil. The clinical decision is the most zealously guarded of the physician's prerogatives and at the same time the most in need of some kind of surveillance for individual and public good. It is, moreover, the most difficult process to evaluate in a definitive way.

In a sense, everyone who works in the hospital, or is associated with hospital decision-making, to some extent also participates in clinical decision-making. The decision of the trustees, for example, to initiate an open heart surgery program, install cobalt therapy apparatus, or to engage a full-time staff, all have ultimate effects on the well-being of patients in a hospital. The same is true of admission and business policies, the decision of laundry workers to strike, etc. Such an interpretation is, however, too broad to produce anything more than a global review of decision-making, which would scarcely be useful to an analysis of the central medical activity in the hospital.

We will, therefore, understand clinical decision-making in this discussion to refer to the processes whereby the most prudent and beneficial actions are chosen to meet the medical needs of the patient when he seeks aid from a hospital. We refer for the most part to those decisions which are made, so to speak, at the "bedside" by physicians, nurses, and other health professionals who provide personal and technical services, and which bear on the patient's reasons for seeking assistance. We include, also, those policies and decisions made at a distance, i.e. by the institution as such and by the community, which alter the context of clinical decisions and impinge necessarily upon the relationship of patient and physician, even though indirectly.

Clinical decisions have traditionally been vested for the most part in the physician and, to a lesser extent, in other health professionals. Today the

*Revised version of paper presented at Conference on Hospital Organization Research, May 22-23, 1970, Institute for Social Research, The University of Michigan, Ann Arbor, Michigan. Edmund D. Pellegrino, M.D., is Vice President for the Health Sciences and Director of the Health Sciences Center, State University of New York at Stony Brook.

context within which even intimate clinical decisions are made has become institutionalized, organized, and more public than ever before possible. Even individual clinical decisions now have implications beyond the welfare of the patient and in the aggregate touch upon society at large. The physician is, in consequence, no longer free to make his decisions apodictically or in isolation from policies, procedures, and goals established on an institutional and societal basis.

It is the purpose of this essay to examine the very drastically changing matrix of relationships which now characterize the context of clinical decision-making (see Chart 1, near the end of this chapter). To this end we shall first examine the expectations of the major participants and the way in which they may confront each other. Then the factors changing the traditional primacy of the physician will be detailed, particularly the intro-duction of the team concept of care and the imposition of institutional as well as consumer controls and accountability. A set of relationships will be described which may provide a reasonable context for decision-making con-sonant with the legitimate expectations of the community, the institution, and the professionals. Finally, the role of sociomedical research on the value choices essential to any rational system of decision-making will be touched upon.

Divergence and Confrontation of Expectations

Much of the difficulty in achieving satisfaction by participants, safety for the subject, and surveillance by society of the decision-making process arises from a failure fully to appreciate the confrontation of expectations within which the decisions are made. Let us first examine these expectations from the points of view of physicians, the other health professionals, administra-tors, trustees, and the patients themselves. Any research into the decision-making process must examine critically this catalogue of expectations.
ᶜexpectations.

The Physician

Within broad limits, the physician sees himself as the central authoritative figure and the final arbiter in the making of clinical decisions. Following the Hippocratic ethic, he is still, by and large, the benign father figure who knows best and who takes upon himself the responsibility for the judgments he makes and even for judgments that a patient might wish to make. The physician's attitude toward the hospital is that it is an instrument designed to serve him and his patient, and that, within reasonable bounds, he has a right to demand the resources—in personnel, facilities, and equipment—he deems essential for the optimal care of *his* patient. From this point of view all other hospital personnel, administration, and the board of trustees become facilitators of what he, the physician, may demand in the name of his patient or what the medical staff as a body may demand for all patients. The overriding responsibility of the individual physician for his own patient is so ingrained in the tradition and history of the medical profession that the doctor's expectations are often expressed within a framework of righteousness which, in the extreme, assumes hieratic proportions.

There is undeniably some justification for the physician's primacy in decision-making in special clinical contexts. In emergency, in the operating room, in technical diagnostic matters, the good of the patient as determined by the good physician must have precedence. What needs examination is the extent to which this primacy in acute or difficult matters is translated to all aspects of hospital operation and to all levels of health care. The physician's expectations must be adjusted to the demands of a democratic society and a highly organized system of health-care delivery. The very goal the physician properly uses to justify his expectations—the good of the patient—is itself contingent upon a restructuring of the decision-making process in and out of the hospital.

The Administrator

The administrator has a different set of expectations for his hospital. He sees it primarily as a complex managerial and societal apparatus directed toward the delivery of health services to patients. His major emphasis is on the aggregate of patients rather than on individual services for individual patients. The administrator expects, in addition, that the hospital will be a community agency, attempting to meet broad responsibilities in the field of health and clinical care. The hospital is also an industry producing a product, namely patient care and services. While the administrator does not participate directly in the definition of the nature of this product, he feels he can and should modify it in nontechnical ways. It is his role, too, to interpret the institutional commitment of the hospital to the community it serves.

For the administrator the physician is the most potent force in decision-making, not only in regard to care of individual patients but in regard to the setting of the policies, goals, and commitments of the hospital. The administrator expects the board of trustees to see the hospital in a broad community perspective and to regard him as the coordinator and manager of the process of production of health care and community services. The administrator easily recognizes the need for a partition of decision-making functions. The technical, medical one-to-one decisions he easily cedes to the physician. But he expects clinical decisions which pertain to the aggregate of patients to be determined in a broader frame. The professional staff may set technical policies, but the managerial, administrative, coordinative implications of these decisions are to be monitored by the administrator and subject to the assent of the board of trustees. Every policy decision implies some priority in resources and personnel, and a rational policy is not the simple sum of individual clinical decisions by individual physicians.

The Board of Trustees

The expectations of the board of trustees, on the other hand, focus on the hospital as a community resource which is committed to provide an optimal quality of care to the patients of the community in terms largely defined by the physicians and implemented by the administrators. The trustees expect the hospital to be managed efficiently and to be fiscally sound. Depending upon their degree of sophistication, moreover, trustees may assume a role of leadership in defining and meeting certain additional social and community needs.

As to the decision-making process, the trustees, like administrators, delegate individual medical, technical, and professional decisions to the physicians. They must intervene when clinical decisions and policies influence the direction of the hospital, especially the distribution of its resources. Trustees see themselves to varying degrees as advocates and surrogates for the community's interests. They implicitly take upon themselves final responsibility for the quality of professional services provided in the institution. But this responsibility is in fact exerted usually only by indirection and by an act of faith in the competence of the professional and administrative staff.

The Nonphysician and Nonprofessional Staff

Another set of expectations intersects those of physician, administrator, and board of trustees, and this is the set held by the nonphysician and nonprofessional staff of a hospital. These groups exhibit varying degrees of expectation with regard to decision-making which are directly related to the intimacy of their involvement in the personal care of patients. Nursing, allied health professions, and pharmacists, for example, expect a more intimate participation than medical or x-ray technologists or medical record librarians. All, however, expect to participate when the process involves those circumscribed areas within which they have expertise. The potent decision-makers—the physicians—are urged to seek out, and defer to, the observations and opinions within the competencies of the other health professions. These professions yield to the physician as major clinical decision-maker in the emergency situation, but increasingly they expect to influence clinical decisions in the nonemergency and less technical facets of patient care. Increasingly, too, they seek greater independence in decisions within their own fields of competence.

This entire nonphysician group expects the hospital to ensure legitimate opportunity for the expression of their professional interests as members of a coordinated and complex health care team. Nonphysician professionals often consider themselves as advocates for the patient against the high-powered technical apparatus of clinical decision-making now authoritatively managed and predominantly controlled by the physician.

The Patient

The patient's expectations are at some variance with those of the physician, administrator, trustees, and health-related professionals, even when these latter so earnestly reassert that all their expectations are rooted in the good of the patient. The patient very clearly sees the hospital as an instrument of specific social purposes. He has every right to expect the needs he feels and brings to the institution to be the focal points around which the resources of the institution must be concentrated. The patient wants to know what is wrong, how it happened, why it happened, and whether it can be treated or prevented. He wants his dignity preserved as a person to a maximal extent possible. He expects courtesy and consideration and understanding. To the degree that he is educated, he will demand an understanding of the technical decision-making which affects his well-being. In the spirit of contemporary participatory democracy, the patient will demand to have some input into the clinical decision-making process as it relates to his illness and to the technical choices which may influence its outcome. Should he be operated upon? Should he take a dangerous drug? Why? What is the cost benefit analysis from his point of view?

The patient also expects the hospital to be available to meet his and the community's emergency needs, on an ever-ready basis, at every hour of the day and night. Moreover, as a member of the general community who only transiently becomes a member of the hospital community, the citizen expects the hospital to ensure the quality of care it provides, to be accountable for the responsible distribution of the dollars which he and others contribute, and to take leadership in providing efficient and economical health-care delivery. The public expects the whole apparatus of the hospital to be pointed to the satisfaction of the needs it feels, and not only those seen by the hospital. The community expects the board of trustees to be its surrogate in making the hospital a responsive and efficient instrument for the improvement of the health of the individual and of the society in which it functions.

When the citizen becomes a patient, he unquestionably wants the decisions to lie with his own physician. As he moves out of the patient role, the citizen demands that the clinical decision-making of the physicians and other health professionals be carried out within a framework which provides safeguards for the patient and for society, In both roles the lay individual expects clinical decisions to be competent and consistent with the present state of medical knowledge. He has every expectation that the hospital will provide access to the full panorama of technical and scientific resources available in the modern world.

The expectations catalogued here are frequently incongruent. Indeed, the confluence of these expectations and the changing nature of medicine in society have vastly complicated the traditional process of clinical decision-making. Clearly we cannot at once meet all the expectations of the physician, the patient, or the administrator in any absolute sense. The self-defined values, roles, and responsibilities of each group are in a situation of increasing tension. We live now in a state of dynamic equilibrium wherein these forces converge at the point of clinical decision-making. This locus continually changes its coordinates, depending upon the shifting strengths of the expectations which converge upon it.

Clearly, any sudden or unexpected surge of force from any one of these directions may perturb the system in dangerous and unpredictable ways. For example, the very strong pressures from minority communities for absolute control of personnel, resources, and facilities to make them responsive to their aspirations regarding health have already perturbed the system of clinical decision-making in certain communities. We can expect further perturbations as other groups grow in political and economic power and come into possession of the levers which can control clinical and nonclinical decision-making within the hospital structure.

The confluence of the variant expectations felt by physicians, administrators, and communities can generate serious confrontations. A new equilibrium between these forces must be established in which some accommodation of diverse goals and subgoals is succesfully effected. In any such accommodation the most serious disruption will occur in the physician's, and society's, perceptions of the physician-patient relationship.

Factors Influencing the Physician's Role

Society up to now has delegated almost all authority to the physician, and for very valid reasons which cannot be ignored as new relationships are generated. Our high regard for the life of individuals and the relief of suffering has contributed greatly to the primacy of the physician in decision-making. The immediate good of the individual patient is thus placed above the more remote good of the group, even in the use of scarce resources. Each patient enters into a personal contract protected by legal and ethical sanctions, in which the physician is expected to protect the patient against harm and promote his welfare under all circumstances. The patient pays the physician, not the hospital, for this service, and the hospital becomes the physician's instrument for its attainment. The patient fully expects the physician and the hospital to respond to his immediate needs, even if it means a disproportionate allocation of community resources.

It is quite difficult and quite impossible for the administrator or trustee to deny the power of this surrogate function assumed by the physician for his patient. This explains too why clinical decisions have been so clearly delegated to the physician and why their structure has been so little studied.

The primacy of the physician and the privacy of his clinical decisions are, however, already being compromised by a number of potent influences which are changing the context of medical practice.

First is the vastly increased knowledge base available to today's physicians. The natural history of many serious disorders can be demonstrably altered; other diseases can be prevented completely; and even noncurable disorders can be effectively ameliorated. Failure to possess or apply a piece of technical knowledge can literally spell the difference between death and survival, or between a useful life and one of disability. The new capabilities of medicine, therefore, make the assurance of competence a matter of social significance and thus subject to closer scrutiny.

To ensure optimal realization of its capabilities, medicine has acquired a larger technologic base and is becoming more organized into a system.

Specialization is inevitable, and where there is specialization there is division of labor. A team of experts must be organized to guarantee that all a patient's needs can be met. In a team relationship the physician inevitably shares some of his decision-making authority with other members and is required to expose the bases for many of his decisions.

Expansion of the knowledge and technological base for medical decisions is taking place in a political atmosphere of egalitarianism and participatory democracy. In every aspect of life the community expects to exert greater influence on choosing the ends to which institutions shall be directed. The valuation of all human services, therefore, depends on the extent to which they fulfill expressed social and public needs. Within this pervading political climate all professions are becoming functionalized and democratized, and all their traditional prerogatives are being questioned as never before. Medicine is no exception; it too must respond by willingness to subject its decisions to the scrutiny of peers and institutions in the interest of accountability. Medicine thus assumes many of the features of a public service and becomes less a hieratic function in society.

We are, in addition, entering an era in which even our much vaunted affluence has proved insufficient to alleviate the social ills of large numbers of our population. Every decision affecting the distribution of resources must face a more rigorous priority review. For the first time in several decades we are forced to choose one social good over another. Health is only one of the desperately needed services which society must distribute more widely. And within health there is a growing public preference for primary preventive and emergency care over the more complicated secondary and tertiary levels of care required by more complex but essentially uncurable disorders. We must consciously support these choices rationally.

These priorities in health care are being established in an era of expanding community control, particularly in disenfranchised sectors of our population. Spurred by the gap between expectations and delivery, and justifiably frustrated by decades of discrimination, our deprived populations are asserting their demands for medical care on their own terms. We are in real danger of the establishment of parallel or competing systems of health care. Well-intentioned community attempts at providing more primary and preventive care for the poor and the disadvantaged can be self-defeating without professional participation.

Contemporary medicine, further, is emerging as the instrument through which the new knowledge of human biology will be applied in society. The capabilities of medicine will then extend well beyond the cure of individual disease states. The potentialites for genetic engineering, control of the reproductive process, eugenics and euphenics, and behavioral modification will place medicine even more clearly in the public realm. Definition of the ends to which this new and potent information shall be directed is of the greatest significance for the human species. Public surveillance and participation in medical decisions in these spheres is essential if physicians and biologists are not to determine the future of mankind by themselves.

To all of this must be added the institutionalization of large segments of medical care. Patients in ever larger numbers contract with hospitals, clinics, and groups rather than with individual physicians. The institution is thus vested with the responsibility for the quality and competence of the decisions made relative to the patient's care. It must fulfill its legal and ethical responsibilities by demanding partnership with the physician in providing health care.

All of these factors must inevitably lead to an erosion of the physician's ancient primacy in clinical decision-making and must also, in consequence, open up those decisions to broader inquiry than ever before imagined possible. There are obvious dangers in this movement and also certain advantages. To deny these trends is to contravene some of the major forces in contemporary life. Even medicine, with its long history and its high value to society, cannot accomplish that, assuming it were desirable. Rather we must acknowledge the existence of a drastically altered context for all medical transactions. New models for decision-making within the hospital apparatus must be devised. The newer models must somehow optimize the making of prudential decisions for the individual patient while allowing for greater participation of other professions and institutions in the process. This means a restructuring of the decision-making apparatus within the hospital and a new relationship between the profession and the hospital, on the one hand, and the community, on the other.

Patient-Care, Medical-Care, and Health-Care Teams

Social scientists have applied many models to the analysis of the social organization of medicine and hospitals. Various paradigms, including the entrepreneurial, bureaucratic, craftsman, professional, and technical, have been applied but found insufficient in one degree or another. In the writer's view the model which seems to fit best with current trends in professional organization and with demands for specialization of functions and services is the team model, regarded essentially as a transitory system. Since the team is so fundamental to the attainment of comprehensive, continuing, and competent mecial care, it should be examined briefly as the essential element in any revised view of clinical decision-making.

Indeed, the central logistic problem in health-care delivery is a human problem: can we effectively organize and coordinate all who have something to contribute to the care of the patient? Only in the resolution of this problem can we find the full capabilities of scientific medicine to every patient in every community in this country. The team is an essential mechanism for fulfillment of the expectations of society for comprehensive health care; it is, moreover, the locus for the first steps in sharing of responsibility between the physician and other health professionals; and it is within its confines that the first movement toward a revision of clinical decision-making can occur.

Despite the inherent difficulties in any attempt to define what constitutes a health-care team, some operational if arbitrary definition must be used.

Generically, a team is any group of persons cooperatively working together for the attainment of some defined goal. When applied to the health care system, the team goal is the satisfaction of certain specific health care needs of individuals or communities. There are at least three levels at which the team can function, and we shall call them as follows: the patient care team, the medical care team, and the health care team levels. These teams are distinguished from each other on the basis of two things: the needs they are designed to satisfy, and the degree of their immediacy of contact with the patients they serve.

The patient care team comprises any group of professionals, semi-, and nonprofessionals who jointly provide needed services which bring them into direct personal or physical contact with the patient and which are part of a program of management for that patient. Doctors, nurses, social workers, dieticians, and aides are examples of members of this kind of team.

The medical care team consists of those professionals, semiprofessionals, and nonprofessionals who provide some needed service in the management of the patient which does not bring them directly or personally into contact with the patient. Examples here would be the operating room supervisor or the hospital administrator, the pharmacist and the laboratory technician, business and purchasing personnel, and others.

The health care team consists of all who are engaged in providing some service or in planning for some service which will improve the general or community health, but which does not require direct or indirect contact with the specific needs of a specific patient.

The number of individuals on any of these teams may be fixed or variable, depending upon the task to be performed. Team composition will change even for the same patient, as the number, variety, and intensity of his needs vary.

Obviously, the captaincy of the team will change depending upon the configuration of the patient's needs at any particular time. The physician will clearly be the captain of the team when the situation is grave, requires highly technical information or skills, and high degrees of judgment ranging over a series of technical considerations. Under these circumstances he will assume the primary role in assessment of the patient's most urgent needs, decide on the order in which they should be satisfied, and work out with the other team members in a collaborative manner a plan of management adjusted to meeting the short- and long-term needs of the patient.

It is equally clear that in the carrying out of agreed upon specific tasks, subteams will come into being, also composed in accordance with the task to be done. Even in the complicated situation these subteams of technicians, pharmacists, nurses, dieticians, etc., often will not include physicians. In that case only the product of their endeavors will come under the physician's surveillance and then only when it is fitted into the total management plan for that patient.

When the patient's condition is less acute, less complicated, or when he suffers from a slowly progressive chronic disorder, the teams may for a period of time be under the captaincy of one of the health professions other than medicine. The captain of the team should be determined by the dominant features essential in the management of the patient. The captain should be the person who possesses the skill and knowledge most consonant with the dominant features of the clinical condition exhibited by the patient.

The patient with a stroke will illustrate some facets of the shifting functions, personnel, and captaincy of teams, and the partition of functions between patient care, medical care, and health care.

When the patient is first admitted, in coma or semicoma, with or without such complications as pneumonia, heart failure, of hypertension, he presents a life-threatening acute medical problem. The physician and other medical specialists, working with intensive care nurses, inhalation therapists, pharmacists, and laboratory technicians, constitute the major team designed to meet the patient's needs. The physician will be captain at this point. Obviously, during most of the day and night the nurse in the intensive care unit will act as temporary or ad hoc captain; she will call for the others as needed. Observations made via instrumentation, nurses, cardirespiratory therapists, and laboratory technicians are fed into the team process continually. Those serving the patient immediately and directly—the physician, nurse, cardiopulmonary technician—constitute his patient care team. Members of the medical care team—those performing essential tasks but not directly or personally involved on a continuous basis—move into, and out of, the patient's ambit as his needs dictate. Examples of the latter are the medical laboratory, x-ray technicians, the radiologist and pathologist, dieticians, and pharmacists. At this stage the health care team, as defined above, will have little contribution tomake to the care of this patient.

In the next phase of illness, as the patient begins to recover from the acute insult to his cerebral functions, his needs change markedly. He will move from the acute intensive care unit to the regular nursing service. His needs now center on treatment of the underlying disorders like hypertension, diabetes, and heart disease. Of equal importance is the patient's rehabilitation, which soon assumes a dominant position as the patient and the family begin to assess the impact of the residual disability. The patient care team now assumes a different composition—physician and physiatrist share the major medical responsibility with the nurse. The physiotherapist, social worker, and dietician move into the clinical context for the variable periods as rehabilitative and long-term measures are instituted and the patient is prepared to return to his own home or a nursing home. Thus some professionals who were members of the patient care team in the acute phase of illness now become part of the medical care team, and the reverse applies to still others.

Toward the end of his hospital stay the patient's chief needs are in the realm of rehabilitation—exercises, speech therapy, learning about diet and the use of long-term medications. If the potential is manifest, he may begin occupational or vocational rehabilitation, and then these specialities enter the circle of care. For extended periods the physician's actual contribution may be minimal, while other health professionals assume major responsibilities.

When the patient is able to return home, the nonphysician services—physical therapy, visiting nursing, social work—all become of even more importance to the patient's well-being. The physician sees the patient less frequently and depends heavily upon other health professionals and the family to carry major responsibilities.

It is when the patient is at home and has in a sense rejoined the community that he becomes a more major concern to the health care team as a member of a group of patients with hypertension who have had strokes and who share common needs. Here the mobilization of community resources to assist in his rehabilitation, welfare, and job adjustment must have been established beforehand by health planners, health departments, and community and governmental agencies. Thus provision of visiting nurse services, home visits by physiotherapists, welfare or sickness benefits, homemaker services, aid in transportation, and a host of other services all are the purview of the health care team, which concerns itself with the larger aggregate of patients and persons of which our patient is one example.

The Team as a Transitory System: Further Questions and Research Needs

Clearly the three types of teams we have described fit best the model of transitory systems, i.e. systems adjusted in composition and captaincy to the needs of individual patients, dedicated to specific tasks, and deriving their existence from these tasks. The patient care and medical care teams interchange personnel and responsibilities as they address the ad hoc problems posed by individual patients. Some teams, like the operating team, are more or less permanent, but they too bear a transitory relationship to the patient which is intensive while he is in the operating room and disappears when he leaves it.

Decision-making in this kind of functional arrangement is increasingly a corporate and cooperative undertaking. Information is continually being fed into the patient care team by its members, as well as members of the medical care and even the health care teams. Teams and subteams address themselves to specific problems, and if the system works optimally each ad hoc team will be assigned the task it is best fitted to perform. Ideally, communication between members and cooperative decision-making can be coordinated for the benefit of the patient.

The key problem is one of coordination, captaincy, and task assignment in a well-formulated and agreed-upon management plan. Most physicians do not as yet accept the idea of a shifting captaincy or of truly shared responsibility and decision-making authority. In more technical situations they can effectively function as team captain—for example in the operating room, emergency room, or cardiac catheterization laboratory. But by and large physicians are not trained for the management role required for more long-range planning for comprehensive management of a patient's problems. This is essentially a job of social and systems engineering, for which physicians and other health professionals must be specifically trained.

The problems attendant upon sharing of authority and responsibility are obvious and difficult to resolve. How does the patient locate responsibility for malpractice? How does he keep from being lost in the tergiversations of irresponsible team members? How does the physician reconcile this sharing of responsibility with his traditional Hippocratic responsibility for the person of the patient? How do we untangle the legal, ethical, mechanical, and personal intersections? These questions are of very grave moment and immediate significance in the current trends toward team care (Pellegrino, 1964). They suggest pressing fields for crucial research by social and political scientists.

The team is a permanent piece of the patient-care apparatus, and we must find the means to make it work efficiently, safely, and considerately at all levels. We must face the full implication of team care, and we have not yet done so. If we wish patients to have the benefit of the coordinated skills of groups of professionals and technical workers in meeting their needs comprehensively, we must radically alter the current system of decision-making. Social and public sanctions must be forthcoming for these alternatives. Ethical and legal responsibilities must be assigned equitably from the point of view of both the patient and the health professional.

We need, therefore, a firmer theoretical grasp of the dynamics of transitory systems, more accurate models, and more experimentation in specific features of their operation. What is the best composition for a given team to enable it optimally to solve the specific ad hoc problems before it? What is the optimal assignment of tasks among existing health professionals and technicians? Are new roles required to carry out necessary tasks now neglected? Who shall be captain and under what conditions? When should the captaincy change? How is that decision made? How do we facilitate the input of all team members, assure consideration of that input, and guarantee that it will be used constructively, regardless of its source? How do we divide responsibility and yet give the team firm, clear direction which keeps it from becoming a mob?

These are some of the questions which the sociologist, psychologist, systems theorist, and operations specialist must confront in their research. Such questions precipitate resistance and anxiety in all current members of the patient care, medical care, and health care teams. But decision-making processes cannot be rationalized and adapted to the changing context of patient care today without provisional answers, at least. The questions will be relatively easy to answer in the case of the functions of an open-heart surgery or coronary care team, for example, but extremely difficult at the other extreme, when we approach the use of a team to provide primary care or comprehensive preventive health maintenance.

We must, in answering such questions as the above, resist the temptation to excessive speculation and theorizing or the incurable itch to collect interminably "more" data. The empirical approach, based on sound theory and soundly applied, is probably the most fruitful one at this juncture. We already have enough information to permit the construction of models built on the hypothesis of a transitory system. The testing of such models in actual patient care situations will validate or vitiate our theoretical formulations.

What is needed in major teaching hospitals, for example, is an experimental patient-care unit in which proper controls can be instituted and in which roles and tasks can be assigned and structured independently of those who now perform these tasks. Freedom to assign personnel based on an assessment of the patient's needs—both his own and the team's assessment—is essential. Only in this way can the usual impediments of professional prerogatives and the status neurosis of professional organizations be overcome.

Each level of care and each team model can be evaluated against one fundamental criterion: what is the effectiveness of the team's output in services, techniques, and skills, in relationship to the needs of those served? For research of this type to be significant, it must address itself to endpoints: effectiveness of care—that is, congruence between team output in service, techniques, and skills and the needs of those served. We must avoid the customary fascination with process and the reluctance to examine endpoints. Process, no matter how titillating to the student of health-care institutions, is meaningless unless it is related to some defined purpose, or outcome, which enhances the health of the people served.

Institutional Controls on Clinical Decision-Making

The entry of the interplay of team dynamics into the previously simple physician-patient relationship has greatly complicated the making of clinical decisions. But an equally potent factor altering the clinical decision-making context is the institutionalization of all aspects of medical care. We can address ourselves here only to the hospital; but it will serve as the paradigm for other modes of institutionalization (like group practices), in which the physician becomes a member of a corporate entity that assumes responsibility for providing medical care through the instrumentality of physicians and other health professionals. In these circumstances the physician must operate within at least two frames of accountability: his duties to the patient, and his duties to the institution to which he belongs.

The hospital is an instrument designated by society to carry out certain special functions which promote the total health of a community. In carrying out this function, the hospital must, by definition, assume responsibility for the quality of care provided, and for the competence of the health professionals it employs or permits to use its facilities. The patient now comes to the hospital most often through the mediation of his physician. In this instance the patient expects the physician to act as his advocate with the institution, to assure the quality of care provided by other health professionals, and to guarantee the safety and adequacy of the equipment and environment to which he is exposed. When, as occurs with increasing frequency, the patient comes directly to the hospital, that institution becomes his surrogate for selection of an attending physician, and it thus assumes a very direct responsibility for the professional care provided.

In both instances, however, the hospital has a responsibility to protect the patient against incompetence or failure of services and equipment. The board of trustees of a hospital is designated by the community to oversee the process of medical care within its walls. The board, like it or not, becomes a silent partner of the physician and the other health professionals and is, by definition, a part of the health care team. The board cannot ease its own conscience simply by delegating medical care to the health professional and forgetting it. It can satisfy the public mandate only by inquiring specifically into the determinants of quality care, examining the end product more critically, and establishing institutional measures to assure that its delegated responsibility is corporately implemented.

This means a new and unfamiliar set of relationships for the physician and the other health professionals, a closer relationship to institutional goals and responsibilities than ever before. It also means new dimenstions of accountability for the professional and the institution in which he works. This accountability is being demanded increasingly by the poor, the deprived, and the minorities in every community. The board of trustees, if it confronts its responsibilities squarely, must establish institutional means for assessing the quality of clinical decisions and optimal use of resources. It is in turn accountable for the way in which it exercises its stewardship for the hospital as a community service.

In exercising its responsibilities the board must be certain first that the professional staff is at least employing those institutional mechanisms of peer review wherein technical and professional decisions can be reviewed knowledgeably, such as tissue and utilization committees. All these mechanisms, if employed conscientiously, are frank intrusions into the comfortable dyadic relationship of patient and physician. Given the conditions of practice in today's hospitals and the demands of the public for an effective voice in quality determination, these mechanisms must of necessity be refined and developed under board mandate. Some of the existing and future mechanisms for board and institutional surveillance of clinical decisions are well known. A few will be selected for brief comment here.

Tissue committees are widely accepted by physicians. When they function responsibly, they provide quite objective means of evaluating the justifiability of an operative procedure and the accuracy of surgical diagnosis. Regular reporting of specific data from such committees and comparisons with data from other institutions of like kind should be required by a responsible board. The chief of professional services or medical director of the hospital has the responsibility to carry out a continuing educational program of the meaning of these statistics for the board. The board members have a corollary responsibility to study these data and to understand them.

One of the most abused areas of medical management is the use of drugs and other medications. The economic cost and the side effects of polypharmacy are incalculable. We have as yet no valid data on drug usage in individual institutions or on the deleterious effects of medications. Some awakening to this problem is the Federal Drug Administration's recent listing of some 369 drugs regarded as ineffective or hazardous (*New York Times*, 1970).

To qualify as rational therapeutics, a drug should be used only when it demonstrably changes the natural history of disease or demonstrably relieves a patient's symptoms. Every medication has the potentiality for doing harm, and the benefit of use in any clinical situation must be carefully weighed against the probability of no effect or of a damaging effect on the patient. Current prescribing practices can scarcely be considered rational by these criteria.

Several important institutional mechanisms which directly and indirectly influence clinical decision-making should be employed in every hospital—the pharmacy and therapeutics committee, the formulary system, and the drug information system—if the problem is to be resolved satisfactorily. These instruments provide institutional surveillance of the quality of therapeutics, as judged by peer physicians and pharmacists (Pellegrino 1965a, 1965b).

The formulary is an essential first step. It is a guide to approved and useful drugs. Only drugs formally received into the formulary can be used on a regular basis or stocked in the hospital pharmacy. Every new agent must be reviewed by the phamacy committee and every usage of a nonformulary item examined critically. In this way useless agents are proscribed, duplication and costs kept to a minimum, and dangerous useful drugs are limited to use by those qualified to do so. A drug information service provides detailed information on all therapeutic agents for use by physicians and others on the hospital staff; it identifies medications brought in by patients; it keeps a computerized record of all medications taken by a given patient, together with the diagnosis, the physician's name, and the side effects observed. These data can be recalled for a variety of purposes: to review the drug prescribing practices of a particular hospital against national norms, to review usage by individual physicians, and to keep an accurate record on indications, side effects, and costs (Pellegrino, 1965a).

The formulary, pharmacy committee, and drug information service each imply a larger and more intimate role for the pharmacist in drug therapy. He acts as director of the drug information service, as permanent secretary of the pharmacy committee, and as a close participant in the taking of drug histories and observing of side effects. He acts as consultant on therapeutics to the physician.

We also need wider use of a medical auditing system which exercises the same surveillance over medical diagnoses and management as the tissue committees do over operative procedures. The central issue here is whether, in a given clinical context, the most prudent or optimal decisions were made, from the patient's point of view: What alternatives were open? Were the best decisions made? How does the management compare with national norms established by peers in the field under question?

Systems of medical auditing are in existence, and though as yet imperfect they offer a reasonable approach to quality control in medical care. These audits can be improved by keeping computerized records of key decisions and diagnoses and their relationship to the patient's outcome. Properly used such data could be an invaluable stimulus to the continuing education of each physician: How accurate were a physician's diagnoses? How long did the patient stay in the hospital for a given diagnosis? Was he readmitted for the same complaint? How expeditiously was the workup carried out? Were hospital, laboratory, and other health personnel involved optimally? Was the patient's need met in terms he can accept and understand?

To answer these questions responsibly for professionals, and to distill from them an assessment of the quality of clinical decision-making understandable to a board of trustees, will require development of national norms for optimal clinical decision-making. This is not as impracticable as it first seems to some clinicians (Pellegrino, 1969). The diagnostic and therapeutic approach to the common clinical problems can be analyzed by a group of peers so as to provide a template of articulated decisions against which individual cases can be assessed. The examinations now given by several of the specialty boards which employ branching logic already make this assumption. We are not calling for a rigidified cookbook format for clinicians, but a comparison between what is done in an individual case by an individual physician against what is the best practice of his peers in a similar situation. Clinicians make these judgments now, but they do so informally, irregularly, and without the opportunity for critical feedback on an individual basis.

Another mechanism which a board can employ to fulfill its surrogate role for the community in the delivery of care is to require evidence of continuing education and periodic retesting, under professional staff supervision and surveillance. This retesting should not consist of the usual regurgitation of factual information. Rather it is the decision-making capacities themselves and techniques used by physicians and nurses which must be periodically evaluated. Obviously, such retesting must be conducted with respect for the person and reputation of the professional. Its results can be judged only by the professional staff, which should assume this responsibility as a corporate duty. We must expect that all the health professionals in an institution will not always perform at the community standard. The hospital as an institution then bears responsibility for providing opportunity and support for continuing education which can enable the individual to make up for the deficiencies.

The clinical care of patients demands intellectual, scientific, and humanitarian fitness which can deteriorate just as physical fitness, athletic prowess, and other highly developed skills deteriorate. Athletes at some point stop being players to become coaches and managers; airline pilots must, in time, relinquish the captain's role. Clinicians, if they really respect the intricacies of their art and its bearing on the welfare of other humans, must accept the inevitability of loss of acumen and knowledge with time. In the protection of his patients, the physician unable to perform as capably as his professional confreres cannot be permitted continued privileges indefinitely. He must not be destroyed in the process; he should be continued as a useful member of the medical community but placed in a position in which his experience, judgment, and knowledge of people are more important than his scientific, technial, and manipulative skills.

I have developed elsewhere the need for an expansion of medical ethics to encompass a more stringent ethics of competence (Pellegrino, in Bulger, in press). The optimal situation is one in which the professional staff of each hospital regards the competence of each of its members as a corporate responsibility, undertakes to assess it periodically, and acts judiciously on the results of that assessment. What the board of trustees must do is to ensure that such a process exists and that it is being conscientiously carried out.

The institutional surveillance of human experimentation is already a well-established fact and is required for funding under grants supported by the U.S. Department of Health, Education, and Welfare. We have here an instance of clinical decision-making subject to prior authorization, post facto review, and auditing (Pellegrino, 1969). The operation of human experimentation committees is perhaps prototypical of the type of scrutiny which will sooner or later be applied in more ordinary clinical situations—mostly on a post facto basis. In any case, the experience obtained in the functioning of human experimentation committees will provide a useful source of information for the social scientist interested in the emerging framework of relationships which surround clinical decisions.

As a board of trustees further contemplates its role in acting for the community, it must also provide mechanisms for measurement of patient satisfaction with the care provided. We will touch on the matter of consumer control and participation in the next section. Within the institution, participation of patients on a patient-care committee is a useful, and insufficiently used, mechanism. Every hospital should have such a committee which addresses itself to the assessment of whether the technical, professional, and human needs of patients are met optimally. This committee must of its nature be interdisciplinary in composition and include physicians, nurses, administrators, allied health professionals, and patients. A member of the board with a special sensitivity for the human responsibilities of his institution should sit on this committee.

The growing pressures for public accountability for medical care will probably not be satisfied simply by participation of patients on a patient-care committee. Some form of patient advocacy organized so that it is free of identification with the professional staff or the board of trustees is a growing necessity. Each board, if it is wise, will establish or encourage such a mechanism of advocacy. Ombudsmen, paid advocates, and other means have been proposed. There is as yet no well-tried format. The need will, however, persist and grow for some advocacy mechanism, and this is separable from the surrogate function which a board can perform if it takes its responsibilities seriously.

These are some of the mechanisms a board of trustees can use to meet its growing responsibilities as surrogate for the community in achieving care which is responsive to community and individual patient needs. I have selected just a few mechanisms to illustrate the way in which they can condition the institutional context and framework for decision-making.

It is very clear that the optimal and efficient use of these institutional mechanisms will modify the ancient dyadic relationship of physician and patient. While many complications are thus introduced, institutional devices are necessary in the complex society which constitutes today's hospital. Through their medium the board of trustees can more realistically fulfill the responsibilities it has undertaken for the community. No longer can it excuse itself by delegating professional care and clinical decision-making to physicians or nurses and other health professionals, and then forgetting them.

What we envision is a new relationship between the professional and the institution which reaffirms the technical and scientific competence of the professional but makes him accountable at an institutional level. This accountability extends from the competence of care he provides to proper utilization of the hospital and other health care resources (Pellegrino, 1968).

For the social scientists a number of very important researchable questions emerge. As these institutional instruments develop, prospective studies can be designed and carried forth on which models are best to ensure fulfillment of institutional goals. Instruments must be developed by social and behavioral scientists to test and evaluate ways in which patient-physician and physician-institutional relationships are modified by the new nexus of clinical decision-making. How can we motivate professionals to assume corporate responsibility for competence and compassionateness of the medical care provided in an institution? How does one act constructively and effectively as a member of an institutional committee dedicated to establishing accountability for the quality of care? How do we motivate individuals to appreciate when their clinical skills are diminishing and when it is necessary to assume other tasks which better maximize their potentialities and capabilities?

Many of the mechanisms suggested here indicate the evolution of a clinical bureaucracy. The many dangers and difficulties in such a system must be studied in the actual context of patient care. The employment of full-time clinical physicians in every hospital in the key departments is a developing trend. Full time physicians are being delegated a major responsibility by the board of trustees: the establishment of standards for the quality of care provided, the supervision of those standards on their services. How do these full-time physicians relate best to the physicians in the community who use the hospital? What is their relationship to the administration and to the board of trustees? To what extent are the decisions of the full-time clinical bureaucracy also surveyed and audited?

Community Participation, Accountability, and Control

The force with the greatest potential impact on traditional clinical decision-making is that of the community, demanding participation in the determination of the quality and quantity of care it receives. The strength and variety of these demands has grown to such major proportions that the initiative for change is being wrested from the professional. No analysis of the social structure of decision-making can be fashioned without inclusion of these new elements.

The demands for control are now most urgently expressed by the black, Spanish-speaking, and other minorities. In an egalitarian society with such sharp differentials in services as exist between the affluent and the poor, these demands will increase in intensity and involve the middle class as well.

Assistance from governments has not been effectual, and more communities will assert their power locally and confront hospitals, boards, and professionals directly. The configuration of any future health care system will in large part be determined by the emerging power of the consumer as he strives to attain medical care on terms he understands for his community (*Bulletin of the New York Academy of Medicine*, 1970).

Admittedly there is confusion about who the consumer is, who represents him, and what is meant by "control." The polarization between professionals and consumers on the meanings of these words is so great that they have become veritable shibboleths. Nonetheless, operational definitions must be sought. Consumers must recognize the values of crisis medicine while simultaneously working for more prevention and primary care; professionals must recognize the limitations in the type and distribution of care they now provide and acknowledge the ultimate right of the community to determine the character of the services it receives.

The whole matter is exceedingly acute because of current limitations on economic resources, which underscore the need to set priorities in the face of growing expectations and needs, and a history of neglect of the minorities and the poor. If the hospital is indeed an institution dedicated to serving community purposes, then the community can demand to determine these purposes. Indeed, more people regard this as the only way out of the incredible situation we are in—growing insufficiency of services at a time when the amount of money and numbers of people and organizations dedicated to providing health care are unprecedented.

We can expect consumer power to be expressed increasingly by direct intervention into judgments previously sacrosanct for physicians, boards of trustees, or health departments and local governments. The community will demand to control such things as location, size, and type of health facilities, the types of care they provide, and the hours they will be open for service. A first priority in most communities is decentralization of primary, preventive, and emergency care and availability 24 hours every day. Consumers are also emphasizing the need for preventive services, for more attention to socially significant problems like drug abuse, alcoholism, nutrition, and mental health, as contrasted with the crisis medicine the professional prefers to practice now.

As communities achieve greater sophistication, they will deal directly with such issues as distribution of specialized facilities, equipment, and personnel. Medical education is seen by many consumers as preparing physicians for crisis and specialized medicine only. It too is already feeling the incursions of the public will. Communities are insisting on more voice in the selection of candidates for medicine, to assure a more just distribution of opportunities among socioeconomic groups. Family practice programs are being legislated, with medical schools acquiescing, rather than leading, and the same is happening with physicians' assistants—all in the attempt to distribute medical care and to make primary care more accessible.

The more insistent communities want more than participation. They want control and accountability and will not support institutions which are unresponsive to needs defined by the community. This control may be exerted through the surrogate functions of a board of trustees or, more directly, through the hiring and firing of professional personnel. The events at New York's Lincoln Hospital are a specific case in point (Kaufman, 1970).

With community control will come more stringent criteria of accountability for quality and safety of care. Stricter licensure requirements, mandatory relicensure and recertification, and more conscientious policing of incompetent practitioners are already being sought. Indeed it has been proposed that the only adequate protection of community interests lies in paid consumer advocates who can take legal means against professionals, boards, and institutions which do not meet health-care needs efficiently, safely, and justly (Cahn, 1970).

These will appear as harsh and drastic measures to the health professionals who have for so long prided themselves on their adherence to a lofty ethic, self-policed and, presumably, detached from personal self-interest. Yet these measures underline the critical and inflammatory state of the health-care crisis today. More fundamentally, they illustrate how the initiative for health care has moved from the hands of professionals and into the hands of the consumer and the community. What shape should the new relationship of professional and community take, if it is to make optimal use of the professional's expertise and yet direct this expertise to socially useful and socially acceptable ends?

This is the central social issue in designing the decision-making structure of health-care delivery institutions in the immediate future. The sociology and social psychology of institutional authority, decision-making, and value determination must engage more of our attention now. Many unplanned "experiments" are already under way and will not await elegant and fastitious designs or neatly designed research controls. Social scientists face an era of "dirty" and rough data accumulation and should make the best of these spontaneous "experiments" in human nature and culture.

Decision-Making Levels:
Some Tentative Relationships

We do not have now a satisfactory model of clinical decision-making which encompasses the full interplay of all the factors we have outlined and which are so drastically altering the context and structure of clinical decision-making in the hospital. It is obvious that we err seriously if we confine our models to the process within the professional staff or within the hospital itself. These formerly "closed" systems are now opened up to forces in the community which are creating serious perturbations, felt even at the level of care of individual patients. The following tentative model attempts to assign levels of functions, differentiation of responsibility, and intersections of authority between professionals and the community. It recognizes the need for disparate elements to work in mutual reinforcement for the good of society and of the individual patient.

The hospital in this schema is understood as the institution designated by society to provide health-care services for a defined community. This means it concerns itself with primary and preventive, as well as secondary, levels of medical care. It must in effect become the community health center and establish decentralized satellites within a convenient time distance from consumers. It is also the backup center for primary care units and provides the wherewithal of secondary medical care: laboratories, specialists, diagnostic equipment, operating rooms, etc. The primary care centers can provide 85 percent of the required care in a region; the community hospital takes care of the remainder, except for 2-3 percent of all cases which must go to a tertiary care center—the university hospital.

In such a regionalized, functionalized, and organized system, decision-making must be organized and functionalized as well. In an ideal system each level of authority would carry the responsibilities most consistent with its capabilities and interests. A possible schema for interrelating and integrating the potentially discordant interests of the community and the professional might look as described below.

The Community-Consumer Interest. Ultimately, the hospital and other health-care institutions are instruments of social purpose, and hence the overall decisions on how an institution uses community resources to serve those purposes must rest with the community. The most likely model for this goal-setting community function is the legislative model. One could envision a widely representative Community Health Authority for each region, as determined by demography, geography, and density of need. This authority would be large enough to comprise representation from all groups within a region, perhaps 100 or more members. The members of this authority should probably be elected, though other means of selection are possible. Its members, it is hoped, could be informed and interested citizens, paid to carry out their health planning and directorial functions for at least part of the year.

This authority would have the responsibility to determine needs for the community and put these needs into some order of priority determined by available funds, intensity of need, etc. The authority would represent community interests, define the goals of its health care system, decide on how much of the community resources should be spent on health, and determine the location of facilities and specialized equipment. It would also see that the defined community goals are being attained efficiently, safely, and economically.

Hospitals, health professionals of all kinds, and other health-related agencies are the providers in this arrangement, and they must also supply the technical and scientific input requisite to defining alternatives and making rational and informed choices among them.

The relationships of the regional Community Health Authority to local and state governments will need exploration. Recommendations for expenditures, for channeling state and federal health dollars, and for committing regional resources must be within legal and other restraints. A model similar to that of transportation authorities in several states may be appropriate. Such capabilities as bonding authority, certification of institutions based on need, and setting standards of accountability would be useful in fulfilling the responsibilities necessary to building a plan, and an organization, for meeting regional health needs.

There is a very acute need for such a unified, regional, overarching authority to produce some coordination of the disparate efforts of individuals, groups, and governments, all trying to improve delivery of health services. The congressional legislation which gave life to Regional Medical Programs and Comprehensive Health Planning was a partial attempt to meet the urgent needs for some vesting of authority for health care planning and implementation. These federal acts have achieved some regional cooperative results in this direction, but as presently designed they are insufficient to meet growing local and regional demands for responsive, comprehensive, and orderly planning and operation of health services. As they now exist, Regional Medical programs and Comprehensive Health Planning should be closely related to any new regional authority, primarily as channels for federal funding.

Hospital Board of Trustees. With the overall goals established, the board of trustees can become the community instrument for implementation of defined community goals in a particular hospital. The board is, then, truly the surrogate of the public in the institution it serves. It is charged with moral and legal accountability for the operation of the hospital. Through establishment of some of the institutional control mechanisms discussed earlier, the board exercises its responsibilities. It must, of course, delegate the technical, scientific, and professional details of patient care to the health professionals on the staff. It depends upon them for expert information out of which it defines alternatives and makes rational choices among them. The board is charged by the community to establish means for accountability in each hospital. Thus it must become informed on measures of the quality of medical care, and it must require continuous reporting from administrators and professional staff on the measures it undertakes and supervises. The satisfaction of patients served is also a major concern of the board and, perhaps, the most difficult to measure accurately.

The board, in short, is required increasingly to provide institutional policies and the organizational contexts within which individual clinical decisions are made. It must provide both for the privacy and confidentiality of those decisions and for a matrix of checks and balances to assure that those decisions are prudent and serve the interests of patients and community, while at the same time the integrity of the professionals who make technical and scientific decisions in the care of patients must be preserved.

The Professional Staff. The physicians, nurses, allied health professionals—all members of the patient-care, medical-care, and health-care teams—must remain always in charge of the technical aspects of decision-making for a particular patient. In so doing they are subject to the continuous review of their peers and colleagues on the various health teams. The professional has the responsibility always to act competently and prudently on behalf of his patient, as prescribed in traditional medical codes. But he now does this in a frame of cooperative work, of shared responsibility, and of mutual constructive criticism and review. His relationship with his patient is still a highly personal one based on trust and confidence. His decisions, however, must become open to auditing, and his state of competence periodically reviewed.

The professional must also fulfill his corporate responsibilities of serving on the various committees and review bodies through which peer review is conducted. In addition, the physician and the other health professionals are required to provide the informed data upon which the community and the board of trustees can base their broad decisions on how best to meet the needs of a particular community. Finally, the professional has a responsibility to make decisions which will optimize the use of hospital and community resources (Pellegrino, 1968).

A diagrammatic view of these relationships might look as depicted in Chart 1.

Goals, Values, and Priorities

If we accept some version of the interrelationships outlined in Chart 1, then it becomes obvious that a major unmet requirement is some system of values which can determine the output of the health care system as a whole. Indeed the energy loss in resolving the divisions of jurisdictional authority among the community, the institution, and the professional, each of which seeks to define the purpose of the health care system, is enormous. The resultant conflict of expectations and prerogatives is the greatest deterrent to the rational, regionalized, functionalized delivery of health care today.

Currently the approach is largely deontologic: each level in the decision-making chain asserts the values it feels should determine the output of the entire system and then identifies those values with its duty to the public. There is as yet no generally accepted theory of values for the health of the nation against which priorities can be set, individual programs evaluated, and resources allocated. Without an explicitly articulated set of values for each community, decision-making is fated to remain a fragmentary process in which the optimal use of resources and the satisfaction of the consumer are growing more difficult to attain.

To elaborate a set of values in the field of health and to establish priorities among them is admittedly a sensitive and vexatious task. It really represents the paradigm of a major challenge of contemporary man: how to make technology and new resources serve truly human ends. Heretofore the response has always been to expand *all* medical services in *all* directions and to provide more of the same care to more people. Other social demands—for education, welfare, environment, civil justice, and order—are now so vast, however, that they must compete with health care for money and attention. How do we choose between the emphases possible in modern medicine? In what direction do we turn our capabilities?

It is staggering to think of satisfying even a partial list of the health

CHART 1

INSTITUTIONAL MATRIX FOR CLINICAL DECISION-MAKING

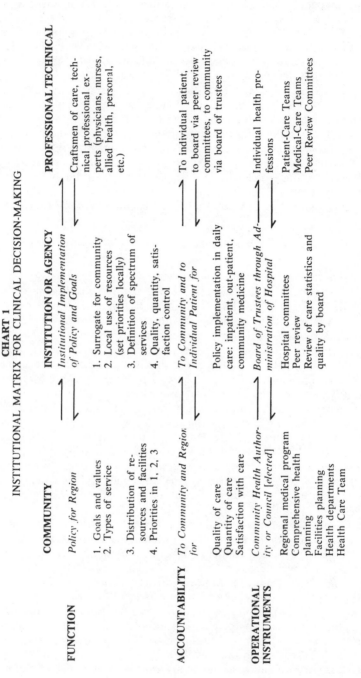

FUNCTION	COMMUNITY	INSTITUTION OR AGENCY	PROFESSIONAL TECHNICAL
	Policy for Region	*Institutional Implementation of Policy and Goals*	Craftsmen of care, technical professional experts (physicians, nurses, allied health, personal, etc.)
	1. Goals and values	1. Surrogate for community	
	2. Types of service	2. Local use of resources (set priorities locally)	
	3. Distribution of resources and facilities	3. Definition of spectrum of services	
	4. Priorities in 1, 2, 3	4. Quality, quantity, satisfaction control	
ACCOUNTABILITY	*To Community and Region for*	*To Community and to Individual Patient for*	To individual patient, to board via peer review committees, to community via board of trustees
	Quality of care	Policy implementation in daily care: inpatient, out-patient, community medicine	
	Quantity of care		
	Satisfaction with care		
OPERATIONAL INSTRUMENTS	*Community Health Authority or Council [elected]*	*Board of Trustees through Administration of Hospital*	Individual health professions
	Regional medical program	Hospital committees	Patient-Care Teams
	Comprehensive health planning	Peer review	Medical-Care Teams
	Facilities planning	Review of care statistics and quality by board	Peer Review Committees
	Health departments		
	Health Care Team		

Note: True "advocacy rule" probably must be outside the institutional framework to avoid conflict of interest.

demands being made today: comprehensive, continuous, preventive care for all; better care for the aged and chronically ill, for children, for the handicapped; more concern for diseases of social significance, like drug abuse, alcoholism, nutrition, the problems of adolescence; the psychosocial problems of living in a technological society; better treatment and prevention of acciidents, occupational, and emotional disorders. The list grows as our capabilities grow. It will not help to say that all are equally important to society, though they may be for the individual. Society may not choose health above other problems of human significance.

For the first time in history, man's enormous capabilities can outstrip his resources. The community and the professional do not always share the same values, and their choices may be in direct conflict with each other: prevention of rheumatic fever against open heart surgery, primary care against care of the complicated medical and surgical problem, applied research or research in patient care against basic investigations, preventive mental health against sophisticated care of chronic and incurable conditions. These are not false dichotomies. They represent real choices which are being made fortuitously now and which must be made consciously, cooperatively, and with full explication of the social costs involved and the values expressed in them (Pellegrino, in press).

Better community and institutional instruments must be developed to bring the consumers, educated professionals outside medicine, and the medical professions to an intelligent discourse on choices. Priorities must be mutually agreed upon and altered as the values of society change. If medicine is a special organ of the body social, how can it promote the health of that society, which is something more than the health of its individual members? Is it possible to think of limiting some of our capabilities in medicine? These value questions grow out of the remarkable advances in medical science. They are only partially answerable by improvements in efficiency and responsiveness in our technological knowhow. For the most part the solution demands a concerted sociophilosophical, socioethical inquiry based on a firm knowledge of the scientific roots of contemporary medicine.

The Medical Sociologist and the Algebra of Values

The history of sociology is one of ambivalence so far as values are concerned. Those who have wanted to make sociology more like the physical sciences have emphasized objectivity, quantification, and controlled experiments. They have eschewed studies of values as too vague or too difficult. In so doing, of course, they have placed the values of science above other values. The younger and more activist sociologists now contravene this view and hold that the sociologist must be involved and must assert his values. Indeed, some have gone so far as to suggest a desire to impose certain values on a too slowly responsive community.

Neither extreme is tenable or responsible in the value crisis which confronts the community and the health professions today. Medical sociologists with a taste for axiology must be more willing to study values and value systems as they condition clinical decisions of professionals, institutions, or community groups. Professor Lewis Coser has concisely stated Max Weber's admonition that sociology itself must be value neutral but not value free. His own view and that of Robert Merton coincide in outlining a position of "detached concern"—one which permits the sociologist to study values while yet not imposing his own on society (Coser, 1969). The social scientists can thus perform an essential task if they will analyze the consequences to society of holding to some set of values or departing from it. Clinical decision-makers need such beacons to warn against the rocks on either side of the narrow straits of clinical decision-making.

Most of the decisions involve an algebra of values—a summation of the positive and negative effects for the individual and for society of any decision or practice. If the goals are determined in advance, i.e. if the output is defined clearly, the algebraic sum of advantages and disadvantages can be assessed objectively. The student of organizational structure should inquire into the consequences for patient care of alternative modes of organization of hospital, community, or professional groups. He can also study the consequences of the intuitive acts of professional or lay change agents, as they try to actualize some special expectation of their own or of the groups they represent. The growing impatience of communities is producing newer and sometimes quite aberrant versions of health care delivery. Each experiment exemplifies some value or set of values whose consequences for the efficacy of the system should be carefully studied. Richard Scott (1966) has touched on some of these questions and reviewed the pertinent literature. So, too, have Georgopoulos and Mann (1962) in their definitive work on the community hospital.

The medical sociologist interested in decision-making and in the organization of patient care systems has a responsibility to sensitize all of us to the need for a more conscious appraisal of the values which underlie any contemplated solution of the health-care crisis. Perhaps the day will arrive when planners, consumers, and providers will carry out the necessary algebra of values in advance, rather than in retrospect. Were this to occur, political strategies might be more effective and legislators more willing to support significant changes in our health-care system.

We need also a better perception and better knowledge of what the expectations of the consumer really indicate. Would he choose the same alternatives if he could objectively appraise the full range of capabilities of medicine against the resources available? The consumer now depends upon the provider for all of his information on alternatives. Would he not be more confident of his choices if, in addition, an objective analysis of the social cost of each alternative were set forth?

These and a variety of other very significant questions are open to the method of sociomedical research. They involve the sociologist in continual discourse with change agents of all sorts—in the community, the professions, government, and institutions. These questions also dictate a deeper involvement than has been customary in action research. The competent pursuit of such studies is essential if we are to understand and then constructively modify the complex interrelationships which now characterize all our decisions in the health care system.

Conclusion

A limited analysis of the markedly changing matrix of clinical decision-making has been attempted. It is clear that the delegation of such decisions to the absolute control of the physicians and other health professions is no longer realistic. Health professionals, as a consequence of contemporary scientific, technological, social, and political forces, must now function in a matrix of relationships becoming ever more complex and more public. The demands of consumers, the requirements of social and institutional accountability, and the capabilities of modern medicine surround the professional with a growing number of direct and indirect constraints on his daily decisions.

Better organizational patterns are needed to ensure that all groups with a legitimate interest in the health care system can exert that interest in a manner which simultaneously balances the integrity of the professional's expertise with the services society needs and demands. We face problems of values, priorities, and goals which entail the establishment of a sophisticated set of relationships directed to closing the gap between the expectations of consumers and providers.

The simplicity of the dyadic patient-physician model can no longer dominate the decision-making process. The health care system is changing and posing new demands. Elaboration of a new set of relationships requires conscious and careful analysis of goals and values and a compromise of demands and prerogatives which will challenge all of us in the health professions for the next several decades.

References

Bulletin of the New York Academy of Medicine. Community participation for equity and excellence in health care. *Bulletin of the New York Academy of Medicine,* 1970, *46*, 12, 1025-1151.

Cahn, E. Discussion of the division of the role of the community in developing improved health care. *Bulletin of the New York Academy of Medicine,* 1970, *46*, 12, 1032.

Coser, L. A. The craft of sociology—letter to a young sociologist. *Sociological Inquiry,* 1969, *39*, 131-137.

Georgopoulos, B. S., and Mann, F. C. *The community general hospital.* New York: Macmillan, 1962.

Kaufman, M. Lincoln Hospital: case history of dissension that split staff. *New York Times,* December 21, 1970, 1 f.

New York Times. Drugs deemed ineffectual or dangerous. *New York Times,* November 28, 1970, 35.

Pellegrino, E. D. Nursing and medicine: ethical implications in changing practice. *American Journal of Nursing,* 1964, *64*, 9.

Pellegrino, E. D. Drug information services and the clinician. *American Journal of Hospital Pharmacy,* 1965 (a), *22*, 38-41.

Pellegrino, E. D. A physician appraises the formulary system. *Hospitals,* 1965 (b), *39,* 1, 77.
Pellegrino, E. D. The physician's role in optimal use of health care resources. In *Financial implications for hospitals in comprehensive health care planning.* 26th Annual Program on Hospital Finance, Accounting, and Administration. Monograph Series, Graduate School of Business, Indiana University, 1968. Pp. 75-89.
Pellegrino, E. D. The necessity, promise, and dangers of human experimentation. In World Council Studies, *Experiments with man.* Geneva: World Council of Churches, and New York: Friendship Press, 1969. Pp. 31-56.
Pellegrino, E. D. Physician, patients, and society: some new tensions in medical ethics. *Harvard University Press,* in press.
Pellegrino, E. D. Toward an expanded medical ethics—the Hippocratic ethic revisited. In R. J. Bulger (Ed.) *Hippocrates revisited,* in press.
Scott, W. R. Some implications of organization theory for research on health services. *Milbank Memorial Fund Quarterly,* 1966, *44,* 4, pt. 2, 35-64.

14

ISSUES AND DISCUSSION OF PART FIVE
Doctor's Role In Institutional Management

Presentation Highlights: R. H. Guest

I approach this subject with some trepidation, for much of what I have to say is probably known by now. I backed into this area and the whole question of hospitals and the medical profession as a result of being intrigued by a study I was engaged in a few years ago. I went off on my merry way studying non-medical organizations but suddenly realized that some of the things that I had been studying had relevance for hospital organization, particularly some of the things I encountered at the National Aeronautics and Space Administration because they have developed some real Rube Goldberg operations there. Griffith asked a very challenging question earlier when he was talking about the organization of the broader delivery of health service and the models we use. That question is appropriate here in terms of the things I have to say. I would also like to say a few words about how some of these things are done in NASA, if we have the time. We may disagree about putting a spaceship on the moon and spending $36 billion to do it, but the way they organize to do things has some real relevance here.

Studying the problem of professionalism and bureaucracy also has been mentioned. We have known about this age-old problem in complex organizations, but in a way this is new in terms of the doctor and the organization he works in. What is discouraging is that, despite all the studies, it does not seem to me that some of the insights we have gained have helped us very much when in comes to doing something about health care delivery. A lot of work has been done on the relationship of the scientist in industrial and other organizations to management. We know that there is a dual role in the professional place, where the professional has his allegiances both to his practice within the organization where he works and to the outside professional organizations to which he belongs. And, of course, we say that this is also true about doctors in hospitals. But in going through the literature concerning the institutional role of the physician I find very little research done with the doctors as the center of focus. There is a tremendous amount of research on administrators but not on doctors.

I assumed that since so much had been done on scientists and engineers in industry, it must have been done in hospitals too. One of the difficulties is that doctors, for one reason or other, simply have been unwilling subjects of research. Perhaps I am oversimplifying here, and this may not be entirely true. It may be that the social scientist has the perception that the doctor is unwilling to be researched. But recently I wanted to have some students do a study of a primary care unit which involved interviewing the doctors, and we had a very difficult job of it. I got flack from the doctors, time and again, about "having these students follow me around on the job." They were complaining about the violation of the confidential relationship with the patient, etc. I am led to believe, then, that there is something to this unwillingness problem.

In my paper I also stated that "some observers have suggested, perhaps irresponsibly, that proposals for research may lead to change and that this traditionally conservative segment of society, i.e. the doctors, while applauding change in medical science and technology, would resist any possible exposure of their own institutional roles." And somebody said to me: "Why did you say 'perhaps irresponsibly'?" I was trying to be nice because I showed this document to some MDs before I came, and I was worried that if I just made the flat statement they would be unhappy. The truth is that when I showed this modest document to five doctors in New Hampshire they all agreed with me. But then one of them called me up, and I thought I must have said something offensive (and so I was a little surprised that it was you that I offended). To my surprise, the doctor wanted to say that my statement was too modest and too mild, and that I did not "blast enough."

My next point goes back to some of the things Straus said earlier focusing on the incarcerated patient and the history of hospitals. I see the same thing. Historically, it is true that the early hospital was not focused on medical care as such. It was a place to throw people in to let them die. It was only in the middle of the nineteenth century that the doctor began to play any kind of a crucial role in the institution. As time went on, with the advances in science and skills, he found that special attention needed to be given to the patient. But this required proper facilities, and the solo practitioner working from his house found that he just did not have the tools to do the job properly.

I often wonder what would have happened if hospitals had developed differently. Most hospitals were not founded by and operated by physicians. Had they been created by the medical profession, perhaps the entire development of institutional patient care might have been vastly different. This is only speculative, of course, but I think what we see today has its historical roots, and it is a fact that the doctor was never an employee of the institution but rather a guest. And yet we have this curious fact that because of professional authority he was at first and has been dominant in the institution. Recently, of course, this has been changing. But Dr. Jaco, I believe you think that in California it still is very much true that the doctor is the dominant factor.

Dr. Jaco: There though it is the California consumers' fault; they let them get away with it. But that is another problem.

Dr. Guest: In any case, I want to go back to Scott's model here because it stimulates thought. Not only was the doctor's authority made explicit by the traditions of the professions, but he was clothed with an informal authority that was accepted by every segment and function in the institution. Thus he stood in marked contrast to the patient—the sick, aged, poverty-stricken, and frequently homeless patients that he was treating.

There were a lot of forces, as we look historically, coming to bear on the medical practitioner in his hospital role, i.e. in his institutional as distinguished from his purely professional role. Medical schools themselves also were growing, and to an increasing extent the student was getting his training in larger organizations. The former apprenticeship system was disappearing. At the same time, the doctor's solo relationship to his patient was becoming more dependent upon his being a member of a hospital staff organization, on interacting with colleagues and administrative units, and so forth. In addition, we now see the growth of group medical practice where the doctor is playing, you might say, a subinstitutional role within the profession.

We also talked earlier about the changing role of the board of trustees in this picture. Traditionally, boards consisted of philanthropists and the wealthy who were the patrons of the institution, and the medical profession was pretty free to act with a minimum of control from above. Since World War II, however, the picture has been changing. Instead of merely being the fund raisers and having the statutory power to appoint the doctors, boards are becoming more concerned with what is going on inside the institution. Along with the growth and professionalization of hospital administrators, we see that boards are taking more interest in financial matters, in controls, and indeed in the quality of patient care. As we look into the next decade I think it will be quite natural that the consumers, third-party people, and the government will be a significant influence upon the hospitals, and particularly upon the institutional role that doctors are playing.

I realize that I did not make it clear, and I am not so sure I am clear in my own mind, whether the doctor ought to play a larger role in institutional management, as distinguished from being more involved in institutional management, even if he did not have a role as a member of management as such. I may have left the impression that doctors really ought to have a say, a vote, or actual direct power in the management of the rest of the hospital, acting in some respects in a managerial capacity. I do not think I meant to suggest that. It scares me when I think of doctors getting into management roles. They do not have time, and I think they are not very good at it anyway. Further, I do not believe you can even train them to be very good at it. What I mean is that I wish, and here I am talking normatively and not as a social scientist, that the doctors would be more sensitive to and more aware of those elements of the total system that are not purely professional.

I quoted a comment, you may recall, from John Gardner, who at the time he made the statement was Secretary of Health, Education, and Welfare. Very briefly, the national committee involved bluntly recommended that appropriate members of the medical staff be directly involved with the administration and developing of the budget and operating plan, and in the achievement of financial and service objectives as budgeted and planned. The committee was convinced that physician participation in the budget and planning areas not only would help the hospital but also would help the physicians' own performance and, of course, the patient. The National Advisory Commission on Health Manpower, just before this other report came out, also found a shocking lack of physician involvement in the management process, noting that: "Although physicians are subordinates in the formal organization of the hospital, they are the leaders in the informal organization that controls most hospital decisions. How to give physicians responsibility commensurate with their authority is a problem. Presently, most physicians feel little responsibility to a hospital because they pay nothing for its use. Neither do they suffer any direct consequences when the hospital gets into financial trouble. Medical and hospital associates should jointly explore means to increase the physician's responsibility for the successful and economical management of hospital operations."

As I said before, I do not know enough about the problem, and I am a little confused in my own mind, but it does not seem realistic to say that physicians should be put on all of the permanent budget committees and be expected to devote great amounts of time to the myriad of things that are involved in administration. But the comments by these commissions seem to make some sense (I am talking about practical things now not so much about research). At least they make sense from the standpoint of emphasizing the need for physician exposure to the larger institutional processes. It is this exposure to the various major facets of the organization which I think is not only terribly crucial for the effective operation of the hospital now, but which is going to become even more important in the years ahead.

The knowledge of clinical practice is owned by the doctor, and that knowledge is his. But the technical tools of his practice, the enormous and complex new technology, are owned to a large degree by the institution which gives him the privilege to practice. Even the doctor's clinical knowledge is being supplemented by the specialized knowledge of other groups and staffs in the hospital, paramedical and nonmedical. And the doctor's role as a member of the hospital organization, as distinguished from his purely professional role, is being made increasingly explicit in bylaws of the medical staff and in written agreements with administrators, boards and outside parties.

We now have to tie the practicing physician, regardless of the type of his practice, into the management of the health care service system. The physician should be deeply involved in the planning and managing of our health services inside and outside the hospital. Already we have seen the proliferation of hospital insurance plans, the expansion of Blue Cross and Blue Shield, Medicare, Medicaid, and other important developments in the health field, all of which affect the physician's role. We are going to see group medical practice growing, and this has further implications. So does regional planning, and the probable development of health service centers. Such centers are going to tie groups of hospitals together, and different hospitals may have to rely on central laundries, central purchasing, central data processing, etc.

In order to prepare physicians in the future for the role that we are beginning to see they are going to have to play, we have to take these changes into account, study their implications, and act accordingly. If we take Garfield's article in *Scientific American* as the basis, for example, we are led to one possible model. Garfield says that we should spin off from the physician a lot of activities he now performs that can be done by paramedicals and others, leaving the treatment of the sick to the doctor; health testing service, preventive maintenance service, and other programs that we see coming along can be performed by others. One implication of this is that if we simplify the physician's task by having others perform these services, this will lessen the pressure on the doctor to assume greater involvement in the management of these institutions. Conversely, it seems to me, the doctors will have to play a greater role in the planning and setting up of training programs for the paramedicals and others. They will have to become deeply involved in the planning of health service in the broadest sense of the word, not just confined to the hospital alone.

And so, on the one hand, if you accept anything that Garfield said, the doctor's role will be simplified because he will not have to perform a number of the time-consuming things that he is now performing and, on the other hand, he is going to have to be involved in the training, planning, and other facets of the system. In talking to deans of medical schools I find that they deplore the fact that men going through their medical training get little exposure, if at all, to anything that has to do with organizational life as such, even though their future life will be in an organization.

I have not said anything about research needs for the future. I do feel that I was quite stimulated by Scott's model. He would be the first to say that this is not the most elegant or refined model in the world, but I could see what he was talking about when he was discussing the power dependency relationship and accommodation that has to take place between the doctors and the management of the institution. We really do not know too much about the dynamics of this relationship; we know it better in other kinds of institutional arrangements. A good deal has been written on power by political scientists, for example, as well as by sociologists. The tension points between the actual managerial structure and the desired structure, desired by professionals and others, bring about conflict. And we know, we have enough research tools to study the nature of tension in hospitals.

But I am worried about how much time we have to get into a great deal of elaborate or, shall we call it, pure research. I may be wrong, but I think we have a revolution coming up in this field, and the whole nature of medical health services is going to change very rapidly. Personally, I feel that we need to structure our research in a way in which it is action research. I think we can test out a lot of hypotheses, we can try models too, and do it all at the same time that we set some goals as to what we hope would come out of this in terms of human beings behaving in a way which will give us more effective health care services. I know that it is fun to go into an organization and do nice, neat, little research jobs, and study some variables and check them out and retest them again, and then take somebody else's work and replicate it and say "yes, now we are really getting some place, we can replicate this stuff." And I admit my prejudice in what I am saying, which is this: let us not be too elegant and too elaborate in what we do, but let us focus on things that need to be done.

We also mentioned earlier that taking the hospital as an organization and focusing on the hospital alone is not going to be adequate as we look into the future. You said the same thing John (Griffith), when we got into that argument about the pressures from the consumer and who was the consumer. We did not really define who the consumer was. Perhaps we have a difference of opinion in our own group here on this. I tend to agree with Pellegrino, however, when I say that there are these pressures growing from dissatisfied consumers of health care, and that their noises are finding their way into the congressional committees. I made the statement that once we get the Southeast Asia thing on the back burner, the thing on the front burner is going to be our whole medical health service problem, and I was told no. Somebody said it is poverty, housing, or ecology, and that health service is going to be lower in priority. But those I know in Congress are not talking that way; they are talking of the health care area as the number one or number two priority.

Discussion

Dr. Scott: I would like to make about fifteen comments but I will make three. I really think that I disagree with a lot of what I take to be Guest's prescriptions for the problem. I think your analysis of the problems is correct but your prescriptions I take issue with.

First, my own view is that there is, and there has to be, a good deal of tension between people who focus on the individual needs of particular patients and those who are concerned about the welfare of patients as a whole. It is very important that there be people with broad administrative responsibilities concerned with moving many people through care systems and with the routine aspects of care. There also ought to be people with some power so say "Hey, wait a minute; this guy needs certain kinds of special arrangements, and the routine will not work here" (I am talking about the doctor or the cure group here.) A certain amount of tension between the two is very functional in these systems. A good deal of power for the administrators at all levels but also a good deal of power for the technical experts and the people who are directly involved in providing care to unique and peculiar patients are both necessary.

Second, I think that many of the kinds of problems which we have seen in the past in the relationship between physicians as a group and the administration are going to work themselves out. We may or may not have time; if you are right, we will not have time. But I think some of the problems are in the process of being solved by the increasing shift of power to administration. The power dependency relations are shifting, and physicians are, to a much larger extent than even ten years ago, dependent upon the hospital, its facilities, and the kinds of things administrators can provide and mediate.

Dr. Guest: I did not think that was happening. But you are quite right that the administrators are gaining the respect of the doctors. The doctors are realizing that administrators can no longer be just little handmaidens.

Dr. Pellegrino: I wonder if Dr. Scott would modify that and say that power is shifting to the institution, because I think there are other phenomena not accounted for if you say administrator.

Dr. Scott: Well, yes. You would want to include the board, and I would not object to that.

The third thing that I really want to speak very loudly about is that I am not sure that doctors, as doctors, have any real competence or expertise to get involved in the routine management of hospitals. And here I argue from analogy. It seems to me that in the present crisis period of the university, when students are causing disruptions of various kinds and staff have to be cut, this is when for the first time the faculty are invited into the halls of power. But I am just very unimpressed with my own ability and the ability of my colleagues to run a university. I think we run departments very well because we are close to the work and we know something about what is required to do that kind of work. But as a faculty body we have meetings, endless meetings and various kinds of committees, and when meeting as larger legislative bodies there are 100-150 people present with 250 opinions about what should be done, because some people are unsure or confused. And I really think that there is just an enormous amount of wastage of people being kept from the kind of work they can do, in our case research and teaching, in the process of trying to give us a little piece of the action in terms of saying what the larger picture is.

Dr. Guest: Could I respond? Remember I said that I am somewhat confused myself. When I used the word "involvement" I was not saying that the doctor should get involved in the managerial processes as such. Then I believe I used the word "exposure." What I am about to say is anecdotal, but it shows the power of informal activities or informal organization. I know of one hospital where two doctors, I do not know for what reasons, were intrigued by a lot of what was going on in the managerial processes. They went out and had dinner with the administrator quite frequently, dropped into his office, looked at the budget, etc. These fellows, who were not the head people or chiefs of departments, acted as informal leaders. They would go back to their staff meetings and when the medical staff was discussing its professional problems, whether it was a discussion of a tissue committee or something else, they would inform and educate their colleagues because of their own personal interest in the administration of the hospital. How one can institutionalize this I do not know, because it came from a personal interest of these people.

Comment (Dr. Jaco): I would like to introduce a foreign note here about physicians being involved in management or in control. There is something inconsistent with some of the other comments we have been making about the physicians, the shortage or the waste of their time, and how important it is that they should be treating patients, for after all, that is what they are trained for, without wasting scarce resources. And now, it seems, we want them to get involved in managing the facility. Much of the experience of our group here I think has been confined to the university or the teaching hospital, which is very atypical when compared to the general hospital in this country. When we consider the private practice of medicine in most general hospitals, much of what we say here might go right past 90 percent of the practicing physicians as nonsense.

What do you suppose goes on in the monthly medical meeting in these hospitals? If the meeting is run properly by the administration, doctors will discuss the problems of the facility, not just tissue committee reports, assuming of course that some of the doctors show up at those meetings. Attendance is pretty poor, bcause they are busy, and they should be busy. Being busy, they have a general tendency to take a dim view of doctors who are messing around in things besides treating patients, in terms of the value system of the medical profession as such. There is a certain unrealism, I think, in some of our discussion about the role of the physician in management. If we are sincere about using the physician's skills properly and more efficiently, the doctor's role should be strictly in the area of treatment, unless we start turning out a different brand of physician and a different brand of administrator. Personally I have just been to too many voluntary hospitals out in the field, and I am convinced that the attitudes of the physicians are too alien and too different from what is being suggested about the role of doctors in institutional management.

Dr. Guest: What research I did was not in university hospitals but in community general hospitals. And I agree with you, although that is not the point I am making, that they do not have time.

Dr. Jaco: I have been to many staff meetings in hospitals; I am sure many of us have, and not just in teaching or university hospitals. I am talking about the MDs in private practice out in the field, who basically have a hostility toward the medical school faculty, anyhow, for what they did to them for four years. This is also part of the reason, frankly, why Regional Medical Programs are phasing out and Community Health Planning is coming in. The doctors are pretty sure that they can control CHP and that they cannot control RMP. But what I am saying is just that the physician is always busy, and he should be busy treating patients.

Comment: I think we need pure research in this area, a great deal of research as to what the impact of various forms of physician involvement is. Most of the many published opinions have the error and aura of unreality Jaco is talking about. There is very little research that undertakes the problem of, for example, a twenty-man medical staff, a ten-man board of trustees, and one administrator, and examines how this constellation can be organized to get reasonable consumer representation, reasonable control of tensions, etc., so that the result is a stable and yet socially functional organization. I do not think that your opinions are any better than the pronouncements of prestigious figures in the health field. We need research.

Comment: I have some observations here on the health system. First, when focusing on hospitals, we tend to forget that a lot of physicians are in administrative positions, particularly in public health. I am not familiar with the specific figures, but if you look to see how many trained physicians are practicing and how many are in administrative positions, you will be surprised with the number of physicians who are managing various kinds of organizations. We seem to believe that putting a man through a medical education does something to him, while subsequent additional training of a different kind does not result in any enlightenment, presumably because it produces a different role (an administrative role) which is at odds with the role of his supposed colleagues (the practicing physicians). Let me give an example. In a recent RMP meeting we turned down a project for a survey screening for stomach cancer in children (80 symptomatic children), which has an extremely small incidence besides being cruel because there is nothing you can do about it if you find it. Even though the evaluation committee, which consisted mostly of epidemiologists, turned this down, a group of practicing physicians on the cancer committee approved it, much to our surprise. In any case, we do have a number of physicians in administrative positions already in the health-care system.

Second, this ritual that we have of training people first in one field and then putting them in another is based on questionable logic. I think the rationalization is that physicians will listen to other physicians, that practicing physicians will listen to administrators who are physicians. I am not quite sure that this is true. But this polarization does result essentially in a situation where the doctor in the administrative position has neither a constituency nor colleagues. This is reminiscent of Floyd Mann's problem when he was working with blacks, dealing with them locally. He found that he could bring them along with him but then those people who were representing the black community lost their community. They finally had to work through tape recorders whereby the representatives of the community recorded the sessions and brought the tapes home in order to bring their constituencies along with them in this negotiation between the community and the organization. It is a very similar kind of problem here.

Comment: Let me return to the point that Scott made. Personally, when I started to watch physicians and study a couple of hospitals, I was impressed by the fact that the physicians did exactly what you report. They knew as little as possible about what was going on, and they avoided understanding what happened once they threw an order into the system. I even have records of physician participation in committees documenting this behavior and showing a fantastically astute way of coming often enough to make one's weight felt but not sufficiently frequently to share the responsibility for the conclusions. And after a year I came to the scientific conclusion that they are despicable. But after the second year, and this is the key point, I came to the conclusion that these doctors are doing this in the benefit of their job. There is a notion here of what you might call the secondary gain of primary ignorance. In effect, by not knowing certain things, the physicians in a sense remain ombudsmen for the cure process. I have never seen a physician go to a head nurse and say, "Miss Smith, do you have time to give fifteen minutes to these patients?" It is the physician rather than the nurse who serves as the patient's advocate, partly because the patient says, "I like my doctor to do it; he is my doctor and I want him to order it if that is what he wants to do."

Comment: That is not true in the Kaiser system though.

Answer: Sure, but that is a very fundamental difference between the Kaiser system and the typical hospital. I am speaking of the typical general hospital where in fact ignorance allows the physician to be the advocate. This not withstanding, there is now a particular movement on the part of some medical schools to actually include some content in their curriculum that tries to accomplish this sensitivity.

Comment: I am struck by the fact that our conference, and this is the second time, has faced its boundaries. We faced one boundary in trying to focus on the hospital apart from the rest of the so-called health-care system. And, I must say, sociologists have not been especially notable for their analysis of the total health-care system. They have focused on the hospital setting, and then they have taken an industrial perspective and focused on the nurse usually much more than on anything else. We have already seen some of the limitations associated with this. But, in addition, here we have run into another boundary having to do with the structure of careers and the whole area of occupations and professions.

I think it is quite clear that there is a revolution going on in the career lines of people and the trends in medical education that will reshape careers in the health field. Although what Guest is talking about might not be applicable to physicians in the mass, it might be extraordinarily important for certain doctors at certain key points in their careers. The whole notion of looking at career ladders, career chains, transformation of careers, and the interaction between changing models of career has not been touched here.

Comment: On the question of research concerning the role of the physician, I know of one insightful master's thesis about physician participation in medical committees, staff committees like the credentials committee, the executive committee, etc. That study found a high correlation between active participation on these committees by physicians on the staff and their admission rate of patients to that hospital. In this particular case there were two very large urban hospitals in the community with a 60 percent overlap of medical staffs in the two hospitals. The doctors, depending on the occupancy situation and other factors, put patients in one hospital or the other. But the patient admission rate per doctor varied with the extent of his participation in committees; the degree to which doctors became involved in administrative matters was correlated with how many patients they happened to have in the hospital. Assuming that there would be more involvement of the physician in that hospital in which he had more patients, he is also more likely to be efficient, because while he is making rounds and seeing the patients he can also stop over for a committee meeting. One implication here is that the doctor can combine his particular role as a curative therapist with administrative tasks more efficiently when most of his work takes place in one hospital, or when he can be at the same place where he sees his patients and also tends to administrative matters. I might add that the only exception to that correlation was the psychiatric staff. For all the other staff divisions in the hospital the correlation held.

Chairman: If a further implication that doctors who combine those two aspects of their work are also more productive were correct, then this would be a very important finding. It might well be that, other things being equal, the individual who is getting involved in the system beyond the core functions of his role expends additional energy in his work, tries to become enlightened about his work surroundings and about the organizational forces and constraints that affect his professional role, and thus becomes a more efficient performer both as an individual practitioner and as a member in the system.

Changing Matrix of Clinical Decision-Making

Presentation Highlights: E. D. Pellegrino

I am going to modify what I had in mind to say in the light of some of the cogitations I have had as you all have been talking. And, since there will be another opportunity toward the close of the session to make some additional comments, I am going to reserve for that time the reversal of the tables. While sitting here more or less as an insect encased in amber as you paleontologists looked at that insect, I had some difficulty suppressing my responses because, to be perfectly honest, some of your observations are phenomenologically incorrect and some of the deductions are open to logcial attack. However, I will give a small dissertation on the role of social sciences in medicine later, if I am permitted to provoke you a little toward the end.

I would like now to make a few points on this matter of decision-making and the ways in which it might be controlled. Dr. Zald, forgive me for getting into the field of control, but as you gathered earlier I am very interested because I believe that we must open up, in a way that is socially responsible, that mystical personal confrontation of a person in need with a person attempting to satisfy that need, and this includes all the health professions, not just medicine. By they way, when I use the word "Medicine," I would like it to be understood as medicine with a large M, i.e. all the health professions. I will be using physician medicine as my paradigm, but I feel that the same things apply to the other health-care professions.

Let me give you my letters of credit, since some of you do not know me and since I will be making statements which sometimes are provocative but which I think can be useful to stimulating some thought. I spent six years in a rural community establishing a rural community hospital which I am happy to say, without blushing, has become a model of what a community hospital should be. I am a product of the work-study program; I study what I do after I do it. And I would say that one of the deficits was that we did not study it as we were doing it. But I come out of that situation, working very closely with a community. This is why I insisted so much earlier on emphasizing the tremendous force of the community, and the way in which community needs and desires are going to be expressed. What I gave you was a response at a time that I see this building up exponentially, and I will not press you further with it except to say that this is one of the areas for which I am going to suggest some kinds of research to you.

From there I went to the University of Kentucky to become chairman of the Department of Medicine, again starting from scratch. I would rather go deductively in the medieval fashion, you see, deducing what is the way to a thing, then doing it, and then asking others to study whether or not it has achieved the purpose it set out for itself. The induction comes first, but I have not preceded this kind of research; laboratory research is concerned with what you do now.

Currently, I am involved, as the executive officer, with the establishment of the new Health Sciences Center at Stony Brook, which includes six different professional schools, two hospitals, and a plan for organizing the health-care services in two and perhaps three counties comprising some five and a half million people. This is not to impress you with what I am doing, but simply to indicate that I am feeling these community forces in a very acute way. I cannot wait; there is no time to wait for the results of research. And I would submit that very likely the research would be better if applied to what we are doing to see whether these hypotheses we set forth deductively indeed have validity.

Now, I want to talk about the area in which perhaps I am a little more capable and competent, and that is the area of clinical decision-making. I am an internist, by the way, and I see patients, work in the laboratory, and teach, and if that does not keep me busy I also participate in the quelling of campus riots from time to time. But let us look at the matter of clinical decision-making at the bedside. I think of the hospital as one unit in a matrix of institutions that are designed to meet the health-care needs of society as defined by society, and not as defined by the professional. This must be absolutely clear. If we see the hospital as one unit in this matrix, then I think the balance wheel of the institution is the clinical decision-making, which I define as follows: the process whereby all of the people necessary are involved in arriving at the most prudent decisions which will result in an optimal solution to the problem presented by an individual patient. This means some technique whereby we assess those needs in terms seen by the patient and then in terms seen by the professional and come out with an optimum decision.

It is very important to emphasize this. Though some of you may see it as labeling the obvious, it is not. I am not talking here about the right diagnosis or about the right treatment as defined by professionals or by myself as an internist. That is an entirely different matter. I am concerned with prudential decision-making, optimizing the mini-max principles so to speak, in the clinical area. That is the aim. One reason why I was emphasizing the short-cutting process is that the people out here are beginning to get a feel for this process. The dissatisfactions today which are often expressed in terms of economics, efficiency of care, and so on, are related to an increasing awareness on the part of an educated populace, the consumers. And, incidentally, let us get that out of the way right now. Everybody is a consumer of health care, present or future, and everybody is concerned and knows that this is one of the areas they have no control over. Everyone will become part of the health-care system at some time. The only other people who have that claim to make are the undertakers. Until we resolve the problem of preventive medicine, we are going to have everyone being a consumer—either potential or actual consumer. Let us not develop a semantic argument over that.

The consumers are the ones who, as you say, are speaking through their legislators and saying: "Look, I know that one of the few rounds left in human life today of which I have no control, and which I must hand over to the competence and trust of another human being, is in this area of the disabilities of my physical body and my emotional disturbances." And there is a great deal of resentment over this. Some of the phraseology that came out in our group here is an expression of something deeper than the health-care system. It is an expression of a disturbance with morality, and we as physicians unfortunately must sop up that aggression as well. And we do; it is part of the job. But I want to keep clear that what we are talking about here is an increasing desire on the part of those for whom this whole system is developed to have some input into that bedside clinical decision-making process.

This process has been held sacred, yes. And I think, you are absolutely right, doctors resent people getting into it. But I think that is wrong. I happen to be with the group who believe that we have got to open it up. We also want to remember some of the history of this, however. First of all, the Hippocratic ethic, which everyone thinks has a very high set of norms for every physician, is insufficient in this regard. Actually, the Hippocratic ethic tends to foster the idea of exclusiveness of this one-to-one relationship. If you look at the five or six books on Hippocratic ethics, those which deal with anything even resembling ethics in the philosophical sense (most is etiquette rather than ethics), you will find that the physician is the authoritarian father figure, the benign paternalistic guy who has all the information and who really assumes upon himself all of your problems, becomes your advocate, and so on. In two places in the corpus, the Laws and the Physician, it says that you ought not to tell the patient what is going on for fear of hurting him and also, quite frankly implied in there if you read between the lines, for fear of the intrusion of the patient into the process.

This is a very strong factor in the medical culture, if I can speak anthropologically for a moment. The medical culture goes back to this set of norms and justifies much of its action on the basis of this. I am just completing a paper now on the disruption we ought to have in the Hippocratic ethic. Some of us are beginning to attack even that sacred outpost.

Second, the doctor-patient relationship is of high value. Hans Mauksch gave voice to this when he said, "When I need a medication I want my doctor to order it," and in one fell swoop he did away with the nurse, the administrator, and all the rest. When you are that person, you place a high value on this. This high value has to be preserved, and yet I think we can still achieve that end without saying the doctor is sole authority with reference to what the others do.

Another thing that has caused you trouble, I think, and on which you must change your thinking a little bit, is that you tie too much to the present system, the entrepreneurial system of medical care. Here I come back to my delineation of what I mean by institution. The contract up to this point has been a highly personal contract between the physician and a patient, including the implied contract to health and not to hurt. Now that contract increasingly is being made with an institution. I do not want the administrator or any other person singled out in the institution. I want the institution; that is where the contract is now occurring more and more. If you go to the emergency room of a hospital, your contract is with an institution; it is no longer with a physician. The physician, then, is going to become increasingly a part of the institution. And we have not yet taken into account still another related movement, the trend toward the full-time physician who is there to serve institutional goals.

Now we can begin to think in terms of the possibilities and the control system of a group of physicians who are dedicated to carrying out institutional goals as defined institutionally, and not as defined in terms of the propagation of their own practice. And there is a tremendous dichotomy between these two value systems. Ergo, once again, do not pick on any particular source of power yet. You have got a way to go in this, because I think you have got to take all these factors into account. These factors have not been sufficiently recognized. While the central practice of the physician has not been the hospital, it is becoming that increasingly. So let us take a look at control and the clinical decision-making process with these things in mind. The doctor-patient relationship is going to have to change, and we can get into this formerly sacred process.

There are some ways in which we can get at this process in terms of control. We can measure how the physician, who has input from a lot of people and who works with those people in the output of prudential decisions, is performing. If we think in terms of prudential decision-making we can do it. A certain amount of pessimism about our ability to measure quality of care was expressed here, and I want to take a stand against it. We can measure the output in terms of the prudent decisions being made. We can ask and answer the question, "Is this the right decision at this time?" And I want to emphasize this point again, because you are not clinicians, and I want to put it across forcefully. A prudential decision may be made by the most nonscientific practitioner in the world. It can be made by a chiropractor, it can be made by a practitioner of Vedic medicine, it can be made by a faith healer, and my thesis is that I do not care who made the decision if that were the prudent decision for that patient at that time. It is the endpoint and the end result that we are looking for.

In the system, obviously, the probabilities of prudential decisions will vary with the nature of the illness. And certainly a Vedic physician can do as well as I can with perhaps 40 percent of the common ills of mankind. Beyond that, society has to decide how much it wants to pay for the insurance of the remaining 60 percent. For the majority of cases that would involve the ordinary practitioner; it is only about 10 percent that you call scientific medicine. I am talking here about competent prudential decisions in terms of action. Whether the care is also administered compassionately and personally is another dimension, and on that the physicians have no corner on the market any longer. We are going to measure that in another way.

Let us go back and look at the decision-making process. It seems to me that these are the things which are coming, and I am not going to worry about the intervening research. What I think you should do is research to find out whether or not these deductions we are making are valid and solve the problem. That is one kind of research which would be useful. In order to assure society, whoever the intermediaries happen to be, we have to be able to provide some answers. We have to be able to examine the individual physician's practice. (When I talk about this among my colleagues I get a lot of response, because I deal with them in a different way than I deal with you, but I do not expect that I will get the same reactions from you.)

What do I mean by this? I mean that we are going to have to institutionalize the surveillance of clinical decision-making, institutionalize it not in the hands of the administrator, as some would like, but in the hands of a group of people properly designated and given the right of surveillance. This is already occuring in some places, and we are beginning to develop a new brand of person for this. But, more importantly, what I would like to see is that the physicians in the institution take it upon themselves as a corporate responsibility transmitted back to them through a chief of professional services, who is not the familiar chief of the medical staff. What is needed is a chief of professional services, institutionally ordained, to see that the things I am going to.talk about actually do occur. The chief of professional services will be working for the board of trustees, for the community people who gave rise to this hospital by putting their money into the hospital because they wanted certain ends to be achieved. This has actually been done, in my own experience; I have personally done it. Ergo, it can work at least in one case.

What are some of the things that are feasible? I am talking about feasibilities in clinical practice. Certainly one of the first things has to do with medications. Hospital administrators will have a dim view, perhaps, of what I am going to say, because they do not have the people in their hospitals who can carry this out and have the muscle to do it at this time. But let us take the matter of prescribing practices, one segment of it. Consider the use of drugs, for example. It is not even three tetracyclines rather than five; you need only one tetracycline available in the hospital. The people who perpetrate most of this extravagance are the pharmacists and the physicians, but the physicians more than the pharmacists—the physicians who somehow hold that the particular brand of drug they are using has a visceral sensation or is a more useful drug.

In our situation we have developed a system in which the prescribing practices of every physician are collated. Every patient, through a drug information center in the hospital (we started this in Kentucky and have extended it further since then), has a card with the diagnosis, the major facts about him, the drugs that are being used at any particular moment for him, and the attending physician and the house staff who are associated with him. I am suggesting that initially we can do two things with the drug prescribing practices. We have done the first of these, which is to call periodically for a review by the appropriate committees or departments of the drug prescribing practices, first en masse, of the community of physicians in that hospital. When you do that, you get into some problems. For example, urologists are perhaps the least intellectual of all the people in medicine, except perhaps the allergists or the dermatologists. And the urologists have a fatal fascination for using dangerous drugs for trivial infections. You could single out individual physicians, but that is not the way to go at this. The way you do it is to ask what are the prescribing practices vis-a-vis urinary tract infections in this hospital. And we can pull this off the record very quickly and find out that for E. coli, for era erogenous, for such and such and so and so, this is what is being done. Then you tally that against the best practice of one's scientific peers, and this is available in such things as the newsletter, the journals, and so on.

So, first, you can check on the practices of the staff as a group, and here is where the lay board can get something that is understandable. It has got to be interpreted by a chief medical official who is serving them, however, and who says: "Look, this is what is happening." Second, you can examine the individual prescribing practices of individual physicians. I think we are going to have to impersonalize their thinking to a certain extent. But we can do this by a computer, and the individual physician can check at any time what he has been doing with his cases as opposed to what the peer optimum decision-making would require at that time for urinary tract infections.

We can devise similarly appropriate programs for most of the major ills of mankind. We are beginning to do it in continuing education. We are interested not so much in the ability of the physician to spew back the latest article in the *Archives of Internal Medicine*—that has a certain intellectual delectation about it—but really we are interested in terms of how he is handling certain situations now vis-a-vis the way in which a group of the best people would handle them. Medicine is an authoritarian group and, believe it or not, they do respect authority when it is well established. And they will respect the point of view of peers whom they know on the handling of particular situations. After all, that is what continuing education is all about. We can review not only prescribing practices but also such things as: "How long does this man keep such and such a patient in the hospital?" "Did that patient come back for the same illness?" "What are this man's workup practices?" These are all technical things that I do not have to explicate to you, but I can assure you as a clinician that we can work out the necessary techniques. We are going to have to do that for individual physicians. This would include the usual reviews we have now which are just minimal and all too often cursory, such as the reviews of tissue committees and all the rest of them.

Another aspect that we can carry out, and it is going to occur without any question, is the mandatory recertification of every physician—and I would suggest at seven-year periods. This is another way in which the group outside can have control over the efficiency of clinical decision-making. In all seriousness, the mandatory recertification route is coming. It is essential, and, again, we are going to have to admit that some people are not able to make the prudent decision either by force of age or disability or whatever. And then we have to do what every profession has to do, namely protect those who are not capable of doing certain things. By protect I do not mean to let them do what they cannot do well, but find alternative pathways for them and have a series of pathways for the individual who cannot measure up. This is the only way society can be protected, and the only way we can get competence. And as I said earlier, competence now becomes a moral issue because we have capabilities. It was not an issue when we did not have capability.

You were looking for national norms earlier, were you not? Well, out of the prudential decision-making process, if we look at it that way, we can develop national norms. And we may get to the point that we can make this a very highly objective sort of evaluation, possibly by physician number. We can begin now to develop a program in which we want to follow the key points in decision-making in individual situations for the individual physician, utilize it, and keep it under his number. Then we can call it back. We could give a monthly rundown by physician number, just as you do with students who do not want people to know what their marks are. We can give an objective evaluation of prudential decision-making against a peer group.

If you want to think about this in terms of research, I think that sociomedical research here is going to be primarily in the area of methodology. Can we devise methods—and this may require more psychology than sociology—which will indeed ensure that we are measuring what we think we are measuring? In terms of the internal organization of the hospital, it seems to me that what is needed is a role for a person who will be responsible to see that this evaluation process goes on. If we create chiefs of professional services in hospitals who are charged with this, as they are at least in some of the teaching institutions, we will take a step in the right direction. It will not be perfection, but this way we can intrude into the physician-patient relationship.

For that role I would use the craftsman model that Mauksch brought up. I think the craftsman model would fit well here. Craftsmanship is definable in relation to the end product. Craftsmanship is required, so to speak, to bring it about. It can be measured, and I think that the model will work in terms of measurement and evaluation.

Another area that I wanted to say something about is the area of the team. Let us look at the decision-making process within a team. Here the suggestion of the transitory system fits beautifully. But let me say a couple of things about the team that are important from a social scientist's point of view. There is no fixed medical care team. That is point number one. And, generically, all I mean by team is that group of individuals who at any particular time are required to bring about the optimal solution to the patient's problem or a medical problem.

I see three levels of teams. There is a patient care team, there is a medical care team, and then there is a health care team. Everybody is on the team, of course, just like everybody is involved in decision-making. The administrator is involved in clinical decision-making if he makes a decision about admission policies, for example, quite obviously. Similarly, the trustees may decide not have an open heart program; thus they are involved in clinical decision-making for a person who comes to that hospital. But let me try to be a little more definitive because the distinction among the three teams has not been made sufficiently clear.

The patient care team is that group of individuals who deal directly, in direct confrontation, with the patient in the solution of a specific problem engendered by a specific patient. The emphasis is on direct personal confrontation with the patient or on a personal service to the patient. Physicians, nurses, social workers, and even the transitory personnel such as the technicians who come in and stick the patient once in a while are members of this team. But the key members are those who provide the personal services. This is the patient care team.

The composition of the patient care team varies with the needs of the patient. Obviously, if you take one end of the spectrum, the surgical amphitheater, there can only be one captain of the team, the surgeon. You do not want anybody else, and I do not want anybody else. But if you take the other end of the spectrum, a patient who is recovering from a stroke, I think the captain of the team need not, and indeed should not, be a physician. If you go somewhere in between, the patient with a medical problem who has recovered from the acute phase, I think the internist is partly the captain of the team, and he too can drop out of it at a certain point. And if you want to go to the next step, you have the coronary care unit where for the most critical moments the nurse is the captain of the team. She is making the decisions as to whether you do or do not call this or that person in.

Thus there is a varying captaincy. The physician is not automatically the captain of the team. Therefore, in your analysis of power structures I think you must take this into account. In the future the captain of the team will not necessarily be the physician. And the power for clinical decision-making or the initiation of it is going to shift, indeed it is already shifting. In long-term units, for example, the physicians now are bowing out in actual fact, and the nurse who is there is captain of that team.

Another team is the medical care team, which consists of all those people required to solve a medical problem but not in direct confrontation with the patient. Here you have all of those people who say: "Oh, yes; but I am part of the team too. I am down in the business office, and I am making it possible." Or, "I am in the laboratory measuring the oxygen saturation." They too are part of the medical care team, but not the patient care team. (I am discussing the three teams in this particular order because I think there is a corresponding hierarchy of values here, and I hope to say something about values later.)

Then there is the health care team, which includes all those concerned with the question of how we plan for the health of the community, how we improve the total health of all the individuals. This is a more preventive concern while the concerns of the other two teams are more curative, but the elements in all are needs, quite obviously. On the health care team you have all of the people in public health, and the people in sociology, and all other people who are concerned about how to make this whole vast system work for the goals which society has defined.

Here is how I see the professional relating to the power structure. The professional in these situations, obviously, is the expert for implementing the overall plan. I agree thoroughly that the physician should not be the one who establishes the goals of the health care system or even the goals of the hospital. If the community decided, for example, that it wanted an outpatient department and did not want to put its dollars into beds, than I think that should be open for discussion between the community and the physicians. The physicians would spell out the alternatives and say what is needed to do the job. But the distribution of resources I think is a social decision which does not lie with the professional. The power there, as far as I am concerned, lies outside the medical system. This is again why I emphasize the forces outside the system. In the area of the individual needs of individual patients, however, the power resides and must reside, on a day-to-day basis, with the health professions, not just medicine but the health professions. The physician, as I have tried to indicate, increasingly will share this power with other health professionals.

The health care team presents a bigger issue, and it would take more time than we have to go into it right now. But for the patient care team we can use the transitory system model. This team is a nice transitory system that could be studied as it is being set up. The goal is specific and you can measure the outputs, I think, reasonably well because you can say: "What was the problem? How did they do it? Did they do it efficiently? Did they use all the people necessary? Did they satisfy the needs? Essentially it is based on the idea of developing a template of needs for each patient when he comes in and then seeing how well that has been filled in. It is not that difficult and can be done fairly rigorously.

The health care team I think is more difficult to evaluate because it gets into the question of values. I do not know how detailed sociologists want to be about values. I know Weber's prescription not to be too value-oriented, to be value neutral. But perhaps you cannot hold to that today as much as you did in the past. He developed that notion because he did not want sociology to be a tool with a political aim, of course. But I think you may have to help, in this way at least, by analyzing the consequences of value decisions for all of us. You have a very important role in this area.

Let me briefly summarize what is just the top of a very big iceberg that I have before me. Simply, I believe that we can think in terms of opening up that sacred one-to-one relationship in medicine. We can open it up in certain specific ways, and I have just touched on some of them, at least superficially. That opening up is going to put the people in the community who want to use the hospital for a purpose in direct, or rather more direct, contact with the hospital and the medical practitioners, short-circuiting the clinical decision-making. Those in between are going to be caught in between unless there is some question of how to satisfy their needs as well. And the research needed, sociologically and in terms of models, would be research that would study the perturbations in those systems as power shifts around among these various groups.

Discussion

Comment (Dr. Scott): I have been involved for some time in work that I think bears very closely on some of the ways in which social scientists could help in doing precisely what you want to do here. We are trying to reconceptualize power and authority and focus on power in terms of its effect on tasks, i.e. the work that is done in organizations. We feel that the only way we can do that is to have some kind of evaluation process. So we begin with a model of the evaluation process.

We have said that there are certain kinds of fundamental components that have to be present before an evaluation can take place, and we have labeled these allocation. A person has to know for what he is being evaluated. There has to be some kind of task definition; some kind of criterion setting is needed. Standards, properties, or dimensions of the task have to be singled out for attention, with appropriate weights, if those values are to be combined in some way. Second, there must be some sampling, some attempt to look at the actual values of the dimensions that you have defined as relevant, and some attempt to look at the actual values produced by a performance on those dimensions. And finally there must be the actual appraising in which you look at the values in the sample and compare them with the values on the appropriate dimensions and the criteria to arrive at a performance evaluation.

What we mean by performance evaluation is that an evaluation is arrived at such that sanctions or rewards and penalites are distributed in terms of how the person scores. One of the reasons why we divided the evaluation process into these particular components is that in complex organizations these components are very often given to different actors in the system. Some people are involved in the allocation of tasks, perhaps a supervisor. There are other people who are involved with criteria-setting; perhaps a unit that is away from the actual flow of work sets standards for these kinds of tasks (and we are talking about groups which could set standards that could be used in publication and so forth). In complex organizations there are very often inspectors who actually gather the data. They do not themselves make the evaluation, but they gather the data or set the sampling frame by which data are gathered about the quality of work being carried out. And finally there is perhaps again a supervisor who compares the sample with the criteria, making adjustments for particular problems and situations, to arrive at an appraisal.

One of the things that we have been doing for the last five years is attempting to map, in a simplistic or loose and descriptive way, the distribution of these rights, because individually each of these has an effect on the evaluation and, therefore, also on the distribution of sanctions. Each can be viewed as an authority right: the right to allocate, the right to set criteria, the right to sample, and the right to appraise.

One of the things we are doing is looking at the way in which these rights are distributed across positions in a formal organization. Once you take this kind of fairly specific model, you can ask very specific questions of people, e.g. "Who does this kind of thing?" The things you then find in a whole range of organizations we have looked at are rather interesting. First, there is very often enormous ignorance on the part of performers. They realize that evaluations are being made, that somehow their work is being observed by someone, but they are not quite sure what the criteria are and they are not quite sure who does the sampling. I think that people who care about the quality of their work, professionals in particular, get very upset and irritated when one begins to talk to them about the evaluation process, because they realize the sloppy way in which these very important kinds of judgments are being made.

It seems to me that one of the ways in which this kind of model can be used is, first, to study the complexity of different systems, simply by looking at the different kinds of positions that become involved or are exercising these different kinds of rights. Second, the model helps one to focus on where the problem areas are and where they may be. It helps one determine, for example, that a certain function is not being performed at all, or that it is not being performed in such a way that it becomes visibly apparent and understandable to the people who are subject to that particular authority system. I think that this kind of research we are doing very much would support your kind of interest here, in trying to say that we can look at these fundamental tasks and then begin to talk about appropriate ways to control their performance.

Question (Dr. Jaco): Would there not be a question though about who decides what the criteria are? A lot of people get upset because nurses get too tired of people telling them what they should be doing but never consulting with people who are performing those tasks about what the standards should be.

Answer: That is why we introduced distinctions like "who actually does it" and "who do you think should do it?" We look both at the actual distribution of rights and the extent to which people believe it is proper, or legitimate, that these people exercise the particular rights. One learns a lot about problems in the system by making just these kinds of comparisons.

Comment (Dr. Pellegrino): In the clinical situation, we are beginning to see ourselves getting to the point where it is going to be a peer group who can establish these things almost on a national basis. Let me give you an example. We had great confusion in the area of diagnosis with the diagnostic criteria of heart disease many years ago. Finally, the New York Heart Association after much effort, and then the American Heart Association, were able to elaborate a set of diagnostic criteria so we are all talking the same language or at least beginning to approach it. It is this kind of thing we do now in certain areas of therapeutics, Dr. Jaco, and I would submit that in the fields I know we can do it with reasonable ease.

Comment (Dr. White): I have two points to make, one of which is informational. This problem of quality of care is of much concern in the medical literature. And the kind of model that you both describe to some extent is being implemented in one or two cases that I know. You might know about Clement Brown in Philadelphia who has had a hospital going for about five years with a system like this, with a computer built in for these kinds of processes. Also, you might know about John Williams' study of a traditional system pointing out to physicians that unexpected positive results on tests were not responded to. The problem they had there, when a kind of authoritarian system was used, was that this was not responded to.

My second point has to do with another aspect of what you have been saying. I think I would agree with you, but would point out some of the difficulties in what you call society. We have a pluralistic society with very little consensus and a number of groups with differential power and ability, so that what comes out of this may not be a rational system. Everyone may be striving for his own type of rationality, but in the collective process it is always hard to tell what will come out.

Response (Dr. Pellegrino): I understand that thoroughly, and yet unless we make the effort to make contact with whatever it is that constitutes the community, we are never going to get the kind of relationship that I think is being demanded. I think you are right, there are those who make more noise than others and therefore have more power or more influence on the system at any given moment.

Chairman: You do not, though, say that the solution would be the net outcome of these inputs. All you are saying is that these inputs should find their way into the focal point within the health care system.

Answer (Dr. Pellegrino): Absolutely, I am thinking of a continuing feedback system. There must be a mechanism for inputs, and here again a student of social organization can help us. Research can be applied to discover what are the best mechanisms for a continuing input, and for creating a sensivitity and responsiveness which we do not now have because our institutions today are so complex and heavy and not responsible. And, I must say that in that first experience I described for you in that rural area, I really felt that there at least we were in contact with the bulk of whatever the community was. And we had much evidence for this—for example, fifty thousand volunteer hours in a small community hospital, more than the Columbia-Presbyterian Medical Center. The number of people who came through and were involved was another kind of evidence.

But, personally, I would suggest that if you want to go beyond this you need something more than a conventional board of trustees. Frankly, I see the board of trustees only as the executive committee of an elected council or some kind of elected Community Health Authority for the health-care institutions. I do not think they are going to become responsible until that kind of power is vested there, perhaps via a legislative process. I know all the dangers. As you probably have gathered, there are not too many people who are as highly individualistic as I am or as desirous of autonomy. Yet within the kind of health system that I am speaking about, we have got to have this kind of reflection and control and responsibility.

Question: Organizationally, what would you recommend? To whom does this chief of professional services report? You say he is an employee of the board of trustees. Is he responsible to the board directly, or to the administrator of the hospital? I think this is a vital point.

Answer: At the risk of alienating some of my administrative friends, I think we are going to be developing a new group of clinical-care administrators who are trained, by-and-large, in clinical medicine and then, as hospitals move to full-time physicians, become the chief officers in hospitals.

Question: Do you have in mind a dual administrative arrangement?

Answer: No. I am talking about the medical director who is trained in both clinical medicine and hospital administration. And, by the way, medical education does not disqualify one from an administrative role.

Question: Do you have in mind the director of medical education?

Answer: No. The trouble with the DME is that he has no power; the chiefs of service have the power. But when you have a chief of professional services, he is going to have power.

Comment: But if he reports to the chief of the medical staff, he would be just a flunky.

Answer: He would be the chief of professional services in the hospital and report to the medical director or the director of the institution. If you want a nonmedical person, that is all right. But what I have in mind is a chief of professional services who is charged with the responsibility as I am, for example, in the university. I am delegated the authority from the president to run the health sciences center, but I still have to report to the president.

Comment: That is something important organizationally, because this role is given authority and power. Many hospitals have just a chief, either of professional education or of some such thing, who does not have sufficient authority or power over medical practice.

Comment: He is a flunky, you are right. And the chief of the medical staff is an honorific position which comes to a man only if he lives long enough. I am talking about a person charged with carrying out the institutional goals; he is the institutional agent.

Question: Would this be the hospital administrator?

Answer: No.

Comment: That is where, I think, you have got a blind spot.

Answer: O.K. Let us get at this later, if we can. May I make my point quickly? We have a hospital board of trustees and then, whatever you want to call it, a Community Health Council. The director of the hospital can be a physician or nonphysician. That is not my point; he can be either one in my opinion. I think he has to have a director of professional services, and I would see all the professional services, including medicine and nursing, under him.

Chairman: You are suggesting some ways in which social scientists might contribute something, Ed (Dr. Pellegrino), and your suggestions raise a fairly key issue in my mind from the point of view of research. It concerns organizational structure. Let me first make some points and then raise a question on this.

To a considerable extent our discussion has been futuristic or prospective rather than retrospective. While we are evaluating the literature of the last decade we are looking toward the future a great deal at the same time. Most of the comments made so far seem to point in the direction of greater openness and more democratization of the health system, greater representation of community interests, more sensitivity to consumer demands, more other-directedness on the part of the hospital and the various professional groups, and greater interdependence among all concerned inside and outside the hospital. You are proposing certain solutions based upon performance evaluation, power relations, and contribution to the clinical decision-making process. It is also historically true, it seems, and our political situation in the current national scene seems to bear this out, that the democratic model based upon elective representation sometimes does not work well unless you have appropriate checks and balances and structural mechanisms that reinforce the democratic process. What are the structural mechanisms and organizational arrangements, or innovations, that one has to introduce into this emerging institutional system to accommodate and reinforce these kinds of new trends, so that what you are proposing would be an effectively functioning system? I think our models, so far, tell us how to study important variables, and some of the variables that we should study, but not very much about the nature of the structure.

Answer: That is right. This is a key question, and it is this kind of research that I would like to see coming out of this. Those of us who are put in my position of taking action now have to arrive at it deductively. But I would hope that you would come up with alternative models of structure, and also study the models that we actually put into practice.

Part Six

15

THE HOSPITAL ADMINISTRATOR AND ORGANIZATIONAL EFFECTIVENESS*

Anthony R. Kovner

The primary purposes of this paper are: (1) to survey that part of the research literature of the 1960s which is concerned with the administrator's influence on hospital effectiveness; (2) to delineate major problem areas in hospital effectiveness for the 1970s; and (3) to assess the hospital administrator's capacity to influence organizational effectiveness in these areas. The literature surveyed is rather limited, because of the difficulties in measuring hospital effectiveness and the administrator's influence upon effectiveness. Those studies and articles reviewed have been written by social scientists and administrators and pertain to American short-term general hospitals. The survey also encompassed over two hundred articles and books to which reference is not made. These were felt to be repetitive of references cited with regard to a particular point or to be either not relevant or not useful. (Complete bibliography of all sources considered is available from the author on request.)

The introductory sections describe briefly some of the goals of hospitals and their characteristics as organizations. The education of hospital administrators, their characteristics, and the tasks which they perform are described next. The major problem areas which are then discussed include: cost control, the sharing of power, organizational structure, manpower utilization, and patient care.

The Hospital Industry

In 1968 there were 5820 nonfederal short-term hospitals employing over 1.7 million people and spending almost $14.2 billion annually. The industry has been labeled "cottage" because of the large number of small units. There has been a trend in the direction of a decreasing number of units, however, and of an increasing size per unit. In 1968 there were 456 fewer hospitals than in 1959. In the same period the average size of hospitals increased from

*Revised version of paper presented at Conference on Hospital Organization Research, May 22-23, 1970, Institute for Social Research, The University of Michigan, Ann Arbor, Michigan. Anthony R. Kovner, Ph.D., is Director of the Graduate Program in Health Care Administration, Wharton School, and Executive Administrator of Group Practice, Department of Medicine, University of Pennsylvania. The writer acknowledges with thanks the suggestions of a number of colleagues and friends, in particular Robert Eilers, Joel Kovner, and Robert Sigmond, who were especially critical and helpful.

116 to 139 beds, and the percentage of hospitals with less than 200 beds decreased from 84 to 79.

Hospitals are becoming more complex and more costly, as well as larger. From 1959 to 1968 personnel per 100 patients increased from an average of 223 to 272, and the percentage of hospitals with pharmacies, recovery rooms, and intensive care units increased from 43, 47, and 7 respectively, to 72, 73, and 42. In 1968 the cost per patient day of $61.38 was more than double that of $30.19 in 1959 (*Hospitals*, Guide Issues of 1960 and 1969).

In 1968, 59 percent of the nonfederal short-term general hospitals were under voluntary auspice, or ownership, 13 percent were proprietary, and 28 percent were governmental. Of the 806,000 beds available in 1968, the voluntary hospitals had 70 percent, the proprietary hospitals had 6 percent, and the governmental hospitals had 24 percent. There has been no great change in auspice since 1959. In 1968, 61 percent of the hospitals and 70 percent of the beds were under voluntary auspice.

Since 1968 business corporations have entered the hospital industry, and the proprietary share of facilities may increase. Thirty-eight companies now control more than 25 percent of the proprietary hospitals and nearly 40 percent of the proprietary beds. These corporations now own 19,100 beds and have planned, as of 1970, to add or construct an additional 14,000 beds (Earle, 1970).

As an organization, the short-term general hospital has certain distinguishing characteristics, including: a high ratio of personnel to total expenses; a diversity of objectives such as medical care and education and research; round-the-clock service; dual authority resulting from the independent status of doctors; a product, health or medical care, which is difficult to measure; and an involvement with problems of life and death (White, 1961; Georgopoulos, 1966). The goals, structure, and technology of particular types of hospitals (e.g. small and rural, middle-sized and suburban, large, complex, and urban), however, may have more in common with those of business or welfare and education organizations of similar size, complexity, and environment than with those of hospitals of other types (Perrow, 1965; Woodward, 1965).

Because of the varying character of hospitals, their goals also differ. For example, large complex teaching hospitals in urban settings tend to set a higher priority than other hospitals upon the treatment of patients who are critically ill, and upon providing comprehensive care for disadvantaged segments of the community (although the latter has had a higher priority only lately). Middle-sized hospitals in suburban settings tend to set a higher priority upon meeting the needs of medical staffs and physicians in their private practice. Small hospitals in rural settings tend to set a higher priority perhaps on financial solvency and institutional survival.

Hospital Effectiveness

Effectiveness may be defined as level of goal achievement. One ideal goal for hospitals would be to provide optimal health services to a given population group. In a statement of the American Hospital Association, optimal health services are described as including the following: a team approach to care of the individual under the leadership of the physician; a spectrum of services including diagnosis, treatment, rehabilitation, education, and prevention; a coordinated community and regional system of health services; continuity between hospital and nonhospital services; continuing evaluation and research on quality (American Hospital Association, 1965).

Such a statement of philosophy does not lend itself easily to measures of accountability and can be challenged certainly on economic grounds. It does represent, however, a strong feeling among some consumer representatives and health professionals that the goals of the hospital must be broadened. Such groups often favor determination of hospital goals by others than providers and administrators. Regardless of the merit of this point of view, there are indications that hospital goals are being broadened. Some of these indications include the establishment of psychiatric units in general hospitals, the provision of home care services, the development of neighborhood health centers, the provision of multiphasic screening by certain institutions, the expansion of family planning clinics, and a growing recognition of the need for local and regional planning of health care facilities.

Recently, Sigmond (1967) stated that the present goals of hospitals were a mixture of: better quality of patient care; better education and research results; meeting the needs of the physicians or medical staffs in their private practice; comprehensive care for disadvantaged segments in the community; financial solvency and institutional survival; and prestige for those associated with the institution. Interest groups within the hospital set varying priorities regarding these goals. The composition of groups which will support different objectives varies according to objective. For example, physicians differ regarding the relative values of care for the disadvantaged as compared with private practice patients, and trustees differ regarding the relative values of prestige as compared with financial solvency.

Governmental and proprietary hospitals have been accused of being ineffective and having inappropriate goals. Government hospitals have lacked adequate financing because of the low social class role of governmental institutions in American society (Elling and Halebsky, 1961). Moreover, they have suffered from rigidity of procedures and organization, and often have had difficulties in attracting professional staff (Klarman, 1965). At least theoretically, however, governmental hospitals would seem to offer advantages of greater accountability to representatives of all the community, and of greater coordination of care through the employment of large numbers of full-time physicians.

Proprietary hospitals have been accused of allowing unnecessary utilization, of providing care of low quality (Morehead, 1964), and of expanding in violation of planning recommendations (Earle, 1970). Proprietary hospitals generally provide routine care to nonindigent patients, leaving the complex, more expensive care of indigent patients to the nonprofit sector (Trussell and Van Dyke, 1960). Nevertheless, according to Earl (1970), proprietary hospitals have adopted recommendations that for years have been directed at voluntary hospitals, e.g. sharing services and facilities, optimizing use of scarce management talent through operation of mulitple facilities, and avoiding duplication of unnecessary facilities.

As to the level of goal achievement by American short-term general hospitals during the 1960s, this writer believes that the level has been high as regards the provision of complex care to critically ill patients; moderate as regards the provision of patient care to those not critically ill and the provision of services in a convenient way to ambulatory patients; and low as regards the systematic provision of a broad range of health services to a given population group or the total population.

The Hospital Administrator

Professional Education

Westfall (1969) has estimated that as many as 30,000 administrative positions are found in the health services industry. Assuming a turnover rate of 5 percent, he projects a need to produce 1500 graduates of health-care administration programs per year currently, and 2000 graduates per year by 1979. The education of hospital administrators is now being carried out within the wider context of medical care or health services administration. The great majority of program graduates are employed by hospitals; of the 5466 alumni of programs, Chester (1969) states that in 1968, 75 percent were employed in hospitals and related institutions.

In 1968, 30 programs in hospital administration issued about four hundred degrees. More than half of the programs were set up in the 1960s, and only nine presently operational were active before 1950. Excluding two large programs (Army-Baylor and George Washington), the average intake per program in 1967 was 20 students, ranging from 12 at Yale and Florida to 32 in Minnesota (Chester, 1969). Most programs are parts of schools of public health or business adminstation. Wren (1967) found no significant differences in program attributed to location in the two types of schools.

Programs in hospital administration have been categorized by Griffith (1967) as focusing on the hospital as an institution, the health care environment, and administrative skills. Thompson and Filerman (1967) have specified areas of coursework related to medical care to include the following: the incidence and prevalence of disease in the population; chronic disease and geriatric problems; the cost of medical care; medical personnel; the history of medical technology and hospitals; health insurance; the hospital as a community health center; hospital planning; the supply and distribution of hospital beds; and governmental proposals for health insurance and public and medical services. Courses considered relevant to hospital or medical-care administration include: public health, biostatistics, epidemiology, environmental sanitation, maternal and child health (emphasized more in schools of public health), accounting, statistics, economics, management, and data processing (emphasized more in schools of business) (Wren, 1967). Elective courses are often available to students in economics, sociology, psychology, political science, management, and insurance and law.

A typical hospital administration student in the early 1960s was characterized by New as having graduated from a small undistinguished college, and as having made two or three major career changes following blocked mobility in small firms or small departments of large firms. The student had perhaps tried another profession after the occupantional experience prior to admission to a program. Such a student desired to work in a small to medium-sized rural or suburban hospital where he would work up to the position of administrator and thus achieve security and respectability in a moderately challenging position (Perrow, 1965; see also Barnett, 1964). Today's prototype is perhaps younger and has graduated from a larger, more prestigious college from which he has directly entered a program. He desires work in a large urban or suburban hospital or in a related health organization such as a planning agency, where he will work up to an executive job which can afford him prestige and status in a challenging position.

There has been some movement among programs toward increasing the academic program from one year to two, with a decrease in the student residency to the three-month period intervening between the two academic years. It would be useful to compare the effectiveness of graduates of programs with short and long residencies, and to evaluate different types of residencies of the same duration (for some of the problems associated with the residency, see Hartmann and Levey, 1964). The relationship between type of education and administrative performance should also be explored, although problems in measuring and isolating the dependent variable will be difficult to overcome.

At present there are few programs which provide training for positions which require less than graduate education but more than on-the-job training. Such positions include those of administrative assistants in departments such as radiology and laboratories, and certain department heads. Efforts in the area of continuing education have been limited. Cost-benefit analysis needs to be made comparing investments in various kinds of manpower training in hospital administration.

Professional Tasks and Characteristics

The chief executive officer of the hospital is known variously as the superintendent, the hospital administrator, the executive director, the executive vice president, and the president (Johnson, 1966). In his study of 356 hospitals in New York, New Jersey, and Pennsylvania, Rosenkrantz (1967) found that 22 percent of administrators were members or officers of the board of trustees and that several held the office of president of the board of trustees. In many hospitals, besides the chief executive officer there are associate and assistant administrators or directors, administrative assistants and assistants to the chief executive officer. In some hospitals personnel officers, controllers, and directors of nursing carry these titles as well.

Mechanic (1962) has emphasized the special expert knowledge of the administrator who is also a doctor of medicine, this stemming from his ability to oppose legitimately a doctor who contests an administrative decision on the basis of medical necessity. Although increasing specialization and rapidly changing technology limit severely the medical administrator's knowledge in any medical specialty, shared training and language probably result in a higher legitimacy of decisions affecting medical staff. It would be interesting to learn whether there is a difference between how medical and lay administrators spend their time, and whether their administrative staff differ.

Special medical knowledge is not an important part of the administrator's job if one accepts Perrow's emphasis that "the increasing complexity of inpatient care and diagnostic medicine, the proliferation of specialists, medical and paramedical, and the dominant role the hospital plays in organizing and servicing a variety of community health services" demand a level of administrative ability and a disinterested concern for community health that goes beyond the socialization and training of medical specialists (Perrow, 1965). The trend is toward a smaller percentage of physicians as a percentage of the total number of administrators, from 33 percent in 1952 to 23 percent in 1962 (Katsive, 1965). This is true for all hospitals, including 2500 long-term and federal hospitals, of which psychiatric hospitals are often legally required to have a medical administrator.

The 1965 Cornell Survey (4000 respondents) characterized hospital administrators as follows: two thirds are between 35 and 55 years old; 79 percent are men; 72 percent are college graduates; 43 percent have advanced degrees; 50 percent have been in their present jobs for less than 6 years, the average job tenure being about 7 years. Forty-eight percent of the administrators of hospitals with less than 100 beds earned from $5000 to $10,000 per year; 69 percent of the administrators of hospitals with 300 to 400 beds earned $20,000 or higher per year (Dolson, 1966).

Connors and Hutt (1967), in studying the five-man administrative staff of a university teaching hospital, found that on the average administrators spent 27 percent of their time in extramural activities, 23 percent in controlling, 22 percent on planning, 12 percent on personal affairs, 8 percent on organizing, and 8 percent on directing and coordinating. The top administrator spent considerably more of his time (37 percent) in extramural activities, planning (26 percent), and organizing (13 percent), and less time in controlling (17 percent), directing and coordinating (5 percent), and personal affairs (3 percent).

Murray and others (1968) used the same format in a later study of 55 Catholic and non-Catholic hospitals. They found that, for the most part, there were no significant differences between the Catholic and the non-Catholic hospitals. Percentages for the non-Catholic hospitals are compared, in Table 1, with those for the teaching hospital studied by Connors and Hutt.

Certain differences in time allocations are explained by size and complexity. Administrators of large hospitals spend more time planning and less time operating. Problems in methodology would seem to account for the significant differences between the time spent on directing and controlling (one fifth as much by the teaching hospital administrator compared to Murray's 55 hospital administrators) and on organizing (three times as much

TABLE 1. PERCENT OF ADMINISTRATOR'S TIME SPENT ON VARIOUS ACTIVITIES

Activity	Connors and Hutt (1967) Teaching hospital	Murray et al. (68) Non-Catholic hos. All in study	400 beds or more	1-99 beds
Planning	25.8	25.5	31.2	23.3
Directing and Coordinating	4.5	24.6	20.7	23.6
Extramural	36.9	20.9	22.7	16.2
Personal	3.4	11.8	13.5	13.9
Controlling	16.5	11.4	8.6	10.9
Organizing	12.9	3.9	3.1	4.1
Operating	- -	1.9	0.3	8.0

by the teaching hospital administrator). But even after combining these two categories, differences remain which warrant further investigation for an understanding of the administrator's job.

Problem Areas of Administration and Organization

The rest of this chapter will examine some areas in which hospital effectiveness is being questioned, and the influence of the administrator in these areas. These include: costs and financing, the sharing of power for decision-making, organizational structure, manpower utilization, and patient care.

Costs and Financing of Operations

Many decisions regarding costs and the financing of operations, such as the level of reimbursement for care of indigent patients and for educational expenses, are not controllable by the administrator. If operating losses are to be avoided, efficiency savings cannot be reinvested in desired nonreimburseable activities. Reimbursement on the basis of cost provides a disincentive to the low-cost producer who is in effect choosing a lower level of goal achievement. For example, assuming that a public relations department provides some of a hospital's community with information necessary to utilize services effectively, the low-cost hospital with no public relations department chooses to be less effective. Current methods of reimbursement favor use of most expensive rather than least expensive medical care facilities and are not sufficient to discourage unnecessary procedures and utilization. (For alternative methods of reimbursement see U.S. Department of Health, Education, and Welfare, 1968; Health Manpower Report, 1967, re: the Kaiser Foundation Medical Care Program; and Perrott, 1966.)

Other decisions are controllable at the hospital level, but the administrator generally lacks the authority to make them. It has been estimated that 10 percent to 20 percent of the patients in the hospital on any one day do not need to be there (U.S. Department of Health, Education, and Welfare, 1962).

Despite utilization committees and additional extended care facilities, this is probably so in 1970. The hospital administrator cannot directly influence physicians to perform fewer procedures and order fewer tests, or readily induce insured patients to utilize doctors and hospital services less. The individual hospital has no control over the supply of physicians in the area nor can the hospital in most cases train or authorize less qualified professionals as substitutes to perform certain procedures. The hospital administrator can do little by himself about securing other hospital affiliations for physicians so that each hospital does not have to provide every service for the physician to practice medicine as modern technology requires (Reder, 1965).

The administrator cannot easily influence the size of his hospital. Hefty (1969) has indicated that in hospitals average cost declines with increasing scale of output for a substantial range of output, and suggests that the point of minimum average costs is between 200 and 300 beds (see also Mann and Yett, 1968). Klarman (1965) suggests that there may be a range of optimum sizes, given the existence of specialized factors of production. It is difficult for the hospital administrator to gain the cooperation of other hospitals to increase interhospital scheduling for small services such as pediatrics, or to obtain the cooperation of his medical staff to close underutilized units, or to increase utilization of special hospital facilities on weekends and evenings. The administrator can perhaps more easily facilitate the establishment of minimal or extended care units which can result in lower unit costs with no decrease in quality. But this usually requires capital funding as it is more difficult politically to convert nursing units presently used for other purposes. In 1968 the national average occupancy rate was 78.2 percent (*Hospitals*, 1969). High occupancy and increased utilization would generally result in lower unit costs or in increased hospital effectiveness (see Long and Feldstein, 1967; Reder, 1965).

What the administrator can do is admittedly less than many administrators desire. He can attempt to influence medical chiefs to develop and implement guidelines concerning the performance of procedures and the ordering of tests. He can try to influence the American Hospital Association and his board of trustees to apply pressure on legislators for facilitation of alternative reimbursement and for removal of legal obstacles barring the performance of certain procedures by properly supervised and accredited nonphysicians. He can work with hospital planning agencies, medical societies, and other administrators to try to systematize interhospital relationships. He can encourage his board to establish minimal and extended care units and to decrease facilities and manpower for underutilized services. The administrator can apply operations research techniques to achieve savings in areas such as inventory, staffing, scheduling, and sequencing of activities (Gue, 1965; see also Fetter and Thompson, 1966, for application to an outpatient department). He can more easily establish interhospital relationships for purchasing and such support services as blood banks, laboratories, and computers (*Hospitals*, June 16, 1969), than for patient care.

There is a strong inference in data collected by Hospital Administrative Services (a service of the American Hospital Association) that administration can do more to control costs. Hospitals selected were of comparable size and were located in the same area. Yet total costs per patient day for hospitals of medium size (100-299 beds) were almost evenly distributed over a range between $43 and $65. For hospitals of large size (300-400 beds) total costs ranged among the twelve hospitals considered from $54 to $110—a twofold difference, which remained even after adjustments for wage and salary differences (Health Manpower Report, 1967).

In addition to controlling costs, the administrator can influence financing of operations by an increase in hospital revenues. More effective fund-raising and collection systems can be developed. Variable pricing could be established for services characterized by low utilization (e.g. scheduling of procedures on weekends). To help finance operations, hospitals can also increase sales of nonmedical services and can tax physicians, for each of whom there is an estimated $70,000 worth of hospital equipment and facilities (Hixson, 1965).

The administrator's influence on cost control is, at least potentially, most importantly exercised in the budgetary process (see Health Manpower Report, 1967 re: the Kaiser Foundation Hospitals). The administrator has greater influence over expenditures for new programs and facilities. Substantial cost savings or increased efficiency, however, can probably be realized through reallocation of existing budgets, and better correlation of budgets to unit performance and not merely to historical cost levels. Performance budgeting assumes some quantifiable output at some given level of quality. Output is quantifiable to a limited extent in hospitals, but measures do exist and can be used, such as square feet of floor waxed, number of major operative procedures performed, or number of disability days per community.

The administrator has perhaps more leverage in the cost area than in areas discussed in later sections. Cost control is seen as a legitimate administrative function by medical staff. As a representative of the organization as a whole, the administrator is seen as a likely mediator between conflicting demands and interests. In-depth studies of the actual budgeting process in hospitals are required to learn the effects of varying participation by medical staff, board of trustees, and administration in budgeting, and the impact of budgeting upon long-range planning and upon integration of powerful interest groups.

Sharing of Power: Consumer Groups and Nonphysician Employees

Those who have power to make and implement decisions in the hospital are generally certain trustees, the medical staff, and administration. This section is concerned with the relationship between those who now have the power and those who in some locales seek power—consumer representatives and the nonphysician employees of the hospital. In this struggle the administrator must play a difficult role. He is part of the "establishment," and must represent his own interest, as well as that of the trustees who employ him and medical staff who must at minimum tolerate him if he is to survive. As a result of his professional training and commitment, however, the administrator is also a representative of the consumer, and, as the chief executive of the organization, of the nonphysician employees whose willingness to participate must be obtained for the organization to be effective.

Consumer groups. Consumer representatives have deplored the high cost of hospital care, the low quality of patient care (in terms of convenience, dignity, and continuity rather than medical care narrowly viewed), and the composition of hospital boards of trustees as reflecting producer interests and not being sufficiently concerned with reducing costs or satisfying patient needs (Burlage, 1968; Strauss, 1969). Hixson (1965) notes the changing composition of boards from the socially elite to business experts, and predicts future change in the direction of a board more broadly and truly representative, to include all geographic, professional, social, political, management, and labor segments of the community served by the hospital.

The representation question is difficult to map. There can be an interest as well as a communications gap between consumer representatives and their constituencies. Perhaps more crucial than any precise quotas for representation is the issue of fixed terms and mandatory retirement ages for at least some board members and criteria for board membership being responsive to problems the organization faces. One must not forget that although hospital boards do not significantly finance hospital operating expenses, other contributions may mean the difference between breaking even and incurring a deficit, and that hospital boards still finance a sizable proportion of new facilities (see Stambaugh, 1967) or can be helpful through contacts in obtaining such support (see Elling, 1963).

Burlage (1968) asks how "voluntary" are institutions when they are dominated by the commercial and professional power structure, and how "nonprofit" are they when they keep large retained earnings for expansion and incur high administrative costs, including large salaries and expense accounts. The administrator can anticipate these challenges and must often develop appropriate strategies in response. In documenting the response of the City of New York to the problems of its hospital system, Burlage concluded that the affiliation program with voluntary institutions reflected a system ideology antagonistic to public sector planning, direction, management, and services leading to abdication of public control.

Despite tremendous expenditures, difficulties in patient care were largely unresolved. These difficulties included a lack of extended care facilities, inadequate service in prenatal care, mental health, geriatrics, dentistry, podiatry, overcrowded emergency and outpatient facilities, unavailability of services at hours convenient for patients, little dignity or amenities, no follow-up for episodes of illness, and a higher priority on education and research than patient care. Many of these same charges can be leveled by consumer groups against many voluntary hospitals. To the extent that the administrator's position is a powerful one, he can use these charges and claims in concert with consumer groups and nonphysician employees as a basis for redefining organizational goals and acceptable levels of performance.

Whether consumer representatives, variously defined, should control hospital boards has become another highly charged issue in some locales. Pomrinse (1969) suggests that the voluntary hospital is already accountable to numerous publics such as its patients and staff through comments and suggestions, its trustees as official representatives of the community, its reimbursement agency through audit, and the government through inspection and audit. He notes that at one institution a one-year count revealed 105 separate required reports to, or inspections by, governmental agencies, in addition to 38 reports to voluntary agencies. Pomrinse agrues that "to claim that hospitals are not publicly accountable implies that the only additional involvement of the public would be in making the detailed decisions that govern the hospital's operation," and that this would in fact turn the voluntary hospitals into governmental hospitals when they would lose all the advantages of flexibility, adaptability, and excellence which have distinguished voluntary hospitals. Pomrinse also argues that advisory committees of consumers are needed, but that boards of trustees can back up their decisions with influence, status, and money, have the necessary education and experience to make decisions, and that professional staffs are not likely to take direction from others.

As with consumer groups, the administrator must anticipate increasing militancy from the representatives of nonphysician employees. Although fewer than one in ten nonfederal hospitals (7.7 percent) had formal collective bargaining agreements in 1967, this was twice as high as in 1961. Union activity is greater in predominantly unionized cities, in larger hospitals, and in government hospitals (Miller and Shortell, 1969). Nurses associations, and even physicians associations, have begun to bargain for increased wages and fringe benefits and for influence over the work environment. For example, the California Nurses Association has obtained by contract the right to determine who, how many, and what personnel classifications are to perform nursing duties (Osterhaus, 1968).

Nonphysician employees. Highly skilled nonphysician employees are increasingly aware of the gap between their knowledge and authority. For example, the nurse often has information about the patient which she thinks the physician should use but which he is unwilling to accept routinely from her. In Georgopoulos and Mann's (1962) study, 29 percent of registered nurses and 46 percent of doctors thought that the medical staff had a very good understanding of the work problems and needs of the nursing staff. Less than 15 percent of the staff nurses interviewed by Mauksch (1966) were aware of the doctor's communications with the patient. Staff nurses and technicians were the most unstable employees in Georgopoulos and Mann's study, in terms of length of service, turnover, job history, and strength of commitment to the organization. These skilled workers need to be better integrated within the organization. One approach would be to include nursing and technician representatives on medical staff committees, at least on those committees which make recommendations affecting their work.

Unionization and professionalization have both disadvantages and advantages for the administrator. The organization will be less effective if the administration yields its leadership responsibility and permits the splintering and unintegration of various worker groups. The organizing of nonskilled and skilled workers, however, can facilitate such integration assuming that there can be mutual understanding and delimited negotation between administration and effective group leaders. Union stewards can help increase overtime by workers, or combat bad safety records, absenteeism, or poor quality work (Kuhn, 1960). Administration can unite with highly skilled workers to improve patient care even when this requires additional demands on medical staff, for example requiring physicians to arrive in clinic on time and remain until the end of the session.

The problems of the administrator increase with the number of bargaining units and the number of unions in any one hospital. Negotiating with unions on an interhospital basis may result in the individual hospital's securing the most expert representatives and in not being "whipsawed" by unions. But such negotiation may also result in contracts which are not tailored to each individual hospital. Just as problems with organized consumer groups have resulted in larger or new departments of public relations, problems with organized labor have resulted in larger or new departments of personnel. At the same time, since both departments are extensions of the administrator, this has resulted in his gaining additional power and authority.

Sharing of Power: Trustees, Medical Staff, and Administration

Bucher (1969) characterizes the professional organization as one in which groups struggle for varying levels of professional recognition, with differential success in different locales. The reward for success is autonomy and influence in defining problems, determining solutions, and monitoring the functioning system. Any claim the administrator might make to have the occupation with the most highly developed body of knowledge to make decisions (Goode, 1969) for the organization as a whole may be subject to challenge by the medical staff and/or the board of trustees.

Wilensky (1962) observes that when the hospital administrator decides to intervene in the use and payment of salaried medical specialists, to control the quality of surgery, to investigate the impact on health of using a new drug or anesthetic, or in more routine matters of scheduling of operations or admissions, or use of proper techniques of sterilization, his authority may be questioned by medical staff. Similarly, if the administrator intervenes in areas of long-range planning, capital financing, selection of or tenure of trustees, trustee participation, or development, his authority may be questioned by trustees. Perhaps his legitimacy in intervening is dependent upon how he intervenes rather than whether or not he intervenes. For example, the impact may differ depending upon whether as a result of an operations research study the administrator presents to the medical staff for implementation a plan regarding changed operating room schedules; whether he asks a medical staff committee to study the matter with suitable staff support; or whether he persuades key surgeons benefitting from current arrangements to benefit less in return for a full-time salary and provision of office suites in the hospital.

Perrow (1961) has traced a general development of hospitals from trustee domination, based upon need for capital and legitimation, to domination by the medical staff, based upon the increasing importance of their technical skills, to administrative domination based upon requirements of internal and external coordination. He cites this as an ideal model, and points to the possibility as well of multileadership—a division of labor regarding the determination of goals and the power to achieve them. Under a condition of multileadership, power relations are generally unstable, there is no guarantee that precarious values (e.g. ambulatory services) will be protected, since these stand by definition outside of the interest of power groups, and there is avoidance of long-range planning which could expose conflicting interests.

Gordon (1961) stresses the informal and negotiative aspects of the administrator's role in reaching agreement with medical staff, but also the formal organization aspects which assure authentication of authority and accountability. In a study of three hospitals, Gordon found a direct relationship between the severity of problems, as cited by the administrator, and formal organizational relationships (for example, perpetuation and superannuation of trustees was a severe problem when there were no bylaw provisions with regard to age or retirement) (see also Guest, in Moss *et al.*, 1966). The writer hypothesizes a relationship between integrating structures, such as joint board-medical staff committees or task force committees, including members of different occupational groups, and organizational effectiveness, comparable to Lawrence and Lorsch's (1967) findings in industry. Gordon (1961, 1962) emphasizes as well the administrator's reliance on interpersonal relationships to influence medical staff, especially relationships with key officers and committee members. Such influence, of course, must be traded off to satisfy the interests of such physicians. But the relative power of the administrator will be increased to the extent that he influences the outcome of who occupies, or does not occupy, key positions in the medical staff hierarchy and on medical staff committees.

Viguers (1961) defines power as the ability to make or influence important decisions. If the administrator is the sole channel of communication between the trustees and the medical staff, he tends to have power (see also Hawkes, 1961). Viguers observes that where a single trustee or a small group of trustees becomes particularly active, the administrator's power diminishes. Such is also the case when trustees assign only maintenance or support tasks to the administrator, and have the controller and medical staff report directly to trustee committees. Viguers suggests that the trustees seldom support the administrator when he needs support; they will pass formal resolutions and vote, but when it comes to taking action to enforce compliance, they will usually seek to avoid the issue.

When the medical staff withdraws its support, the administrator almost inevitably loses. The community is not organized for any effective action, and usually is not close enough to the situation to know what is going on. The employees are not organized, do not have good lines of communication to the trustees, and are afraid of losing their jobs. The administrator is, in Gordon's term, "a stranger"; his functions and behavior are not clear to many trustees and medical staff members. If some trustees or doctors constitute barriers to the administrator's influencing organizational effectiveness, he must, if he is to persist, gain allies among other trustees and doctors. With regard to the medical staff, this should not always be difficult since, according to Georgopoulos and Mann's (1962) findings, the highest level of tension in hospitals is among doctors.

If, on the other hand, the administrator can, as Viguers indicates, please the public, keep morale high, satisfy the medical staff, and secure adequate financing, then his success will breed power. The most difficult task is probably to gain organizational momentum. Sometimes only a crisis can realign authority so that sufficient momentum may be gained. The best opportunities for rapidly increasing administrative influence are therefore in new institutions and in those whose survival is threatened. Before assuming responsibilities for "turning an organization around," the administrator can insist that his authority to stimulate and implement change be legitimated by key segments of the trustees and the medical staff.

Organizational Structure

Structure refers to the organization of tasks, of task groups in units, of units in the organization as a whole. Perrow (1965) states that organizational structure often does not change appropriately in response to rapidly changing technology. The writer hypothesizes that in hospitals organizational structure has lagged behind technology, and that this lag influences significantly the quality of patient care, especially in larger, more complex institutions. Work is still largely organized in hospitals by department rather than by unit or, in March and Simon's (1958) term, by "process" or skill differentiation rather than by "purpose" or task differentiation. While the numbers of differently skilled workers at the unit level have multiplied, official coordination remains centralized, usually and primarily by the nursing hierarchy. Activities are carried out at the unit level by an abundance of doctors, nurses, clerks, housekeeping aides, dietary aides, messengers, and escorts.

Official coordination which is centralized often results in a lack of authority, responsibility, and operative coordination at the unit level. As Mauksch (1966) suggests, "if the distribution and quality of patient care, beyond being a specific component of medicine and nursing, is to become a concern of the whole institution per se, the coordinating functions of the hospital must be endowed with managerial rather than mere communicational power." As tasks have grown more complex, as the patient's expectations for service have increased, the need for unit coordination has become more urgent. Many new units have been developed which are often managed more or less on a purpose basis, such as intensive care, cardiac care, and acute respiratory care units, but this pattern has not generally spread to the majority of patient care units.

Demonstration programs in decentralized coordination have been carried out at the university hospital at Ohio State and the University of Florida, and at the Gouverneur Health Services Program in New York City. Howe (1969) describes the Ohio State system in which the hospital is divided into eight patient-care areas—medical care, surgical care, operating room, delivery room and obstetrics, pulmonary disease, psychiatry, physical medicine and rehabilitation, and ambulatory care. Each area is organized along the lines of a separate hospital with its own administration. Reporting to each patient-care administrator is a director of nursing, a housekeeping suprvisor, a nutrition supervisor, and a social work supervisor. Medical staff joins with others on a patient-care committee. Departmental directors such as the director of nursing care are responsible for education, research, and policy development.

At the Univeristy of Florida, a doctor, a nurse, and a ward manager are responsible for coordination of care for each 64-bed unit. The ward managers are responsible to hospital administration. Problems which are not resolved at the unit level are referred to functional supervisors or, if necessary, to the executive council—a patient care committee made up of the hospital administrator, chiefs of staff in medicine, nursing, and health related activities (Taylor, 1962).

Kovner and Seacat (1969) discuss a similar organization for a large ambulatory care program in New York City. Primary care family health units are composed of internists, pediatricians, psychiatrists, nurses, nurse aides, social workers, clerical staff (one of whom functions in a manner analogous to a ward manager), and assistants to social workers (there "social health technicians" function as service links between providers and low-income consumers; to a lesser extent the clerical and nurse aide staff also perform this function). Each units serves a subdistrict of the total area served by the program and has a physician team leader who supervises the day-to-day activites of all team members. Department heads such as the chief of medicine or the director of nursing set professional standards, recruit and train departmental staff, and schedule unit coverage in consultation with team leaders.

Research is needed concerning the advantages and disadvantages of departmental versus unit coordination and of various types within these categories. For example, units can be coordinated by the administrator, as at Ohio State, by a threesome of doctor, nurse, and ward manager, as at Florida, or by the doctor as at Gouverneur.

Another important question of structure concerns how patients are assigned to care units. Such assignment has great implications for the organization of nursing staff. Under progressive patient care, patients are assigned to care units largely on the basis of the degree of skilled nursing care required. Progressive patient care has been widely praised but implemented only partially (see U.S. Department of Health, Education, and Welfare 1962, 1963; Griffith *et al.*, 1967; Weeks and Griffith, 1964). In 1968, 42 percent of the nation's short-term hospitals had intensive care units, but only 5 percent had self-care units (*Hospitals*, 1969). It would appear that a large proportion of the patients in intermediate care units do not require nursing service by registered nurses. In a personal communication, Hardy has estimated that 50 percent of admissions to the department of medicine's units in the North Carolina Baptist University Hospital are to a self-care unit (see also Walker, 1964). The present organization of units, largely by medical specialty rather than by complexity of the technology and stability of the patient, results in some nurses providing services for which they have not been trained, and others doing routine tasks which could be delegated to less highly trained workers (Kovner, 1966).

Coggins (1965) describes the successful operation of a 52-bed self-care unit in a 250-bed Florida hospital. To be admitted the patient must be capable of providing for his own bodily needs or have a family member rooming with him who can do so; his illness must not be life-threatening; he must require no intravenous or intramuscular medications or oxygen therapy; and he must assume responisiblity for oral medication. Licensed practical nurses, who are on duty 24 hours a day, report patients who appear too sick to remain in the unit to the nursing supervisor, who can then call the attending physician.

The administrator has generally lacked the authority for program coordination. Even as a facilitator, by posing relevant problems for his medical staff chiefs or unit leaders to solve, however, the administrator can influence the development and implementation of formal programs of coordination (see Georgopoulos and Mann, 1962). These in turn may influence nonprogrammed coordination by relieving problems otherwise inherent in the flow of work which frustrate pleasant interpersonal relationships.

Manpower Utilization

In 1900 three of five health professionals were doctors. In 1960 one of five health professionals was a doctor, and seven of every ten doctors were specialists. There are over 200 health occupations, and increasing numbers of medical technologists, medical record librarians, physical, occupational, and speech and hearing therapists in hospitals. New Health occupations since World War II include those of inhalation therapist, nuclear medicine technologist, radiological health technician, cyto-technologist, and medical engineering technician (Kissick, 1968).

Demonstrations in the successful delegation of functions from the more highly paid health workers to less highly paid workers include programs for medical emergency technicians at Ohio State, physician assistants at Duke, pediatrician public health nurse practitioners at Colorado, unit managers at Florida, nurse clinicians at Kansas, and social health technicians and family health workers in New York City (Kissick, 1968; Wise et al., 1968; Lewis et al., 1968; Adelson and Kovner, 1969).

Gilpatrick and Corliss (1969), in studying the occupational structure of New York City's municipal hospitals, urge career ladders for entry level employees as a solution to the critical chronic shortage of skilled technical and professional manpower. Presently the "shortage jobs" have no articulation with entry level jobs and must be filled by persons who have received specialized formal education and who can pass examinations (see Hale, 1968, re: the necessity of such requirements). Gilpatrick and Corliss recommend sequential education to provide exit credentials at various levels reflecting individual differences in abilities and aspirations.

Through job analysis, skills, jobs, and the knowledge required to perform existing tasks (with existing technology) can be identified. This can result in a clustering of tasks into related skill and knowledge families. Job pathways can then be designed so that changes in output and technology can be handled by rearranging job structures and selecting appropriate job populations for assignment of new or different functions. Rather than increasing the numbers of formally trained students with little or no work experience, Gilpatrick and Corliss argue for making more rational use of existing skills and knowledge. They have divided jobs into three categories: information, human interaction, and plant, equipment and material. Career ladders are sketched out as, for example, from nurse aide to practice nurse to senior practical nurse to staff nurse to nurse specialist to assistant physician; or from office skills trainee to clerk typist to steno-typist to special typist to executive secretary to support services manager to junior hospital administrator.

The administrator does not control professional associations which have constructed educational and licensing barriers to performance of certain tasks (see Somers, 1969), nor can he initiate formal educational programs to meet the needs of working adults who must be accredited to get ahead. But demonstration programs with educational institutions can be conducted to show that tasks can be safely delegated downward, successful demonstration programs of others can be replicated, and jobs which do not require accreditation can be restructured to fit organizational and individual goals. Intrahospital constraints to the development and implementation of such programs include lack of reimbursement for training, and opposition by those (for whom training is also necessary) who must cease performing tasks themselves that may have been routine but pleasant, and who are now being asked to supervise and work effectively with others.

Patient Care

The accrediting of hospitals and the change in malpractice laws (see Somers, 1969) have certainly increased the administrator's claim, as chief executive of the total institution, to responsibility for patient care, and have facilitated minimum necessary changes in the evaluation of care. The administrator can be held accountable for implementation of a system that facilitates high quality care for all patients. This would include establishment of a formal evaluation unit or medical staff committee. It is easier to establish such a unit, of course, than for the administrator to hold accountable supervisory or senior doctors for significant deviant performance by their staff (see Donabedian, 1969, for scope and timing of formal evaluation activities).

Serious deficiencies exist in the care provided in hospitals. Donabedian (1969) cites these among other examples:

1. On a given day, 40 percent of long stay paitents were judged not to require services in a general hospital (Van Dyke, 1963);
2. Only 22 percent of municipal and 1 percent of independent hospitals in New York City were "consistently good" in identifying accurately, in both bacteriology and chemistry, specimens of known characteristics submitted to them (Schaeffer, 1967);
3. The management of hospitalized illness for families of workers belonging to the Teamster's Union in New York City was judged to have been fair or poor in a little over 40 percent of cases (Erlich et al., 1962, and Morehead et al., 1964);
4. In the outpatient department of a teaching hospital, routine procedures were not carried out in 15 percent of cases, and abnormalities were not followed up in 22 percent of cases (Huntly et al., 1961).

In their study of a teaching hospital, Duff and Hollingshead (1968) found that communication regarding personal and social maladjustment was limited or nonexistent even though these factors were related to the hospitalization of 26 percent of patients, and that the care of patients, especially the personal aspects of that care, was not controlled directly or effectively by the hospital or anyone. Strauss (1969) diagnoses the weak point of medical organization as the "vaguer" residual areas of care, which include "much nursing care, various kinds of instructions to patients about their regimens, along with general evaluation of and communication about progress or retrogression after patients leave the hospital." The poor have special problems in obtaining hospital care, such as their inability to negotiate the hospital system so that they can get seemingly important things from hospital staff. The middle-class bias of skilled hospital workers often results in issued orders which are not understood and cannot easily be followed (see also Roth, 1969).

Neighborhood health centers have had varying success in reorganizing ambulatory services for the poor to include attention to psychosocial needs and to the patient's family and community, participation of the community in decision-making, membership on policy-making committees of staff other than physicians, training of community persons as liaison staff between professionals and consumers, sending staff out into the community, providing evening clinics and transportation systems, and instituting appointment systems (Light and Brown, 1967; Montefiore, 1968). Neighborhood health centers have been criticized as well for inefficiency and ineffectiveness, if not in the literature, by those familiar with these programs (see Shostak, 1969, re: participation in decision-making).

The responsiveness of hospital employees can be increased by establishment of units in which patient feedback is encouraged and in which patient complaints are recorded and chronic offenders identified. By confronting employees and their supervisors with written transcripts concerning unresponsiveness, or by confronting them with complainants and their representatives, the administrator may influence the behavior of employees.

Concluding Comment: The Administrator as Change Agent

Bennis (1966) has outlined the necessary elements in a consultant's implementing change as follows: the client system must understand the change and trust the change agent; the change effort must be seen as self-motivated and voluntary; and the change program must include emotional and value elements as well as cognitive (informational) elements. A change agent is more likely to be effective as a facilitator rather than as a director. The administrator, because of his training, position, and responsibilities, is for many hospitals the person most qualified and most likely to act as change agent. And yet if the administrator is to be increasingly held accountable for hospital effectiveness he must also be able to hold program and subunit heads, including doctors, similarly accountable.

Because of increased specialization, changing technology, and increased expectations of consumers and nonphysician employees, hospitals require increased coordination and organizational adaptability. The administrator's expertise is that of an integrator structuring the perceptions among producers, and between producers and consumers, so that change can be effected without destroying organizational integration. The administrator requires authority appropriate to his responsibility. This writer suggests that some administrators can gain sufficient authority to influence hospital effectiveness through successful performance as facilitators and integrators, and as a result of increased demands from the hospital's public for changed goal priorities and higher levels of achievement. With appropriate authority, as Hill (1969) suggests, administrators can be held far more closely accountable for poor results as well as good ones.

References

Adelson, G., and Kovner, A. R. Social health technician: a new occupation. *Social Case Work,* 1969, *50,* 395-400.

American Hospital Association. Statement on optimum health services. Chicago: American Hopsital Association, Publication S-17, 1965.

Barnett, E. D., and Heiser, R. B. Characteristics of some students in university programs of hospital administration. *Hospital Administration,* 1964, *9,* 16-28.

Bennis, W. G. *Changing organizations* (ch. 9). New York: McGraw-Hill, 1966.

Bucher, R., and Stelling, J. Characteristics of professional organizations. *Journal of Health and Social Behavior,* 1969, *10,* 3-15.

Burlage, R. K. The municipal hospital affiliation plan in New York City: a case study and critique. *Milbank Memorial Fund Quarterly,* 1968, *46,* part 2, 171-203.

Chester, T. E. Graduate education for hospital administration in the United States: trends. American College of Hospital Administrators, Chicago, 1969.

Coggins, W. J. Hospital ambulant unit: report of an experience. *New England Journal of Medicine,* 1965, *272,* 837-842.

Connors, E. J., and Hutt, J. C. How administrators spend their day. *Hospitals,* 1967, *41,* 45+.

Dolson, M. T., *et al.* Study reveals what administrators earn. *Modern Hospital,* 1966, *106* 103+.

Donabedian, A. *Medical care appraisal: quality and utilization.* The American Public Health Association, 1969.

Duff, R. S., and Hollingshead, A. B. *Sickness and society.* New York: Harper & Row, 1968.

Earle, P. W. The nursing home industry. *Hospitals,* 1970, *44,* 45-51, and 60-66.

Ehrlich, J., Morehead, M. A., and Trussell, R. E. The quantity, quality, and costs of medical and hospital care secured by a sample of teamster families in the New York area. New York: Columbia University, School of Public Health and Administrative Medicine, 1962.

Elling, R. H. The hospital support game in urban center. In E. Freidson (Ed.) *The hospital in modern society.* New York: Free Press, 1963. Pp. 73-111.

Elling, R. H., and Halebsky, S. Organization differentiation and support: a conceptual framework. *Administrative Science Quarterly,* 1961, *6,* 185-209.

Fetter, R. B., and Thompson, J. D. Patient's waiting time and doctor's idle time in the outpatient setting. *Health Services Research,* 1966, *1,* 66-91.

Georgopoulos, B. S. Hospital system and nursing: some basic problems and issues. *Nursing Forum,* 1966, *5,* 8-35.

Georgopoulos, B. S., and Mann, F. C. *The community general hospital.* New York: Macmillan, 1962.

Georgopoulos, B. S., and Matejko, A. The American general hospital as a complex social system. *Health Services Research,* 1967, *2,* 76-112.

Gilpatrick, E. G., and Corliss, P. K. The occupational structure of New York City municipal hospitals. New York: Health Services Mobility Survey, 1969.

Goode, W. J. The theoretical limits of professionalization. In A. Etzioni (Ed.) *The semi-professions and their organization.* New York: Free Press, 1969. Pp. 266-315.

Gordon, P. J. Top management triangle in voluntary hospitals. *Journal of the Academy of Management,* 1961, *4,* 205-214; 1962, *5,* 66-75.

Griffith, J. R. Educational challenge for the programs and the practitioners: the new role of the administrator. *Hospital Administrator,* 1967, *12,* 127-142.

Griffith, J. R., et al. *The McPherson experiment: expanding community hospital services.* Ann Arbor: University of Michigan Press, 1967.

Gue, R. L. Operations research in health and hospital administration. *Hospital Administration,* 1965, *10,* 6-25.

Hale, T. Para-medical crazy-quilt needs more than just patching to mend staffing crisis. *Modern Hospital,* 1968, *110,* 82-87.

Hartman, G., and Levey, S. Preceptor attitudes towards the residency. *Hospital Administration,* 1964, *9,* 37-48.

Hawkes, R. W. Role of the psychiatric administrator. *Administrative Science Quarterly,* 1961, *6,* 89-106.

Health Manpower Report of the Advisory Commission on Health Manpower, Vol II. U. S. Government Printing Office, 1967. Pp. 197-228.

Hefty, T. R. Returns to scale in hospitals: a critical review of recent research. *Health Services Research,* 1969, *4,* 267-281.

Hill, L. A. Financial incentives: how they could reshape the health care system. *Hospitals,* 1969, *43,* 58-62.

Hixson, H. H. Hospital governing boards and lay advisory boards: the challenge of the future. *Hospital Forum,* 1965, *8,* 20+.

Hospitals. "Guide Issue," Vol. *34,* August 1960; and Vol. *43,* August 1969.

Hospitals. Innovations in hospital management. *Hospitals,* 1969, *43,* 73-96.

Howe, G. E. Decentralization aids coordination of patient care services. *Hospitals,* 1969, *43,* 53-55.

Huntley, R. R., et al. Quality of medical care: techniques and investigation in the outpatient clinic. *Journal of Chronic Diseases,* 1961, *14,* 630-642.

Johnson, E. V. Continuing evolution of the hospital administrator. *Hospital Administration,* 1966, *11,* 47-59.

Katsive, J. A. Vanishing medical hospital administrator. *Hospital Topics,* 1965, *44,* 41+.

Kissick, W. L. Health manpower in transition. *Milbank Memorial Fund Quarterly,* 1968, *46,* part 2, 53-91.

Klarman, H. *Economics of health.* New York: Columbia University Press, 1965.

Kosa, J., *et al. Poverty and health: a sociological analysis.* Cambridge: Commonwealth Fund, Harvard University Press, 1969.

Kovner, A. R. The nursing unit: a technological perspective. Doctoral dissertation. University of Pittsburgh, 1966.

Kovner, A. R., and Seacat, M. S. Continuity of care maintained in family-centered outpatient unit. *Hospitals,* 1969, *43,* 89-94.

Kuhn, J. W. Does collective bargaining usurp the manager's right to manage? *Modern Hospital,* 1960, *95,* 70-73.

Lawrence, P. R., and Lorsch, J. W. Differentiation and integration in complex organizations. *Administrative Science Quarterly,* 1967, *12,* 1-47.

Lewis, C. E., *et al.* Activities, events, and outcomes in ambulatory patient care: nurse clinics. *New England Journal of Medicine,* 1969, *280,* 645-649.

Light, H. L., and Brown, H. J. The Gouverneur health services program: an historical view. *Milbank Memorial Fund Quarterly,* 1967, *40,* 375-390.

Long, M. F., and Feldstein, P. J. Economics of hospital systems: peak loads and regional coordination. *American Economic Review,* 1967, *57,* 119-130.

Mann, J. K., and Yett, D. E. The analysis of hospital costs: a review article. *Journal of Business,* 1968, *41,* 191-202.

March, J. G., and Simon, H. A. *Organizations.* New York: Wiley & Sons, 1958.

Mauksch, H. O. The organizational context of nursing practice. In F. Davis (Ed.) *The nursing profession: five sociological essays.* New York: Wiley, 1966, Pp. 109-138.

Mechanic, D. Sources of power of lower participants in complex organizations. *Aministrative Science Quarterly,* 1962, *7,* 349-364.

Miller, J. D., and Shortell, S. M. Hospital unionization: a study of the trends. *Hospitals,* 1969, *43,* 67-73.

Monetfiore Neighborhood Medical Care Demonstration: The Early Experience. *Milbank Memorial Fund Quarterly,* 1968, *46,* part 1, 289-409.

Morehead, M. A., Donaldson, R., *et al. A study of the quality of hospital care secured by a sample of teamster families in the New York area.* New York: Columbia University, School of Public Health and Administrative Medicine, 1964.

Moss, A. R., *et al. Hospital policy decisions: process and action.* New York: Putnam, 1966.

Murray, R. T., *et al.* How administrators spend their time: a research report. *Hospital Progress,* 1968, *49,* 49-58.

Osterhaus, L. B. Union-management relations in 30 hospitals change little in three years: second survey. *Hospital Progress,* 1968, *49,* 72-77.

Perrott, G. S. Federal employees health benefits program: utilization of hospital services. *American Journal of Public Health,* 1966, *56,* 57-64.

Perrow, C. Analysis of goals in complex organizations. *American Sociological Review,* 1961, *26,* 854-866.

Perrow, C. Hospitals: technology, structure, and goals. In J. March (Ed.) *Handbook of organizations.* Chicago: Rand McNally, 1965. Pp. 142-169.

Pomrinse, D. S. To what degree are hospitals publicly accountable? *Hospitals,* 1969, *43,* 41-44.

Reder, M. W. Some problems in the economics of hospitals. *American Economic Review,* 1965, *55,* 472-481.

Rosenkrantz, J. A. Should administrators serve on hospital boards? *Hospitals,* 1967, *41,* 63+.

Roth, J. A. The treatment of the sick. In Kosa *et al.* (Eds.) *Poverty and health: a sociological analysis.* Cambridge: Commonwealth Fund, Harvard University Press, 1969. Pp. 215-244.

Schaeffer, M., *et al.* Clinical laboratory improvement program in New York City. *Health Laboratory Sciences,* 1967, *4,* 72-89.

Shostak, A. B. The future of poverty. In J. Kosa, *et al.,* (Eds) *Poverty and health: a sociological analysis.* Cambridge: Commonwealth Fund, Harvard University Press, 1969. Pp. 265-292.

Sigmond, R. H. Health planning. *Medical Care,* 1967, *5,* 117-128.

Somers, A. R. *Hospital regulation: the dilemma of public policy.* Princeton: Industrial Relations Section, Princeton University, 1969.

Stambaugh, J. L. A study of the sources of capital funds for hospital construction in the United

States. *Inquiry*, 1967, *4*, 3-22.

Strauss, A. L. Medical organization, medical care, and lower income groups. *Social Service and Medicine*, 1969, *3*, 143-177.

Taylor, C. How unit manager system works for us. *Modern Hospital*, 1962, *99*, 69-73.

Thompson, J. D., and Filerman, G. L. Trends and developments in education for hospital administration. *Hospital Administration*. 1967, *12*, 13-33.

Trussell, R. E., and Van Dyke, F. Prepayment for hospital care in New York state. Albany, New versity, School of Public Health and Administrative Medicine, 1963.

U.S. Department of Health, Education, and Welfare. Elements of progressive patient care. Public Health Service Division of Hospital and Medical Facilities, 1962, p. 65.

U.S. Department of health, Education, and Welfare. The progressive patient care hospital estimating bed needs. Public Health Service Publication No. 930-C-2, 1963.

U.S. Department of Health, Education, and Welfare. Reimbursement incentives for hospital and medical care: objectives and alternatives. Research Report No. 26, Social Security Administration, 1968.

Van Dyke, F., Brown, V., Thom A., *et al.* "*Long stay*" hospital care. New York: Columbia University, School of Public health and Administrative Medicine, 1963.

Viguers, R. T. Politics of power in a hospital. *Modern Hospital*, 1961, *96*, 89-94.

Walker, R. A. Evaluation of a minimal care center. *Hospitals*, 1964, *38*, 75-78.

Weeks, L. W., and Griffith, J. R. (Eds.(*Progressive patient care: an anthology*. Ann Arbor: University of Michigan Press, 1964.

Westfall, R. Educating for the future: bringing various administration education programs together into one school of management. *Hospital Administration*, 1969, *6*, 81-94.

White, R. F. Contributions of social science to hospital administration. *Hospital Administration*, 1961, *6*, 6-25.

Wilensky, H. L. Dynamics of professionalism: the case of hospital administration. *Hospital Administration*, 1962, *7*, 6-24.

Wise, H. B., *et al.*, The family health worker. *American Journal of Public Health*, 1968, *58*, 1828-1838.

Woodward J. *Industrial organization*. London: Oxford University Press, 1965.

Wren, G. R. Graduate education for hospital administration: a comparison of public health and business school programs. *Hospital Administration*, 1967, *12*, 33-64.

16

ISSUES AND DISCUSSION
OF CHAPTER 15

Presentation Highlights: A. R. Kovner

I would like to begin by saying that I disagree with Dr. Pellegrino in three basic areas. I only have time to comment on one, but I will mention the others. First, I disagree with his analysis of consumers and their impact on the system. Second, I do not feel that there is an economic solution in today's world of medical care for implementing the clinical decision-making system that he discussed. My third point of disagreement concerns his organization of hospitals. That is what I will speak about here.

At the outset, I would like to say that I do have a bias because I am an administrator, although not a hospital administrator at present. I am engaged currently in directing a graduate program of health-care administration, and I am also executive director in a group practice, in an academic group-practicing department of a school of medicine. This is my orientation.

Some people have apologized for not reviewing the literature in their papers as completely as they intended. I would like to apologize for trying to do the hopeless task of reviewing the research literature on hospital administration and organizational effectiveness. In trying to do this, I have not made as much progress as I would have liked toward synthesizing our knowledge in the area. This was done much better by most of the other papers. Consequently, while enjoying an advantage I also suffer from the defects of what I did.

I suffer from still another problem because of the nature of my topic. And part of the problem in looking at this has to do with the question of how you measure organizational effectiveness. I think this is an exceedingly difficult thing to do in the hospital field. When we talk about organizational effectiveness, we talk about goal achievement. But how do you put together into one figure or one representation the total goal achievement of a hospital? Similarly, how do you measure administrative influence on organizational goal achievement? In either case, I do not know where this has been done successfully—either measuring the organizational effectiveness of a hospital or measuring the influence of the administrator on hospital effectiveness.

I feel that there has been very little research on the administrator as a change agent in the hospital. There has been a lot written about administrators and about what they do, and there have been even some time studies on what they do, which have not been satisfactory to my view. These studies have just put the time in certain categories which really do not tell you very much in terms of relationships between time spent and outputs in any significant way. If I have an overall plea in this area, it is for research on what the administrator does. For example, nothing has been done in terms of how many administrators there should be in hospitals under varying circumstances. Or, if you have so many administrators in a hospital, what is the logical way to divide up the work that they would do? You would think that this would be elemental, that it would be the place to start if you were looking at the administrator. But of the work that I know, there is very little on it.

Regarding the question of hospital effectiveness there is some literature but it is not very helpful. There is a definition by the American Hospital Association, for example, in terms of what optimal health services are. These include such things as team approach to care under the leadership of the physician, inspection of services, coordinated community and regional systems of health services, continuity between hospital and nonhospital services, continuing evaluation, research on quality, and so on. But this statement deals only with process; it does not deal with outcomes. Even dealing with process, I think you will find very few hospitals that have any of these things.

Bob Signet has written on the actual goals of the hospital. These goals include high quality of patient care, good education and research results, meeting the needs of the physicians, of medical staffs and their private practice, comprehensive care for disadvantaged segments in the community, financial solvency and institutional survival, and prestige for those associated with the institution. With respect to each of these goals, however, you find that different people are benefiting and consequently it is very difficult to take a unified look at hospital effectiveness. One major problem with hospital goals or hospital effectiveness is that there is disagreement among the various interest groups as to what the priorities are or should be. Different groups have different goals, and there are shifting coalitions around different goals, and these change. You do not find the same forces for something or against something. Because of this, when examining goals, it is perhaps useful to think of the hospital in terms of a negotiated order. I will return to this point later.

If I could sum up what the research shows about hospitals and their goal achievement, I would say that, generally speaking, hospitals have a high level of goal achievement in terms of taking care of the critically ill. They have a much lower level of goal achievement when it comes to patient services or patient care, or when it comes to providing ambulatory services in a convenient, accessible, continuous, and warm and friendly way. And when it comes to providing health services for a given population, their level of achievement is fairly low, because hospitals have not chosen this as their goal yet.

It may be useful in trying to see what is happening in hospitals if we take a look at the hospital industry. I will do this only very briefly. First, I would like to just say that when we discuss hospitals actually we are talking about many different kinds of organizations. When we talk about hospital administrators, for example, we must keep in mind that the administrator of a large urban teaching hospital compared to the administrator of a small rural community hospital has a different job. The organization is different, even the technology may be different, and we just cannot speak of hospitals as one homogeneous kind of institution from a managerial point of view. This is not saying that one job is more difficult than another, only that it is different. I think what we are seeing in the hospital industry is that individual hospitals are facing a more unstable environment and are becoming larger, more complex, and much more costly. I will consider the implications of these trends in a moment.

First, what is happening to the administrators of hospitals? The number of health-care or hospital administration programs has doubled within the last ten years. I think that better students are going to schools of health care and hospital administration, and generally they are receiving a better or at least longer education. Many of the programs are moving from a one-year to a two-year curriculum. And the students who enter these programs, I think, have higher expectations and are more action-oriented than the tradtional hospital administrator.

Next, what are some of the constraints which prevent the administrator from influencing organizational effectiveness, and what are some of the opportunities to influence the organization? Many of the factors here are dual in nature. For example, when you look at the activity of unions, you can say that this is a constraint upon the administrator because he has got to react to something and a lot of his autonomy is taken away from him. But if you look at it from another point of view he has got a structure to deal with and he can work with the union toward organizational effectiveness, as well as be stymied by it. I am only going to discuss three problem areas here, although I have covered more in the paper.

If the administrator has a legitimate role in the hospital, I think it is around the cost area. He is generally seen as the person who should have some knowledge about costs. If this is so, why has not the administrator done something about costs? In looking into this I found that he does not have any control over many of the problems in this area (I am not saying by this that there is not much that administrators could do). One of these problems is the way that hospitals are reimbursed. Another concerns the procedures of physicians. A third concerns the utilization of health services by consumers. A fourth one has to do with the legal regulations of particular states as to what kinds of people can perform what kinds of procedures. A fifth problem is that the administrator by himself cannot very readily engage in interhospital cooperation around such things as closing down underutilized services, for instance, so that the hospital can have a higher occupancy rate.

There have been studies by the Advisory Commission on Health Manpower showing that the administrator probably could do a great deal about costs, because for hospitals of the same size they have found a twofold variation in costs. Such variation makes you suspect that there may be a great deal of inefficiency in hospitals, and that something should be done about it. Part of the influence that the administrator has in this respect, however, is only indirect. He can try to pressure, influence, cajole, or persuade the medical staff to be concerned with quality standards and such things as Dr. Pellegrino discussed, for example. Or he can pressure legislators, through the

American Hospital Association and through the board of trustees, to get the laws changed so that people who are not physicians can do the tasks for which they are adequately trained.

What administrators have been able to do is primarily to work out programs in the support areas of the hospital: the dietary department, among others, where the administrator is seen to be legitimately in control, and the housekeeping department, where there have been many innovative programs for reducing cost. One neglected aspect of the cost picture has been to find ways of increasing revenue as well as reducing costs. Generally speaking, administrators have not been very imaginative in terms of thinking up ways of increasing revenue, although some might say that this is not a goal for hospitals.

I think that one of the greatest means for increasing the ability of the administrator to influence the organization is the budgeting process. Yet until very recently most of the budgeting in hospitals has been on a very rudimentary level. Even those hospitals that have budgeting today seldom do it in terms of performance but rather in terms of new projects. If a certain department has had a certain number of dollars in last year's budget, for example, they usually are not asked to justify getting the same amount this year, with a given cost increase, in terms of what they have actually done or in terms of what their actual output is.

Another subject that I would like to discuss is the power situation. Traditionally, what we have had in hospitals is a situation with the "ins" being the inner triangle of trustees, doctors, and administrators, and the "outs" being the consumers and the nonphysician employees of the hospital. But we are seeing a change in the power situation, which has been alluded to many times in our discussion. The consumers are not satisfied with the service they are getting; the taxpayers are not satisfied with the benefits they are getting for the money they are paying; and the nonphysician employees are not satisfied with their rewards, either in terms of what they do or in terms of their status.

Where does the administrator's power base come from? Unlike the many other kinds of people who work in a hospital, there are only a few administrators and there are only a few levels of administration. Part of the administrator's power base, I think, is coming from the staff services now required in complex organizations to deal with the environment. The unstable environment and the much expanded impact of federal health programs are forcing hospitals to develop separate departments of accounting and controlling. It would be interesting for somebody to do a cost analysis of the cost of the Medicare-Medicaid legislation per patient day, just in terms of the accounting depatment costs of the institution in order to comply with the regulations. Some say that the administrative costs are only 2-3 percent, but this ignores the complete burden of the paperwork pushed on the hospitals. Other recent developments with a similar impact include the creation of departments of personnel, new construction, and public relations. All these developments are giving the administrator the information which he alone has in terms of the organization as a whole, and are increasing his potential to influence the system.

Going back to the matter of shifting coalitions, I think that within the inner triangle of board of trustees, medical staff, and administrator, not enough attention has been paid to the divisions within the board of trustees and within the medical staff. Dr. Georgopoulos says in his work that the most tension in the hospital was between doctors and other doctors, not between doctors and administrators, doctors and boards of trustees, or doctors and nurses. I think much of the actual power realities of any particular institution develop from the coalitions between the administrator and one part of the board, or one part of the medical staff, versus the others. Certainly this is the kind of situation that an administrator must be able to deal with if he wants to implement change.

With the arrival of new actors on the scene, such as the union, the nonmedical professional groups (e.g. the nurses and various technicians), the consumer groups, and the financing agencies, the administrator increasingly has to represent these groups to the board of trustees or to the physicians, to explain the hospital to all these groups and to explain all these groups to the inner power structure of the hospital, and to act as an integrator of the system. This increases his role in terms of influencing the organization. Such influence is reflected in the increasing status and salary of administrators. There are many cases where the administrator is actually on the board of trustees, and in some hospitals he is in fact president of the board.

The next subject I want to discuss is organizational structure. I have very strong feelings about this, perhaps a little wishful, but I believe that there must be coordination at the unit level if the hospital is going to achieve its goals, especially the goal of patient care. The present organization of hospitals is inadequate to the task. The technology has changed completely in the last fifty years, but the organization has remained much what it always was. The division of labor within the hospital has greatly increased, tasks have become more complex, patient expectations have increased, etc., but still the hospital, especially at the nursing unit level, is organized to do the work on an inappropriate basis.

What this means at the unit level is that on any given day the patient can have walking into his room fifty people who are not coordinated at the local level. They may be self-coordinated to some extent or they may be coordinated by a central department of nursing, a central department of medicine, or some other central department, at a distance, but not at the unit level where the work is being done. As a result nothing is adequately coordinated, and I personally believe that in many hospitals the patient care and the service at the unit level stinks.

Recently, with the development of new kinds of patient care units in hospitals, we have seen a switch to unit organization. In the intensive care unit, for example, there is usually coordination at the work level. This is also the case for special respiratory units, rehabilitation units, and some psychiatric units. Either because of a shortage of physicians or because the demands of the tasks are so clearly evident there has been a unit organization in these cases. And I would venture to say that the level of goal achievement is higher in these units than it is in other parts of the hospital. This process has been extended out of these special kinds of units on a demonstration basis. I know of three programs where this has happened. But further research should be done on the advantages and disadvantages of varying systems of organization within the hospital.

In the University of Florida there is a tripartite system where a nurse, a physician, and a unit manager are responsible for a unit 24 hours a day, with the nurse having the coordinating responsibility. At Gouverneur in New York we put into effect, for ambulatory care, a family health unit system in which we made the physician the manager, responsible and accountable for everybody who worked in that unit. Everyone had two bosses, the physician and the director of nursing or director of medicine or pediatrics. The directors laid down standards, recruited, evaluated, and were responsible for training. This suggests, I believe, that the physician may be perfectly able to be a manager at the department level. At the unit level we found that this seemed to work out. It was not carefully evaluated, but at least it was accepted.

The other great problem, in my view, with the structure of hospitals is the way patients are assigned to care units. This has very little to do with the technology. The literature has a great deal to say, for example, about the movement toward progressive patient care. According to this concept, those patients who need the most nursing care supposedly would go to intensive-care units; those who need moderate care would go to intermediate units; and those who need little or no care would go to a self-care unit. This seems to have worked well as far as intensive-care units go, because 42 percent of the hospitals around the country now have intensive-care units. But as far as the self-care units go, it may have not worked well since only about 5 percent of the hospitals have such units.

The intermediate-care units in hospitals could be completely reorganized into routine and nonroutine care units, with a great savings, perhaps on a three-to-one ratio basis. Nurses could probably take care of three patients with routine problems for every patient who requires a good deal of nonroutine care. By putting more nursing in the nonroutine units and less nursing in the routine units and organizing them differently, hospitals could realize tremendous savings in the utilization of nurses. In most nursing-care units now, I would argue, the majority of nurses are underutilized, while in a few units you have people who are not registered nurses doing tasks for which they have not been trained.

Where does all this leave us with the administrator? I see the administrator as a potential change agent in the organization. Of course, there are administrators, and there are administrators, but I would like to think of the administrator as having a vested interest in change. If he is increasingly becoming that person who is looked upon as the manager of the entire organization, he should be concerned with change. And I believe that in terms of the organization's survival or success, increasingly he is going to have to see that substantial change occurs. I believe he sees this and he knows it already, but he just does not know how he can go about it.

Finally, what is the administrator's responsibility going to be? I do not see the administrator as being primarily responsible for coordination; he does not have the knowledge to coordinate. Yet the administrator's responsibility is more than just that of a facilitator of change. I see the administrator responsible for creating the atmosphere in which change can be carried out, but also as having a control function and integration functions. Goals have to be set on a mutual basis, and I would bring physicians into the system too because, if we are going to hold the administrator accountable, he has got to be able to hold his subunit heads and program heads accountable. He cannot hold them accountable, in my view, unless we move into a unit or program style management where everybody who works in a particular area is responsible and accountable for the output, for the outcomes, and for everything that goes on in the area.

Discussion

Comment (Dr. Neuhauser): I like your general statement that there has not been any research on the impact of administration in the cost area, because that is what I have been doing for the last year or so. I tried to look at thirty community hospitals in the Chicago area. For a measure of efficiency I used cost-based indexes per standard patient day. For the impact of administration I used three different measures: the extent of rules and regulations imposed on the employees in the hospital; the extent of operating and financial reports; and the degree to which the administrator is aware of the performance within his hospital.

In general, I am finding that administration does make a difference in the costs at which I am looking, but it is rather small. Apparently there is a great deal of cost in all hospitals that can not be controlled by administration. You made the point that there are extremes in costs among similar hospitals, a twofold difference in extremes. That may be the wrong thing to look at. The question, I think, is: Given the average level of administrative performance, what can we get with a reasonable improvement? And the range I am finding from the average to a reasonable level in improvement is in the order of about 15 percent savings in cost. Most of that comes from lowering the number of man hours rather than increasing the occupancy rate.

Chairman: Your study indicates that, in those thirty hospitals at least, this is the maximum cost improvement you normally expect, on the average, given the present organizational structure of these institutions.

Answer: That is right. Change the structure and then it can be quite different.

Comment (Dr. Straus): You mentioned self-care or minimal-care units, Dr. Kovner, and the fact that only five percent of hospitals have these. I think, and I am guessing here, this is a reflection of current values within the system. The more critical problems are those which are getting the attention, and even where these units have been planned, as at Kentucky, most of the space was preempted for other things. We were able to salvage the concept in pediatrics and the care-by-parent unit (which is not completely minimal care because some of these children are pretty sick, but the criteria had to be that their care could be entrusted to their parents). We have done some pilot studies in the area of communication on this unit which I think are rather impressive. We are finding that the amount of communication that takes place between the responsible physician and the parent in the care-by-parent unit is necessarily a great deal more than in other pediatric units, and this apparently has a very positive effect on the parents' understanding of the problem.

Question: Did you say a great deal more?

Answer: Oh, yes; ever so much more. In the traditional unit a lot of communication might be intended, but it simply does not take place. It does not take place, probably by default, because nobody seems to be completely responsible for doing it; the child's needs are taken care of, but the why and wherefor simply never gets communicated. Without trying to evaluate the hospital experience, we are conjecturing that the posthospital impact of the care-by-parent unit may be significantly better than the impact of traditional care. We have also looked at the experience of students and found that here too communication seems to be much better, and students are learning a great deal more about the problems of the patients and what is being done for them, and why, on the care-by-parent unit than on the traditional floor.

Comment (Dr. Jaco): I certainly would support the suggestion that the role of the administrator be studied and supported a little more research-wise, whether he is a mediator, a coordinator, an instigator of change, or whatever. I would also suggest, however, that the concept of coordination implies that the administrator should be an agent of change. Certainly, this is a widely held view both in educational administration and in hospital administration. Ideally, I would like to see the hospital administrator as a leader in the medical care community. He is in an ideal position to be in such a leadership role.

But I think behind the notion of mediator, the whole idea of what change goes on in a hospital needs to be reevaluated and further examined. We use the word "change" just casually, as if we are all communicating the same thing. A great many hospital administrators think that their job is putting out fires. They think they have survived, and that survival is an accomplishment on their part, by keeping all these loose ends and competing forces still working together at the end of the day. There is some truth in this, of course, because the administrator often has no time to worry about providing leadership in the medical care community. He has an equal excuse to not have time for anything, just like the doctors claim they are too busy all the time. But I think he should be concerned with leadership as well as coordination and change.

When we are talking about change, however, we should be clear as to what kind of change we are talking about, because there are so many forces in the hospital situation. Is it change just to expand a service, or to institute parent-care service (this is going on all over the country, and many hospitals are doing that sort of thing)? Is that change, or is it innovation, or is it just expansion? Precisely what do we mean by change in the hospital? I do not think that has ever been delineated into all of its dimensions. It would be a very worthwhile area in administrative research and operations research to be more clear about what we mean by change. System innovation is something new in the picture, and it may mean changing the whole structure of the hospital itself. This too should be watched. Research is also needed to ascertain the extent to which built in mechanisms are available to evaluate and to promote change in a planned and orderly fashion. What you probably mean by saying that the administrator can be a change agent or a planner of change is that he can give it some guidance, systematic direction, and some rationale, and that he will protect the existing facility so that it will not be destroyed by too excessive change. I do not know whether this is correct.

Answer (Dr. Kovner): There are two areas where change comes in. Change has to be done in terms of coordinating what goes on in the hospital, and also in terms of integrating what goes on there. I think these are the two areas where the administrator can make himself particularly felt. As far as specific changes go, I am particularly interested in structural changes. One of the structural changes that I suggested was to change the way in which care units are organized in hospitals. Another would be to build into the system some kind of consumer feedback. We had it at Gouverneur; it did not work subsequently, but while I was there it seemed to work out very well. What we had was a patient advocate who was responsible to a community councilman and who was helping the patient negotiate with the system and services utilized.

Comment (Dr. Pellegrino): I want to comment on Neuhauser's statement regarding the impact of the administrator on costs, which I think is very interesting, and which brings us back to the question of structure within the hospital. His study indicates something that we all know, namely that the greater part of the cost lies within the professional service itself. The clinical decision-making process is what generates the cost. To reiterate a point I made, we have to enter into this process. I am very dubious, however, that this could be accomplished without some instrument within the institution of the kind I indicated. Someone who has credibility with the professional people is needed, and I doubt that the administrator will have that kind of credibility. This no reflection on him, but I think the successful change agent, by and large, is a person who is obsessed with an idea, who is capable of communicating that to other people by persuasion, and who has credibility in their eyes and in the system.

Comment (Dr. Kovner): I question one thing you said, that the major cost is in the area of decision making. I do not think that it is. It is in the area of manpower, unless you want to call manpower clinical decision-making.

Answer: Yes; it is involved in how you handle that situation. I think you and I have a difference in language which probably, if analyzed, is not as great as you think. I really believe that is the case; we are using words slightly differently. What I want to say is that I think we need some agency within the institution that can effect drastic changes in the way clinical practice is carried out. And I can only see that coming from a person with credibility in the clinical area who has then moved into another area. Granted he has got to be prepared for that, and so on. But I think you miss an important point unless you build that into the structure somewhere. You may want to argue about who is the director at present, and I think that is of some significance. But the key point is that we need to pull together the professional services.

Dr. Kovner: I would not disagree with that.

Comment: We do not have such a thing in most hospitals today. And I do not think that real changes will occur until we do that. That is the only thesis I am contending.

Comment (Dr. Mauksch): I think this is exactly what we just heard in the dialogue between Pellegrino and Kovner. Let me link what has been suggested and what we said earlier. What we have seen is a demonstration of what I call three principles of the complexity of instituting social change and creating social knowledge. There are these three principles: the principle of multiple truth; the principle of cognitive differentiation; and the principle of semantic conservatism.

First, it is pretty obvious that many of us, even within the same community of social scientists let us say, have said many things in different ways, and yet none proved the other wrong. There are multiple ways in which we can state the truth about a complex universe. The truth that we are looking for, presumably as scientists, is, as we announce it, segmental. It was very appropriate and, I think, very telling—I use myself as a victim here—that when I made my earlier comments several of you reacted very promptly and very appropriately, because of the fact that what I was saying was segmental. I was aware that it was segmental, and I agree with their reaction. I would defend what I said recognizing that, in saying only part of it, I was wrong. This is, I think, an important point as we are trying to get out varying knowledge together.

The second thing which is rather obvious, and also very profoundly true, is the much observed concern about the development of cognitive styles and cognitive differentiation inherent in the socialization of multiple individuals. This is one reason, incidentally, why I have a point of concern, not necessarily disagreement but concern, with some of the things Pellegrino said. We have talked about systems. We have even talked about cultures. We have not talked very much yet about individuals who become physicians, sociologists, nurses, cleaning women (who may be one of the most profound observers of the system), and so forth. We must recognize the fact that cognitive differentiation, even as we have seen it here, is a profoundly important thing in our work and for what we are trying to do.

This is not unrelated to the third principle, that of conservatism. The very dreams that we announce, the very solutions that we suggest, and the very notions that we wish to test—either in practical policy-making or as social scientists in terms of how we create our experiments—are all based on previous experiences and synaptic connections which create funerals for ourselves. We are linked to our own past, and these three principles are part of the fundamental baggage that we individually carry with us. I would also say, somewhat facetiously, that the only thing that would really mitigate the problem is a continuous shower of self-ridicule, so that we take ourselves profoundly not serious as we try to negotiate.

Comment (Dr. Christman): I would like to support the point that Pellegrino has been making about a director of professional services from a different point of view. I have a couple of articles in which I just speculate about the effect of the administrator on hospital nursing practice. Most hospital administrators tend to employ as their director of nursing a person who is their alter ego, a captive in spirit and mind of the hospital administrator, and not a person who is going to direct a strong nursing program and who may have a lot of confrontation with the administrator and give him many uneasy moments. A large proportion of directors of nursing are selected in this fashion. Another group of directors of nursing fit the bureaucratic type. They just run the department according to all the rules, regulations, and policies, and change occurs only when the policy allows for change. Under the captive system change occurs only if the whim of the hospital administrator allows that change, whether this is rational or irrational. A third type is the charismatic director of nursing, a person who may have preceded the hospital administrator in his appointment or who has a long continuity in that particular hospital and holds the nursing force together by personal charisma. No one is likely to disturb or ruffle this person—an autocrat or a lovely old lady—and change occurs only according to the charisma of this person.

The smallest group of directors of nursing in the country are nurses who are clinicians, who understand practice, and who innovate change from a clinical, rational viewpoint. They are the ones who get into the most trouble. Hospital administrators have a tendency to fire them because medical staffs get uneasy about them. These nurses know as much about patient care as the medical staff does, and they make the physicians awfully uneasy because they are always showing them where the holes are in the care system and making everybody uncomfortable.

These areas have not been researched, but I believe my statements would stand up because they are based on empirical observation over a long period of time. In any case these problems have not been researched, and one could extend these to other clinical department heads as well. The hospital administrator is a gate-keeper and he tends to pick people for these positions who do not, for the most part, disturb him or who disturb him and the medical staff the least.

Comment: I have a feeling that Dr. Pellegrino's and Dr. Kovner's disagreement over who should be the change agent is a kind of false dilemma, because the critical issue is not who should be the change agent, but rather under what conditions and in what situations will change occur. If you take either of two well-trained, professionally motivated, and knowledgeable people and put them into a situation where the whole structure is stacked against change, they will fail, and only the great will be able to succeed. Most administrators do not fit the great man model.

Comment: They will not accept that kind of a job, if they want change.

Answer: That is right. There are some charismatic people and some great leaders who can go into almost any situation and move it partially. But for most of the world, most of those 7,000 hospitals out there, the average change agent is going to fall by the wayside. In order to bridge the gap, we need an analysis of the combination of change agent and change situation. It is the combination of the credentials and skills of the change agent in relation to the characteristics of the change situation that must be taken into account.

Comment (Dr. Scott): One of the points made again and again by many of us is that the hospital structure is, in fact, enmeshed in a much larger system of health care, and that we isolate it at the risk of doing considerable damage to the phenomena we are trying to investigate. I, for one, am very reluctant to talke about *the* hospital structure, because what we have in fact is a very complex series of structures. In our own research, using the kind of evaluation model that I talked about, we have been forced by the nature of the phenomena we are trying to understand to constantly make those structures task-specific, realizing that given performers are enmeshed in not one or two but in a number of structures. This is one of our measures of complexity, the number of kinds of structures that are generated around a task. My university colleagues, for example, often think of the very different structure that controls their research operation as compared to their teaching.

I would conclude by saying that we should never underestimate the power of social structures to create reality, i.e. to provide goals, motivations, etc., for participants in the system. One of the ways in which we really can change behavior fairly efficiently is to create new structures. For example, the creation of a position of the chief of professional services who has some clout, who is able to make certain kinds of demands, and who has some control over rewards and penalties can in fact affect the performance of large numbers of people. Simply trying to persuade the same people on an individual basis to change their behavior will never work as well. Therefore, never underestimate the power of social structures to create these changes.

On the other hand, never underestimate the inventiveness and the cussedness of individual members and, particularly, of work groups to redefine, to change, and to use these structures to serve their own ends. Consequently, the search for some kind of absolute perfection in structure is always going to be an illusory search. We are going to create structures, and these structures are going to have both intended and unintended effects, and then we are going to have to create new structures to deal with those unintended effects, and so on. We really have to keep in mind both of these inevitable kinds of processes.

Dr. Zald: I would like, if I might, to introduce a modification of my earlier comments. We have talked about organizational models, mostly about open-system models of organizations. We have discussed certain concens about what the boards of directors and the administrators do. We have talked a lot about power. And we have talked a lot about economic problems.

Now, I want to talk about the approach to organization that I have been taking over the last four or five years. I think it does help us bridge, within one conceptual framework, the problem we have been battling around about who are the consumers, or under what conditions consumers have influence, and the problem of board power, or the problem of the interplay between the board of trustees and the executive, on the one hand, and the outside, on the other. This is what I call the political economy framework for the study of organizations, and all I mean by the phrase "political economy," which has a long history, is let us not talk about systems in general.

Let us instead talk about two key sectors of an organization: its polity, or its power-distribution and goal-setting mechanism; and its economy, or its task-production system and the process of transforming raw materials into some finished product. Actually, there is a fourfold problem: the organization's internal political situation; the external political problem; the internal economic problem of the organization; and the external economic situation. One can talk about these both in structural terms and in process terms, and one can have change between the internal and the external situation and causative agents going in both directions. One can have a massive external economic problem of inputs, or of procurement of resources, which affects the internal political process; and one can have external political groups bringing pressure to change the internal polity or economy of the organization, and so on.

In the work I am doing with this model I have not been especially interested in hospitals, but in the effect of goal setting and power distribution on task structure in organizations—the YMCA in this case. I have also looked at social movements in this manner, and I really run this idea of political economy very hard and maybe into the ground. I talk about constitutions of organizations; about the fundamental normative constraints of organizations; about a whole set of political processes, like succession processes; and about various other phenomena, including demand aggregation. Here we talked about unions, for example, and about the question of how to weigh different groups in an organization. You have here what political scientists and economists both speak of as a demand aggregation process. An individual, who is weak transforms himself into a larger power block via connection to groups.

But these have not been tightly drawn together, and they have not been done enough on a comparative basis so that we can start looking for structural variation and power bases. This political economy approach, however, helps us do two things. First, it helps us bridge the environment problem. We no longer talk about the environment in general but about key elements of the environment and how those elements aggregate into critical choice decisions. Second, it helps us look at the interaction between control process and production process in a way that I do not see (though I may be wrong, it may be just my hangup) in the traditional literature on organizational analysis. I just wanted to refer to this approach as another line of research that is going on and that may be useful in hospital studies.

Comment: That is interesting; you go back a hundred years or more.

Answer: That is right. And from that I move to the nation-state. When I look at organizations now my first question is not how do organizations function, but how do nation-states function and what are the ranges of variation out there. It is really a kind of analogical theorizing. What is the range of variation that one might have in nation-states, and then I ask the question of the range of variation in organizations.

Comment: Perhaps this application may have been overlooked because many researchers came to hospitals after having started with commercial and industrial firms where polity questions were not anywhere near as significant. But in hospitals today the polity questions are very important.

Answer (Dr. Zald): I know that and I know this literature, and yet if you look at the negotiated-order idea it is clearly political. I think that there are two parts of my line even there. First of all, a negotiated order by itself has tended to refer to an internal process. You take a group of professionals and watch them interact. But then Pellegrino says that we have to look at this changing crisis in the external situation, and the negotiated-order people have stopped short of that. By and large they have not dealt with the external political aspect. As I read Anselm Strauss and others, for instance, I feel that they have focused on the internal polity, but we also need a mechanism in the theoretical framework that will include the external political dimension (by political I mean only power processes and goal-determining processes.)

Comment (Dr. Mauksch): The negotiated-order approach is not necessarily alien to it. In fact, to go back to the kind of model I presented, you can say that within the hospital there are worlds and stages. You can also say that the hospital is a stage of a larger set of worlds which are external and which move into the hospital. This is also consistent with Scott's point that there are many structures that make up the hospital organization.

Comment (Dr. Scott): There is one difference. To amplify your remark, much of the concern with the environment is relatively recent. As White indicates, social problems instead of being solved are frequently superseded. Anselm wrote his paper at a time when hospitals were relatively stable. Since that time the OEO has had its impact, legal decisions have been made, and so forth, but the environmental dimension can be comprehended by the same kind of thing.

Comment (Dr. Mauksch): But even in those days, in talking with Anselm particularly about some of these things, I can say that he did not campaign for it because all research limitations are arbitrary.

Comment (Dr. Pellegrino): In your political economy model, which I find very attractive, Dr. Zald, I think you are going to have to account for another policital fact. And that is the revolution which I think we are seeing in the health-care systems. Effective changes will be probably drastic and discontinuous.

Answer (Dr. Zald): Let me comment on one of our earlier points of difference because I think it is resolved. When you talked about boards and their coming power, one of the things you said was that their power may come through a technological change, e.g. through a computerization process which now changes the information basis on which boards can act. If you look at the history of boards of directors in the United States, one of the reasons that they got out of phase and toward the business corporation model of organization is that they did not have the necessary information—they did not know what to deal with. Now, however, you have an economic and technological change that feeds back to the power distribution potentials of different groups of people. I would say then that under certain conditions boards can be powerful and under other conditions they are bound by the situation to be weak. This would allow us to get on the same wavelength.

Comment: I think, in relation to Pellegrino's comment one of the interesting things here is that the style of negotiation also is that the style of negotiation also is changing. Even the conflict theorists sometimes forget that they are basing their theories on a Marxian analogy. The Helelian model includes the goal of synthesis, whereas much of contemporary confrontation is a non-negotiable kind of confrontation. This changes the flavor and meaning of a negotiation very considerably.

Comment: Much of the negotiations today are truly discontinuous. I think that is the key point.

· **Comment:** There is also a literature now emerging in terms of structured confrontation. There are consumers on some boards, for example. Looking at this in terms of decision making, to see who makes what kinds of decisions in this byplay between the professionals and the consumers, would be very important.

Comment (Dr. Pellegrino): I just wanted to ask Dr. Kovner not to initiate a debate. Really I do not delight to do that, and the others would be bored by it. But since the term "consumer" is being used again, and since he took issue with me on this term without explaining the difference, I wish that he could clarify now what he means by consumer as opposed to the way the term is being used within the group.

Answer (Dr. Kovner): I think that when we talk about consumers who actually utilize a particular service, such as the local delivery unit, we are talking about a different kind of thing than when we talk about consumer representaives and professional consumer representatives. The impact of the two is different. Further, the concept of a consumer representative is a very complex thing, and I like very much the idea somebody mentioned about the use of tape recorders to bring the discussion back to the constituency. I find that most consumer representatives really do not have any communication with the people they are supposed to represent, either in terms of bringing back to them the information that the group needs or in terms of bringing up to the institution the real problems and needs of particular consumers. So, when you speak about electing consumer boards, it frightens me. I am not saying that it cannot work in some cases, but I would guess that in a rural situation you might have a much different kind of problem in relationship to consumers than you would in an urban ghetto area; it is not the same thing because you do not have a community in the urban situation. At the same time I would like to make it clear that I am all for the increased participation of consumers.

My attitude about consumer participation is that the consumer should not be concerned with all the decisions. The professionals who have been trained for years to make these decisions should have some knowledge as to what these decisions are, assuming of course that the system is running fairly well. Now, obviously, this is not the case today. The situation is not running well, and I think the consumers should get concerned. But they should not get concerned with the division of labor within the institution. The consumers have other jobs and other work to do. And looking at it from an economic point of view, this would be a poor use of the consumer input. When there is something drastically wrong, you know, there are a lot of reasons why things are wrong. You do not need a Ph.D. to figure out what is wrong with the system. Much is wrong, and there are many problems, and these call for some slashing of the Gordian knot, and I think that the consumer can help slash the knot.

Comment (Dr. Pellegrino): Well, as I suspected, I do not find myself in disagreement with anything that you have said there. The consumer can be considered the consumer in the macrosystem when we are talking about the political changes at the federal level in which health-related legislation is coming out. And when we are talking about the consumer as a person or as a member of the general populace who at some time will use health services he can be considered a consumer within the microsystem of the hospital. You sound like a man who has been burned by a blowtorch and afraid of blowtorches, and I know precisely what you are talking about because I have dealt with it too, both in a rural area and in an urban area. The similarities are greater than the differences between the two, and the basic problem is about the same in both areas. It is always different in some respects, of course, depending on the character of the community. I agree with you thoroughly on that, and about all the problems of dealing with it. But all I was trying to put forward was that, realistically, if we are going to lock in today with the most potent forces in our society, and I am not considering the economic aspects, we are going to have to find a way to solve the problems of dealing with the consumers, which you I think have delineated very well.

I find an interesting parallel between the sensitivity of the administrator and the sensitivity of the physician whenever the word "consumer" comes up. Somehow, I do not share that, although I have dealt with consumers across the table and I know what you are talking about. It is difficult, you are absolutely right. Who, for example, represents the student body on campus? This is a similar problem. But at some point you have to assemble a group of people who are willing to stand forward and then work beyond that.

Comment: I wonder, Dr. Zald, if we could add another dimension to your scheme, namely the professional dimension.

Answer: I treat the professional as an economic input, as a characteristic of the labor force. It is a labor characteristic, and the labor input into the organization may feed back through the political dimension. In most economic analyses you have capital, labor, and technology inputs. But the problem with economic analyses is that they tend not to take into account the quality of the labor force, its ideological aspects, and things like that. And, obviously, I would insist upon these.

Comment (Dr. White): Let me comment on the remarks made earlier about consumers and why, perhaps, we have some difficulty with Pellegrino's definition. If you look at the traditional organization of the hospital, considering the ideal model, trustees are certainly consumers. But we are talking about a new phenomenon which involves the direct consumers, and particularly the disenfranchised consumer. We are looking at mechanisms by which these people can have some effect on the organization. This would apply somewhat on a national level, but it is very useful to make distinctions at all levels.

Comment: Just very briefly, I would like to expand this point. There is sort of a "park at both of your houses" kind of comment to be made when you listen to physicians and administrators discussing consumers. There is one frequent assumption made, that of consumer involvement in this disenfranchised sense. Underlying this dichotomization of the board and the disenfranchised is the assumption that these people participate as we do, being primarily concerned with solving health care problems, when in fact frequently these are means to an end in terms of solving other larger issues of concern to the disenfranchised. In other words, the health care system is seen as a means to an end, and this is a problem to which we have not even addressed ourselves.

Comment: Yes, I would agree with that, and also wonder if an age-old distinction that used to be made in the professional literature still is not relevant here, but in danger of being forgotten, the distinction between client wishes and client needs. It seems to me that one of the great problems with the organization of consumer groups and the increasing power of consumer groups—and I am talking about students as well as patients—is that these groups come in having a very clear notion as to what goals they would like to have served, but very often they are not fully aware of what the nature of the system is or what the possibilities are. In this light the problems involved in consumer education are overwhelming. The usefulness of a good many things that we do, both in universities and in hospitals, may not be obvious or directly apparent to the people who are supposed to be paying for these services.

Chairman: That is certainly right. And the distinction between client needs and client wishes is a good one to keep in mind. We must also recognize, however, that the needs and wishes of consumers are not uncorrelated. If we make a sharp distinction between client wishes and client needs, and emphasize the latter while neglecting the former, we run the risk of becoming defensive and avoiding the complete issue.

Comment: I agree, but the plain and painful fact is that the health system, the university, and everything else is going to have to march to a tune now that is called in terms of goals elsewhere. And the thing that we, who regard ourselves as experts in society (and that includes everybody here), can contribute is work and knowledge that would help to make the decisions as rational as possible.

Question: Would you change one word? When you say as rational as possible in relation to the hospital, could you use the words as clinically as possible instead?

Answer: In the largest sense of the word, which implies rational decision-making, I would.

Comment (Dr. Straus): This is unfairly personalized, Dr. Pellegrino, but having watched you operate as chairman of a university senate and in numerous other capacities, I think that some of your optimism, and I do not mean to be a pessimist myself, may be based on your own unusual ability to sense the needs of a large group, interpret these in terms of existing techno-logical and scientific knowledge, and feed these back in an effective way. The reason that I am being personal here is that I think this is a process which you are saying we need to develop but it has not really been explicitly defined. This is not going to happen without skillful leadership of a responsible and informed and perceptive nature. It is not a process that just is going to happen by creating a milieu in which the consumer can have a voice. Somebody is going to have to provide this effective feedback of the scientific and technological element into this decision-making process of the organiza-tion.

Comment (Dr. Pellegrino): One closing remark. I agree with your theoreti-cal analysis. On the other hand, I do not think we are going to develop the process until we get into it, and we are going to have to start very soon. That is really all I am saying. People are going to have to respond in a way that you indicated. Whether we have done it successfully or not is another point. But I think that there are people around who surely can do it.

Chairman: Our discussion of Dr. Kovner's paper, I think, suggests that in addition to being concerned with the environment and the consumer we, as social scientists, have to be concerned with a least three other major aspects in our analysis of the hospital: the internal structure of the system and the organization's decision-making arrangements; the kind of work and work processes that are going on in the organization, and how well care tasks and other functions are performed; and the leadership, including but not limited to administrative or medical leadership, which helps move the system by in-tegrating the motivational bases of participants that activate the work process with the task requirements of the organization.

17

POSTSCRIPT

Chairman: For our closing session, I have asked Drs. Christman, Pellegrino, and White if they would make some observations on our work from their respective vantage points. They have agreed to make a few remarks. Then, each of us will have the opportunity for a final comment.

Observations by P. E. White and Discussion

Dr. White*: I am not well versed in hospital studies, except for those that I encounter randomly and those that border on my research interests. What I would like to speak about is the field we are working in, which is interorganizational relationships in health.** Obviously, we have gotten into a number of areas during the discussions that are directly in the field of my concern. Let me see if I can make some sense of of this.

I was trying, as I listened to the discussions, to put some of these things into a framework that people in interorganizational studies are turning to use. Much of the discussion seemed to be influenced by the fact that we are in a rapidly changing society, one that I call the innovative society in the sense that there is very little in our current social mechanisms that ensures continuity. Many of the funding agencies will now fund innovative programs. They all want to give up anything that is not "innovative" even if it has proved effective. Some excellent research programs are having difficulty getting funds because the society is allocating everything to innovation.

This has implications for discussion of the hospital because traditional studies have looked at the hospital as a system and at the balance of power within the hospital structure itself. As your discussions progressed, it became clear that many people are now interested in what impinges on the hospital. This does not mean that there is no place for studies of hospitals as more or less self-contained systems. I do not think that at all. But there seem to be several kinds of research models involved here.

One is a model of structure. This enables you to look at an organization with definite boundaries. You stipulate what the qualities of the variables at the boundaries are, and then you have good reason and rationale to study what happens within the system. The current trend toward comparative studies, where you look at different kinds of systems for the kinds of processes that are occurring internally so that you can begin to manipulate variables within the system, provides a good example of this approach. The

---

*Associate Professor, Department of Behavioral Sciences, The Johns Hopkins University.

***Editor's note:* See P.E. White and G.J. Vlasak (Eds.). *Interorganizational research in health: conference proceedings.* U.S. Department of Health, Education, and Welfare, 1971.

ideal models that were proposed and discussed here also are very much in that order. Clearly, then, we can think in terms of planned change. We can think of the kinds of ideal situations that we want and compare these with traditional systems as widely diverse as those traditional systems are.

In interorganizational studies, on the other hand, the main focus is upon the process of change rather than the operation of a particular system. Consequently there is a great emphasis on innovation, and on the kinds of sanctions, incentives, and manipulative variables that can be used in a situation in order to change it. This, it seems, is very much related to hospitals, but the aim is to get to the ideal state once you have discovered what it is. If we find out, as in Dr. Jaco's study for example, that a particular structure or innovation is a good thing, then how do we get individual hospitals to adopt such a change?

Obviously there is still a place in our search for valid studies of hospitals as more or less closed systems. All of the quality-of-care studies, the economy studies, and so forth are quite valid within the framework of particular organizational structures. But as soon as we get outside of individual structures, we are in a different area in which a number of you are already beginning to work in terms of the hospital. Dr. Zald's paper on social control, Dr. Pellegrino's concern for the consumer, and a number of other issues in our discussions here fall within the interorganizational research framework.

One of the premises of traditional organizational studies was a structural-functionalist bias in which one looked for variables that would maintain the equilibrium of the system. A byproduct of this was the idea that organizations will not change unless something comes to upset this equilibrium. The assumption was that most organizations, such as hospitals, had achieved this equilibrium in one way or another for a good number of decades, so that it would take powerful outside forces to upset the balance. We are beginning to see these outside forces on the horizon.

In terms of the research models that have been used, aside from the traditional structural-functional models, I would like to elaborate on the process models. Dr. Scott spoke about allocative decisions and the whole process of adjustment of decision making within the hospital. This is a model much used in interorganizational studies and in effect one that probably helps to get away from the pure paradigms of bureaucracy, professionalism, and so forth. A number of us have been thinking in terms of dropping these as paradigms and treating them as forces, valances in the field, and then looking at how they affect individual decision making. Allocative decisions receive a great deal of attention in this manner.

At our conference on interorganizational research, in New York earlier this year, we had a number of people using this kind of decision-making model. The work being done now by James Coleman on collective decisions is also very interesting in this connection, because, speaking of rational models, the collective decision-making model he uses is a rational model in which you get irrational results. The model does not necessarily yield irrational results, but it offers one way of explaining outcomes by combining the various kinds of interests and controls of actors in a situation, their power to effect decisions, the trade-offs that go between them, and the problem of absorbing the social cost of such transactions. Obviously some of these factors are not rational. In any case, there has been a good bit of work that has been done in collective decision making, particularly in communities. This approach is being applied now to community participation in health organizations, and it is definitely related to the kinds of models that you are using in studying individual hospital systems.

One other model being used with increasing frequency is the Neuhauser and Andersen kind of model, which relies on a survey approach and on proxies or indirect measures. I think we have considered the kinds of difficulties this approach entails. It probably represents a more risky business than some of us engage in, because very early in the game those who take this approach have to put their bets on measures that all of us will attack later once they have gotten their results. Any criticism that I may have of that approach is taken with this in mind. Sometimes it pays off very well, and subsequent study allows one to focus more intensively on the variables under investigation. But it does involve major risks, although the study by Neuhauser and Andersen was a very interesting endeavor.

Question: Could you give an example of the use of the collective decision-making model, or a concrete example of its application?

Answer: We are using it in a study of Regional Medical Programs where we are looking at one particular process, that of grants. We take the grants that have been approved and disapproved at the local level. Then we have a number of hypotheses about why grants are approved or disapproved in terms of the system, in terms of the characteristics of the grant, and the kinds of activities or innovations that they are going to fund. These are our dependent variables. Then we have a model, which is essentially an interest matrix model, where we put the characteristics of the actors in the situation—who they are professionally and organizationally, where they are located, and so forth. Then we try to compute scores for the different actors in the scene and relate these to other things, such as the power they have on committees, their positions on committees, whether they are on the National Advisory Council, which has some impact, etc. Finally we weigh these characteristics and come out with different outcomes. It is a little more complicated, but it is like the problem of votes where you have interest in an issue and you try to weigh people's interest in issues and weigh their power according to the size of their constituencies or some other kind of variable. Drawing directly on what Coleman is working with, we have come out with some very interesting things with this in terms of getting a predicting model for who will get grants funded and who will have them turned down.

Question: Would you use the characteristics of an approving body that turns over each year in your model? This might foul up your future predictions, because the people who approve and disapprove turn over every year. I know of a program which already has changed three executive directors in two years.

Answer: We do it also by cycles. We are looking, for example, at such things as: How, in a federated organization, does the headquarters exert control? How do you control the headquarters? There are two ways essentially. One is by directive. Every time the director changes in the division, or the health service as it is now called, a new policy is expressed. And the locals will respond to that or not respond to it. The other way is the granting cycle of the council. We look at what happens in cycle 1 and then we find that, if certain kinds of grants are granted in cycle 1, similar applications will be submitted by the locals in cycle 2. They are responding very much to this kind of control, as it were, but we have not figured it out completely as yet. Essentially, the collective-decision model is useful because we have pluralities of interests and we are trying to figure out what happens, for example, when you get a medical society, a teaching hospital, and, say, a public health school represented on a set of committees.

Comment (Dr. Scott): I suspect this is a terminological quibble, but going back to your comments about it being very useful to treat the hospital as a closed system, I have a problem with the use of "closed system." If I reinterpret that in the following way, I would like to have you comment whether it is acceptable. I would say that the whole message of the open-system model is that human systems are, by definition, open; that no human system is self-sufficient in terms of its resources, that no human system consumes all of its products. Instead, every social system is dependent upon something outside itself, and the actors are involved in other systems than the system that you are looking at as well. On all these kinds of grounds, human organizations are open systems.

If that is the case, in view of your comment about closed system, you have to say, "I am interested in certain activities or functions of this thing and therefore I have to decide what the system is that I want to analyze." And, in effect, the burden of proof is on the analyst. If what I want to focus on is that system which is bound within the hospital, I have to prove that in fact it is an analyzable system. I cannot simply take that on some kind of arbitrary basis anymore. It is after I have taken into account a sufficient number of the things that affect the thing which I want to understand that I can say, "This is my system for the particular purposes of my investigation." And I think this is a different statement from saying we can still study hospitals as "closed systems."

Answer: Yes, we are differing in terms. I think I was affected by one article which was sort of anarchistic, and which stated that there were so many forces that it was impossible to focus on the hospital as a system. I think that is nonsense. Any system can be bounded with whatever you want to bind it as long as you stipulate what the boundary values are. At the same time, we have to be very much aware of what different actors in the situation are representing in terms of what they bring in from the outside, because these aspects affect the system. That is why I was speaking of a "closed" system. We are on the same wave length. I am sorry I used that term. What I was reacting against was the idea, and this may be purely an impression I got, that studies of hospitals as structural units somehow are not as valid as studies of hospitals undergoing change. The study of change is part of the temper of the times now, but I do not see that such an assumption follows.

There are a number of experiments that can be done to discover what structures will produce the results you want, and this is a different kind of problem than the problem of change to an ideal state.

Comment (Dr. Mauksch): This is rather fascinating. It reminds me of something that I grew up with professionally, and that is the influence of Herbert Blumer. Blumer was a sociologist who was so concerned with, and represented so strongly, the differentiation of individual process experience, that some of his students who took him literally developed an incapacity to do research because of the peculiarity of that model. And reading some of the open-systems literature, I found Blumer revisited on the opposite end. I am a great admirer of Blumer, but this risk exists.

Dr. White: I think, in a somewhat unorganized way, this is what I have been thinking about here.

Observations by L. Christman and Discussion

Dr. Christman:* I will focus my comments on nursing and hospital nursing organization. First, I will just take a few minutes to go through a review of why nursing is in the kind of position that it is today.

If you look at it historically, most nurse training occurred in small isolated hospitals drawing students from the same neighborhood year after year. The faculty too was coming out of that same neighborhood, so that there was much provincial inbreeding. There were no other inputs or interaction with other students, and trainees were socialized into the acceptance of two authority structures—one being the physician dictate, and the other the whim of the hospital administrator. The literature shows that the nurse was, and is, more of a captive of the administrator than of the physician. Everybody is nervous now about the nurse becoming a physician's assistant, and how dastardly and unholy that is, when in fact more than half of the effort of most nurses is involved in doing the work of the hospital administrator.

Then, if you look at the way nursing got into universities, some other interesting things come to light. Johns Hopkins, when they built their great physician model after the Flexner report, turned off nursing and did not want nursing involved in university programs. They developed a separate hospital school program that kept nurses in a different category than all the other students on campus. Columbia allowed nurses to come in and get training but at a price of going through Teachers College. They had to meet the requirements of the Teachers College rather than those of the more demanding liberal arts school. They learned all this simple stuff of how you do it, how you teach, how you build curricula, etc., which has nothing to do with clinical practice. They got degrees in nursing administration and nursing education that did not teach anything about patient care. But since these were the only university trained people, they went out and fanned out all over the country, becoming heads of departments of nursing education and directors of nursing all through the system.

---

*Dean, School of Nursing, Vanderbilt University.

These people took the teachers model instead of the clinician model into their practice. This history is not broken up yet by any means, except that now there seems to be some movement toward the clinical orientation. As some of you may know, there is a kind of a Flexner report on nursing being put together now that may or may not have the same effect on nursing as the Flexner report had on medicine. I doubt whether it will, because the establishment is strong, and many physicians may not accept it. There are a lot of other outside constraints against it. The hospital administrators are not happy; they want to keep their little chiefdoms. Some physicians want to keep it the same way too. But this gets us to the point of saying that we can depart from the traditional model.

A countermovement has in fact developed, now about fifteen years old. I was on the first national committee that attempted to develop the nurse clinician at the graduate level. We started out with psychiatry because that was the most vulnerable. The bulk of the patients were in public-supported institutions and physicians did not care who took care of them. There were not enough psychiatrists to go around anyway. But graduate training programs in psychiatric nursing were established in some schools, and the movement subsequently was extended to medical-surgical nursing, community mental health, and other areas. It is now going on; it was not there before.

In the model we adopted at Vanderbilt, what we tried to do was to look at what the patient needed instead of what was good for nursing, the physicians, or the administrators. We decided that we would try a simple model, because part of today's problem with patient care has to do with the fact that too many hospitals try to get into unnecessary organizational complexity instead of simplicity—at least that was our belief. We decided that there were two main elements of care: the clinical or the therapy, and the nonclinical or all the supportive services. We defined clinical as all those activities that assist in preventing, reversing, or arresting pathological states in patients. And the residual, by definition, comprised the nonclinical or supportive activities. Stated differently, the nonclinical activities are all those activities that the patient could do for himself if he were well, while the clinical activities are those things that the patient could never do for himself without the advice and supervision of clinicians, even if he were well and wanted to maintain himself in a state of good health.

Then we looked at the organizational problem of how to get these two services to the patient with the greatest simplicity. By definition we took this to be the role of the hospital administrator. Most of the early hospital administrators coming into the field knew very little about health. They came out of industry and business, where every time you can get a task routinized and get a worker doing it you do so; that is the way to solve a problem. This approach created a whole host of workers on the nonclinical side. But anyone who knows anything about coordination strain knows that the more workers you put into a system the greater the coordination problem. Coordination difficulties grow not arithmetically but geometrically, and this leads to an enormous organizational problem.

Hospital administration and nursing have both contributed enormously to this problem. The nurses, when we had the shortage after World War II, invented that euphemism called the nursing team; this is just a euphemism because it is a form without the substance of health care delivery. At any rate, they invented a lot of specialized workers and categories of nursing personnel. But patient care can be no better than the training of the persons giving it; people cannot use knowledge they do not have. (That is another of the suppositions that we have built into our model.) If a physician or a nurse were to devise an elaborate care program and then turn it over to the nurses' aide (who has only six or eight weeks or two months training) to implement, then inexpert care is all that this patient is going to get. Regardless of how well the plan was devised, it would lose all of its clinical ingredients in the implementation process.

Considering these problems, and the fact that most nurses spend the majority of their time in nonclinical activities at the hospital, we attempted through our model to create some order out of this chaos and give the patient better care. Everybody is talking about nurse shortages. But if we could get nurses being clinicians 100 percent of the time, we would have two or three times the current nurse supply without training a single additional nurse. It would be an enormous social gain for the country even if we could only make a dent in the nurse's nonclinical activities.

In any event, we decided to collapse all of the aide types—dietary aide, nurse's aide, etc.—into a general health worker, who would supply the nonclinical or supportive services to the patient, to the physician, and to the nurse. So instead of the numerous persons who used to serve the patient, now we have only three in direct interaction with the patient—the physician, the nurse, and the general health worker. And to ensure that there be continuity the same team of these three individuals takes care of the same patients day after day. The nurse and the general health worker were assigned to the same patients and the same physicians as a team. No matter which shift they were on, they rotated on the same patients. When they were working on days they had the same patients as when they moved over to the afternoon shift, because these two people moved as a team and they kept the same set of patients. You can see how much information gain there is about a patient in this model, without the huge communication problem that is constantly found in hospitals because physicians and nurses do not talk with each other under the typical pattern of organization.

To tie these three roles together we used what clinicians call the activities of daily living. These are not exactly clean—there has to be some fuzz—but the clinicians, rightly or wrongly, took two or three of these activities that they thought are crucial to the management of the patient and added them to their role. Those activities then not taken by the nurse were given to the general health worker. The division was left up to the clinicians. These activities of daily living were a little different from team to team, but the constancy of the physician-nurse-general health worker trio working together produced a different and more desirable impact on patient care than had the former system.

Question: You used to call them something else, I believe, but now you call them general health workers.

Answer: Yes, but there is something else here; there are a lot of other workers being collapsed into this role besides the nurse's aide. And there is a great reduction in organizational strain, plus the fact that under this system we do not need head nurses and supervisors. This is another great gain in nurse manpower that I have not even talked about. If you look at what I call the system of watchers of watchers in the hospital (aides, LPNs, and RNs, nurse-team leaders, head nurses, assistant supervisors, supervisors, assistant directors, etc.), you find that most of these people are just in surveillance of each other rather than doers. There are all kinds of gains, then, that come out of the new model, and the staffing pattern itself comes out of a severity of illness factor rather than from extraneous considerations. The model is fluid enough to take in the whole range of ways in which illnesses are arranged and managed in any particular hospital, if you use the severity of illness as the cut-across dimension.

We also have hospital administration in the model, but at the action level, because we have instituted the service unit management system. For many years the nurse was responsible for coordinating all patient care activities, and she was held accountable for this but without the requisite authority to do such work. So, we said, if hospital administration does not want to give up its authority to nursing, then they had better get down there and take the responsibility and accountability through an extension of themselves to the service unit manager level. And, of course, as far as we are concerned, we are happy that they are doing it this way. This is what these service unit management people are trained to do and can do. The nurses and physicians—I tend to agree with earlier comments—are not trained for this and do not want to do it. Most of them have no interest in administration. They have a great deal of interest in clinical management activities, and they can do these well. But to worry about arranging the scheduling of a patient, x-ray, and laboratory tests, and all these other kinds of things, or having to fight with the pharmacist, because he does not have the drug out and the nurse is getting locked into arguments between the pharmacist and the physician over what is the right dosage of the drug, and similar other little games that go on, would be wasteful of physician and nursing time.

Our model provides for a relatively simple patient care team structure that we think is functioning efficiently. The problem with most past efforts to reorganize health care delivery at the patient unit level in hospitals might have been resolved, if attemtps to make an inefficient system efficient had been abandoned in favor of developing and testing new models such as the one that I described. The model itself comes out of the same kind of transient team phenomenon that we have discussed here, a phenomenon that can be observed also in other areas. Look at who flies the airlines, for example, from the stewardess on up to the pilot. They are a transient crew for each flight. They may never work together again as a whole, complete crew. The same thing happens over the management of any one patient in the hospital. A particular social worker, nurse, and physician get together, either by chance or by assignment, to bring certain kinds of skills into the situation. But then they disperse after the management of that patient, and they may not get together in quite that same form again for some considerable length of time.

We also have another small innovation that I should mention and that you ought to know about, because others are also attempting to do it elsewhere, but I will spare you the details. Very briefly, we got a grant to develop a family nurse practitioner, who is going to be trained to work primarily in rural areas and with the urban poor. This is all that I wanted to bring to your attention. I tried to complement the previous discussions and, in the process, I realize that I have departed somewhat from commenting only on the things already discussed.

Comment (Dr. Jaco): I think that one very interesting, innovative concept that you mentioned at the onset, that the patient can perform certain tasks by himself, is very new. This is something that would have been heresy ten years ago, except perhaps in army hospitals. There have been some studies done in mental hospitals of what patients can do in the area of care for themselves, or in a group situation, but not in general hospitals. It is in the long-term care facility, I think, where a patient culture evolves around the care problems, that this sort of thing can work.

I am concerned about another trend going on in California that might sweep the country. It may be good or bad, but we have started so many bad innovations out there. I know that in some recent nursing negotiations for wages, salaries, and fringe benefits, nurses were demanding that they get in writing a voice in nurse staffing patterns, in nurse-patient ratios, and they were saying such things as: "You have got to have a head nurse, you have got to have so many RNs per patient," and so on. They would lock in and prevent this innovation that you are talking about unless you get through to them there in a hurry some of your results.

Answer: There is a large group in California watching this. I can tell you this much.

Comment: That is good, because I think this is one of those external forces that are locking in and crystalizing and hardening, and preventing future innovations along these lines, just like unionization is doing and like professionalization is doing.

Comment (Dr. Pellegrino): We worked on such a system some years ago, and one of the problems there as well as for your system is that as you multiply patients and you have different attending physicians, of course, you rock the scheme a little bit. As we move toward full-time physicians, however, I think this will become more feasible and, therefore, you will have a clearly defined team that stays together all the time.

Answer (Dr. Christman): Yes, It would be much easier if we had full-time physicians, but even without them we can implement the model as long as it is the same physician communicating with the same nurse.

Question: I wanted to ask how you handle the pressures, say from the lab, when you have laboratory technicians come to the unit.

Answer: They still intrude because we do not want the nurses and physicians spending their time collecting lab specimens. But they come into the system only as it is necessary, and they do not deal much with the psycho-social life of the patient. It is the three people that I talked about who are dealing with the patient, and I can tell you that patient satisfaction in this unit is enormously different than any place else in the hospital. The satisfaction of physicians also must be high because they are banging the doors trying to get their patients into this unit, even though they do not always understand what is going on.

Comment: I would argue a little with the point that the lab technician, for some patients at least, does not meet psychosocial needs. Some patients may feel that the technician does meet such needs.

Answer: Well, that is another dimension of the problem that should be studied.

Question: About how many intruders, like lab technicians, do you have to tolerate in this system?

Answer: We could work on that problem if we could get funded to work on the whole hospital as a system. Remember that this experimental unit still is a microcosm within a huge medical center complex, and some of the things that generate problems for this unit have their sources in the larger system. We still have to work at that.

Question: How many patients are in that unit?

Answer: Twenty-three.

Question: How many nurses?

Answer: A total of 14 nurses for seven days a week, round the clock. One of the other interesting things that we found out when we introduced this model was that we had to interview 119 nurses in order to get the 14 needed, simply because this was such a radical departure from what nurses did historically.

Question: How many nurses are usually there on any one shift for the 23 patients?

Answer: Three or four, I think.

Comment: If you compare that with typical staffing patterns, that is a lot more nurses.

Answer: Another thing to compare it would be the severity-of-illness factor These are rather severe cardiovascular patients and brittle diabetics. We have a high severity-of-illness factor on this unit so that this is not a bad staffing pattern at all; I think it is too skimpy.

I got lost in something I wanted to add about the macrocosm having swallowed up a lot of the fine edges that we might have developed in this model, because there was resistance within the big system toward this kind of change. As to our recruitment problem, it turned out that of the 15 nurses that we were able to get eventually 14 were young graduates from university programs. These were the only ones who had courage enough to give it a try. The hospital school graduates were least likely to accept it because they said that is not what nurses do. They could not conceptualize it because of their traditional role induction in those small, provincial-oriented schools which offer little opportunity for the student to see any alternative role models.

Question (Dr. White): May I raise a point of information? You mentioned the family health nurse or some such thing.

Answer: I referred to the family nurse practitioner.

Question: Do you see these family nurse practitioners replacing public health nurses and doing some kind of comprehensive health nursing? I have a second question, also. Do you see, in the future, the hospital as the center for the local-care system including public health nursing?

Answer: I see some radiations out. The hospital might be the backup with the technology and with the hot-line information for first-line practitioners, who could be physicians, nurses, or maybe some new team.

Question: Would you absorb them into the system?

Answer: Yes, but use them properly. The thing that we have now makes for too much costly duplication. If you just look at Nashville, for example, there are four open-heart surgery units in the city, and Nashville could have only one. They cannot even keep one such unit going, but each of four hospitals insists on having its own unit, because its medical staff with all their parochial and provincial pride must have their own. So they all do one or two operations a month, and that means that the whole team is deteriorating at high cost to society, high cost to patient care, and not very good clinical results. I think you have to agree with all these kinds of things.

Question: I could see, for example, one of the transition periods where we would have in the community visiting nurses who do bedside care, public health nurses doing prevention and health education, and your family nurse practitioners working out of the hospital. That might be a little chaotic.

Answer: No; that is not what I am talking about. I think we can cut and simplify the system. Everybody is trying to make the system more complex, while what we are trying to do is to simplify the system.

Question: Do you think this is politically feasible?

Answer: Yes, it is. I think Zald is correct in saying that society is going to force it. The economics are going to become the politics, to a great extent. We can train manpower to do this much more efficiently than we are training manpower now. If we get better system utilization, in other words, we will not need to train all those people that the Surgeon General's report recommends. The recommendations of that report are not rational, because they took the old system and used the old system as the base for arriving at the recommended numbers when it is obvious that system was obsolete twenty-five years ago.

Observations by E. D. Pellegrino and Discussion

Dr. Pellegrino:* First, I would like to express my sincere pleasure at being able to sit in on your cogitations. I hope I was not here as a representative of medicine. I did not mean to be, and if I was then I misplayed the role. I had a somewhat different role than the other participants, and I hope that was useful. Certainly, one observation which comes across our discussions and which needs to be reemphasized has to do with the need for closer articula-

---

*Vice President for the Health Sciences and Director of the Health Sciences Center, State University of New York at Stony Brook.

tion between the social and behavioral sciences, on the one hand, and medicine and the health sciences, on the other. We have spent the last hundred years cultivating the interplays between the physical and biological sciences. For the next decade or two or three, or perhaps for the next fifty years or whatever it is going to take, we need to cultivate the interfaces with the social sciences.

As I listen to your discussions, it is obvious to me that we need some kind of ongoing mechanism at the local levels whereby we can become familiar with each other's language, each other's formal point of view, and each other's way of thinking. And I believe that you need much more input than you have at the present time from those who are dealing with the on-the-line problems in the health-care field. This is not to say that you spend all your time in talking to us the practitioners, but I think that the sorts of things that are happening in some medical schools need to be forced further, especially the development of a cadre of social scientists who have an interest in, and a commitment to, the models that are represented in the health-care systems as typologic of complex social systems.

Second, in all sincerity and as a friendly critic, I am impressed also with the fact that there are phenomenological misconceptions about the clinician functions which I think would come out of this dialogue. I would suggest perhaps a biopsy of the clinical situation as you begin to develop your models and begin to analyze them. I would suggest a little more roll-up-the-sleeves, so to speak, not for this group but in general, with that balance wheel that I was talking about as the focus, in which the clinical decision-making at the bedside of the individual patient gets to be kind of a pivot for the whole business.

Third, I would hope for a greater development of the sociology of values. And here I may be in that area of ignorance that Mauksch spoke about, but somehow we need to develop our knowledge of values in a formal way. I think that the attitude of the last thirty or forty years in which one steps back and is value-neutral is useful, and I do not want physicians or social scientists to pick up the cudgels for a political point of view. But I do think that we need someone who can analyze in a formal way the consequences of value decisions in institutions as they exist now, and who can point out what a value decision means in terms of the output and the goals of an institution.

Again, I must confess to a very strong strain of being devoted to the end of what an instrument or social unit is designed for. I am not that much process-oriented; I am end-oriented. That is a personal bias. But I do think that this kind of analysis, which is not going to come out of medicine and which I do not see coming out of philosophy either, is very much needed. I do not know the state of the art in the sociology of values, but I think that one area for research should be that of values as they affect institutions, social goals, and purposes. It may be that such research is going on, but I am not aware of it. Nor do I detect this is the presentations made. Here again I am being an *amicus curiae* trying to turn the cart, so to speak. Medicine has been examined by you; now let me examine your work.

I do not want Dr. Scott to leave what he is doing—I am taking him as a type—because his model development and the analysis in his paper is the sort of thing that I delight seeing. It gives a point of view which we cannot and do not bring in medicine, except in our analysis of physiological systems. I would like to see, when we develop the dialogue, that the social scientist maintains his position and his point of view as a social scientist. One of the grievous things I have seen is that as social scientists become too closely enmeshed in the medical-care process, they then become lost to social science. This I think is a great error because what we need in this human endeavor is the light of another mind, looking from another point of view, and out of this getting greater illumination. Each of us ought to explicate our point of view clearly and then see what new lights we can shed on your work, and yours on mine. I also think that the junior, amateur sociologists who grow out of medicine are just as dangerous on the other side, and we as physicians ought to maintain our clinical stance. But while maintaining our respective position, we must improve the understanding between us. This sounds hortatory, but I think it has to be because I feel a great need, as I move into the sorts of things I must do and other people in my situation must do, to have the kind of critical review that I think social scientists can bring to bear.

This leads me to another aspect of hoping that more of you would become interested in, in a sense tacking onto, the activist kinds of people like myself who are deductively oriented and who are willing to devise a model, as Christman is doing, and then analyze it within the framework of your own conceptualization. We need very much to have such models analyzed in terms of their internal probity because otherwise their translatability and applicability are always open to question. Is what we did in our rural experience, for example, translatable? That is an open question, because we did not study the model as we were developing it. In a sense you would have to commit yourselves to studying what some of us who are activist-oriented practitioners are doing. I am just as cogitative on other realms as you are, but not on this one; I cannot be. I therefore need your point of view and contribution.

There are a whole host of questions that go into what I would like to call not a calculus of values, but the algebra of values, because we are really looking for the algebraic sums of positives and negatives that determine particular outcomes. In your analysis, Dr. Jaco, of the round versus the angular unit, there is an algebra of values involved in that we could have added up the different values which we attach to the various factors that you studied and you could have told us which was the better arrangement. It is this kind of algebra of values, going beyond architecture and into the design of the system itself, that ought to be developed.

There may be some models which are being developed by practitioners like Christman and myself that do not fit any of your standard models. And you all have a typology of models—the bureaucratic, the professional, the open-systems model, etc. Here at the conference, moreover, you began to add a few new ones. I think that is what is needed. It may be that there is something unique to hospital organization—the hospital model may be a genre of its own—and that too ought to be looked at.

These are the main points that I wanted to make. I found it very exciting and intellectually stimulating. Time was too short, really, to come in contact with your minds, and I do not think that our dialogue was sufficient to develop a mutual language or a complete understanding of our respective positions. So I am simply calling for some kind of a hortatory message to come out of this discussion about the need for such dialogue. Although this has been stated before, it comes out very clearly here. I would also hope that, in future cogitations, there might be more characters from the medical underworld, like myself, to engage with you in this kind of discourse. I thank you very much for the opportunity of being able to speak freely and throw some of my views at you. I learned much much more than I contributed.

Comment (Dr. Mauksch): The whole socialization of the sociologist into the medical setting which some of us have experienced, and I wholly agree with you, Dr. Pellegrino, carries with it certain risks. The medical world is used to bringing in the biochemist, the microbiologist, and so forth. And, after the rituals of interviewing, the appointment, and the welcoming tea, they build him a $50,000 laboratory, he gets a key, and that is the last they see of him except for his publications. We social scientists are different, and we fit what I call the decorator syndrome—the parallel being that of the housewife who begs the decorator all year long "Will you please come and paint my apartment?" And he is really wanted and needed, just as physicians and nurses have welcomed us. But, on the third of May, when in fact he comes, we have to roll up our rugs; he tramples all over the place, he makes a mess, and although he is wanted, he is at the same time a nuisance and an interference. He really destroys the system in a certain sense. It is the foolish sociologist, then, who comes in and gets shook by the fact that he is not as welcome anymore when he does do what he was asked to do, because in a sense he disturbs the system in the process. I think this is a fascinating issue, and an issue that has to be taught and resolved before our research really could be effective.

Dr. Pellegrino: What you perhaps are reacting to is the fact that, in a sense, I was giving you one view of the medical world. You have met other medical people, I know. But in relationship to these particular questions I am sure you realize that I am at a particular end of the spectrum. You also need to keep in mind some of the more real world which I am trying to change. But I agree with you thoroughly about the socialization of the social scientist into the medical setting, and I am very concerned about that. I have been dealing with it for fifteen years, and I think you are right. The reaction is always predictable; I can see the symptoms after the third of May. What I am really saying to you is bear up with it, and I am not a romantic about the social sciences. I do not think you are going to solve all the problems of the world. My expectations of you are quite realistic. What I want is another mind against which I can test my own ideas, one that can be critical and can stand up, and not come over to my side of the fence and start being a sort of semi-doctor. It takes a very secure social scientist to do it, and this is one of the problems. By and large those who have tended to slip into these medical sociology positions and then get swallowed up, not those of the group here, have been shaky sociologists.

But, regarding the issue of values, is it improper to just quickly ask if there is a rich and thriving field of the sociology of values? I tend to find and read much more about values in the philosophical literature than in the literature of the social sciences.

Answer (Dr. Scott): I think that is somewhat of an overstatement. A few sociologists have misread Weber and they are saying that you are not to study values, whereas that is not what Weber said; that is not it at all. As you know, Weber said that you do not commit yourself to a value position because this interferes with your analytical ability to investigate. It seems to me that it is hard to talk about the analysis of almost any system without getting into the different value positions, that we sometimes call goals, of the various actors involved. I think that in the old structural-functionalist model a great deal of value analysis occurred, particularly under the notion of latent functions, i.e., values which are being realized through the system although they were not formally legitimated. There may not be a thriving sociology of values, although some work has been done in this area. But I would be hard pressed to show you without too much difficulty that there are enormous numbers of points at which value issues are taken very seriously and analyzed.

Comment: Implicit in what you say, Dr. Pellegrino, is some limitation on the part of the social sciences, an important one. And that is one that Alvin Gouldner, I think, has formulated very well, when he talks about social scientists who focus too much on "what is" and pay too little attention to "what can be," not what should be but what can be. It seems to me that we really have been too limited in our formulation of models in terms of trying to describe what in fact is going on without beginning to devote more attention to what are the alternatives possible, given a particular situation.

Closing Comments

Chairman: I would like to give the floor to Dan Walden. He might want to make a few remarks about our deliberations in his role as director of the Health Care Institutions Branch of the National Center for Health Services Research and Development, which is sponsoring this study and Paul White's project among others.

Dr. Walden: I may comment on my silence. It is not that we are not intensely interested in what has been going on here these two days, because we are. It is just that I do not see myself applying this knowledge in my work the same way that you do in your research. One of the questions I would like to raise with you, asking your advice to me and to the Center, is whether you all find this kind of thing a useful process for furthering the kinds of goals that the National Center has. I have a good idea as to what your feelings might be on this matter on the basis of my watching you all interact. And I have a good idea about the judgments that were made by the Center about supporting these kinds of activities, which I just picked up and helped carry through. But the Center finds itself in a kind of dilemma, either taking research on the organization and delivery of medical care sort of as it comes, or taking a more active role and trying to stimulate different kinds of thinking. If any of you have any comments on this, whether you wish to share them with us now or later, I would really appreciate it.

Dr. Jaco: I could make one suggestion for future meetings. This conference was both similar and different from one that the Milbank people had a few years back. All the participants were sent copies of the papers in advance of the meeting, as we were here, but a formal discussant was assigned to discuss each paper. He went through what he thought was important and reacted to the paper. Then the conferees discussed the discussant's comments in light of their own experience. It was a productive conference. It was also one where they brought in people from different disciplines, and that I think was a key factor. They had a geneticist, psychiatrist, internist, social scientists, and administrators, each with a different point of view, and from their expertise a number of new concepts were generated for research. I would like to see more opportunities of that kind in the future.

Dr. Straus: I would respond very positively in terms of the state of experience and thinking in this particular field that we had here. I am very impressed with what I think we have learned from each other. I think the balance of thoughtfulness that went into preparing for the conference and the willingness of each person to synthesize the key ideas from his paper made for a very useful start. I was going to say this before Jaco made his comment. In our particular context it probably was very useful for us each to comment on ourselves. I have been in that kind of setting, Dr. Jaco, and it can work well; but I have also seen the discussant distort and divert the intent of the original author with the result of a great deal of loss.

I would also like to comment on the size of our group. I think that, fortunately, this has been a very useful-sized group in terms of where we are. And, again, I do not know what thinking went into the distribution of disciplines, but it seems to me that there was some advantage here in having several disciplines represented but not too many. And this is an important factor in terms of the number of divergent frames of reference that a group like this can absorb in one meeting. In hindsight I credit Dr. Georgopoulos with a great deal of foresight in planning this. I think it has been very good.

Dr. Mauksch: I would like to come back to one point that Pellegrino made, where I have some concerns. I think the intellectual process is a funny one, and this links in with what Straus just said, namely that the mix in this group was just right. This conference is also a system that had a purpose. I would like to compare it to another conference. There, at a previous time, we brought together a group of sixty people, half of whom were social scientists and half physicians. The social scientists were psychologists, sociologists, and anthropologists, and one lone biologist. And what we found, which for that conference had some more legitimacy because it was a conference devoted to planning action rather than to synthesizing knowledge, was the closest real life experience I have ever had with the Tower of Babel. I never thought I would live that long. It was a total groping of languages, with the real discovery that not only the social scientists could not communicate with the physicians, but they could not communicate among themselves. There were so many schools of sociologists and psychologists that they were in a world all by themselves.

I am being a little facetious, but it was a failure. The second time around, we came together to happily sit apart, because the way we structured the conference was such that for two thirds of the time the physicians sat together, the psychologists sat together, and so forth, and I believe we then came together. I do think that there is a legitimacy to the tremendous diversity of our own research endeavor. The knowledge-seeking endeavors, not necessarily the evaluative and what you might call programatic endeavors, but the accretion of knowledge and systematization endeavors that are simultaneously aimed at growth and use, may be more than the system can bear. So I am almost tempted to say that the most important thing about the emerging situation is not to "lose your cool" but to go slow.

Comment: I just wanted to say something that Pellegrino and others have said, namely what a pleasure it was to participate in this work, and thank you for my being invited. While we are struggling away with some of the notions that we are, there comes a time when there must be some dispatch, reinforcement, and a fresh kind of look at what we are doing. These kinds of meetings do help that. I appreciate the kind of helpful "teasing view of ideas" that went on here.

Chairman: Perhaps the best way to use the remaining time would be to give each individual an opportunity for his overarching statement, if he has one, or at least for a comment that he might like to make on any of the presentations.

Dr. Scott: Well, I cheated; I made mine this morning. I did try earlier to summarize my general impressions of what I thought the central issues were.

Dr. Pellegrino: I made mine too. I only express the tragedy that just as, I think, I begin to understand and make contact with some other minds, we have to discontinue it, but that is part of the game.

Dr. Straus: I think anything I would say would be anticlimactic.

Dr. Mauksch: There is one thing that I would like to add. It would be really nice if this group, and maybe another ten or fifteen other individuals, no more than that, could take a whole month and continue this work. This is what we need, but we do not have time to regroup according to needs. Otherwise, I am not necessarily against sin. But I think this was an extremely useful conference.

Dr. Andersen: There is one thing that concerns me, and that is some of the kind of research that I think we are being asked to do. I think Dr. Guest said that we do not have to be so elegant, we do not have to devise our models and replicate the work we do. But if we divide the kind of research we do into theory building and testing, evaluation, and, could I say, prescriptive studies or devising means to attain ends, the latter two are really much more difficult to do than is the former, which is the kind that social scientists traditionally do. In a sense you are putting yourself and your discipline on the line when you tell people which are the optimum means to attain given ends or to evaluate an on-going program, because there are tremendous pressures to do research on on-going programs in a way that will validate what has gone before. And we have designs and methods to fight against this but, still, to do the objective kind of research and use an objective frame of reference to study values, or to study on-going research, is a very difficult thing to do. To tie in to the activist is not an easy job. It is much harder than the kind of traditional research that we have been involved in. I know it has to be done, but I am just saying that it is a tremendous and risky undertaking.

Mr. Siebert: I have little to say except, as another spokesman for the National Center, to express our pleasure with the quality and general scope of the papers and discussion, and our gratitude for your participation and, moreover, for your obvious interest in this area.

Chairman: Before adjourning, I would like to thank all of you once again, and tell you how appreciative we are for your contributions and for making this such a stimulating research symposium. I am delighted with the discussion, as well as with the papers, and anticipate much good use for the ideas and analytical concepts that were presented and examined here.

APPENDIX:

Background Material

In large measure, this book owes its genesis to a unique collaboration by contributing authors within the context of a more encompassing research effort. In May 1969 Dr. Basil S. Georgopoulos, Institute for Social Research, The University of Michigan, submitted a proposal for a "Critique and Synthesis of Hospital Organization Research in the 1960s" to the National Center for Health Services Research and Development, U.S. Department of Health, Education, and Welfare. Research Contract HSM 110-69-207 was subsequently awarded, on this basis, for "A Critical Review and Evaluation of Hospital Intraorganizational Research." In the original proposal, special provision was made for holding the invitational research conference on the work of which the book is partly based. The technical section of the proposal was made available to all those subsequently invited to write working papers, along with an accompanying request that they examine a research area of their personal professional interest within the context of that document. The excerpts presented below defined the scope and nature of the project for the invited contributors.

> The purpose of this study is to carry out a careful and systematic review, critique, and synthesis of a certain body of organizational research literature, and thereby appraise and evaluate the current state of dependable knowledge contained in the works studied. More specifically, the scientific literature reporting social-psychological and organizational research conducted in American hospitals by social, behavioral, and administrative-management scientists and scholars during the decade of the 1960s (1960 through 1969 inclusive) will be examined and assessed.
>
> Empirical studies (sociological, social-psychological, psycholocial, and administrative) of internal hospital organization, intergroup relations, and social structure and functioning will be carefully evaluated from the standpoint of (a) substantive content, (b) theoretical orientation and contribution, and (c) research methodology. The major findings of reviewed hospital studies will be summarized at three different levels, as appropriate: (1) the total hospital as a complex organization or problem-solving system; (2) the sub-system or collectivity level, which encompasses interrole, intergroup, and interdepartmental concerns; and (3) the individual member level, with emphasis on organization-member relations, member goal attainment, and member integration into the system.
>
> Empirically substantiated propositions now scattered throughout the research literature studied (e.g. propositions concerning

such areas and their interrelationships as organizational coordination, the allocation of effort and human resources within hospitals, management and administration, intraorganizational strain and conflict resolution, decision-making and problem-solving, organizational innovation, output and performance, organizational integration and member integration into the system, and other aspects of hospital functioning and of the organizational effectiveness of the system) will be meaningfully integrated, using an open-system theory conceptual framework, and topically summarized.

The state and gaps of social psychological knowledge about hospitals and hospital organization, and about the efficiency and effectiveness of the hospital as a complex organization and problem-solving social system, will be thus assessed, research trends, strengths, and weaknesses will be specified, and unmet research needs—substantive, theoretical, methodological—will be noted.

The project should make a major and unique contribution to hospital research and to the study and understanding of complex organizations more generally. Just as metatheory is an important aid to science development and to theoretically-oriented research, "research on research" of the kind here proposed should greatly facilitate future research and practical application of research results in hospital settings . . . . Potentially, the results of the project could set the tone for much future social-psychological research in the health field, guide the funding of hospital organizational studies, and even significantly affect the behavior of hospital administrators and other practitioners interested in organizational innovation or in improving the functioning of their organizations on the basis of dependable research findings and knowledge. . . .

Since the mid-1950s when modern studies of the kind to be reviewed by the project began first to appear, the volume of social-psychological and related organizational research conducted in hospitals has become very substantial. During the 1960s, in particular, numerous studies have been carried out using different theoretical orientations and different methods and approaches. The volume of such research continues to increase, moreover, at an accelerated rate, but apparently without corresponding efforts toward systematic evaluation and integration of cumulated findings, with the result that adequate assimilation and intelligent use (by practitioners, researchers, research sponsors, and the public) of the amassed body of knowledge in this field are exceedingly difficult and not commensurate with the expended research effort.

Yet, for hospitals as for other large-scale organizations, sound organizational planning for the future, no less than proper action, depends very greatly upon the study of past experience and upon ready availability of factual, useful, and dependable knowledge. In the absence of such knowledge, in suitable form, effective organizational action and planning, rational program development, decision-making, and problem-solving, and efficient research effort to produce additional relevant and dependable knowledge, are all seriously impaired and inhibited.

It is hoped, therefore, that apart from its scientific merits and contribution, . . . this project might also help resolve or mitigate some of the above problems. By making available to all concerned, through its results, an important means for tackling these problems on a rational and systematic basis, and on the basis of verified and dependable knowledge from current organizational research, it should at least help hospital practitioners, scientists, and government officials to overcome some of the difficulties which they now face in the above problem areas.

In short, the project is a major study of available organization research literature, particularly social-psychological, sociological, and administrative studies conducted in hospitals during the 1960s, and of the current state of knowledge in this field, as reflected in the research literature. In addition to published studies, important unpublished works will be covered if available, and completed as well as partially completed research will be evaluated, and the trends, merits, and defects of the past decade of hospital organization research will be specified in the process.

The proposed study constitutes "research on research," having as its main objective the systematic review, critical evaluation, and integrative synthesis of the above body of organization research literature. In addition to summarizing the major findings scattered in this literature, the study will inventory the empirically substantiated propositions which emerge from the findings, specify significant unresearched problems, unmet needs, and inadequacies—substantive, theoretical, and methodological—and consider the need for and methods of future research on hospital organization and internal social relations . . . .

In terms of appropriate content focus, it is anticipated that the project will encompass hospital studies dealing with such areas as the following:

hospital administration problems, and problems in the area of management of human efforts and organizational resources; medical staff organization, and hospital board characteristics; patterns, problems, and mechanisms of organizational decision-making; related authority problems and issues, and the distribution of influence and control among key organizational groups and roles; participation in the affairs of the institution by different groups and members; the articulation and coordination of functions, tasks, and efforts, and their convergence toward the solution of work problems or the attainment of organizational objectives; patterns of specialization and work interdependence; staffing concerns, and the allocation of organization resources, facilities, and personnel; the effects of organization requirements upon the participants, and member compliance and adjustment; the professional values and orientations of different staffs and members; member motivation, involvement, identification, and commitment to the organization; problems of strain, conflict, and interrole or intergroup tension; the utilization of human assets, skills, and talents, and innovative behavior patterns in the system; nonadaptive behavior; mutual role facilitation among interacting groups and members carrying out interdependent roles and functions; role performance, group and departmental peformance, and organizational effectiveness; and other social-psychological aspects of the problem-solving capacity and social and work efficiency of the system.

Relationships among the various substantive areas and problems would, of course, also be appropriate, as would the correlates and determinants, and antecedents and consequences, of variables studied.

Selection of Contributors

The initial intent was to invite a small group of competent and well-informed individuals, perhaps five or six, who had done substantial organizational research and creative work in the field, who represented different theoretical orientations within the social-behavior and management-professional sciences, and who had also had some administrative experience either in academic or in health care institutions. Eventually, twelve persons were invited, by the principal investigator and also by the project officer (Mr. Dennis F. Siebert) on behalf of the National Center for Health Services Research and Development, on the assumption that probably half would accept the task. All but three agreed to participate (of those who did not, one was going abroad on sabbatical, one had undertaken heavy commitments that conflicted with the timing of the effort, and one declined) and write the requested papers. In part, this somewhat unanticipated but fortunate response made the present volume possible.

Prospective authors were given maximum freedom in the choice of their topics and in the manner that they wished to accomplish the task, but they were asked to stay within the broad framework of the research proposal. Furthermore, they all consulted with the principal investigator prior to deciding on a particular topic, so that important problem areas were covered in a complementary fashion and unnecessary duplication was avoided. In the interests of integration, moreover, authors were given certain general guidelines in the form of a lengthy letter. This read as follows:

Dear————:

With the support of the Health Care Institutions Branch of the National Center for Health Services Research and Development, we have recently launched what we consider a rather unique and challenging research effort. This is aimed at a systematic "Critique and Synthesis of Hospital Organization Research in the

1960s." The enclosed . . . document, which is part of the technical proposal, describes the study in some detail (see Appendix). I am hoping that you will find this project sufficiently interesting and worthwhile, and be free, to take an active part in it by accepting my invitation to contribute some of your stimulating thoughts and insights.

I would very much like to include you in the small group of . . . reseachers described in the attached proposal. More specifically, we would like to have you select a particular aspect or problem area of your choice from among those indicated in the proposal that may be of special concern to you, and share with us your observations and ideas on it, in the form of a . . . working paper. The individuals who contribute these working papers will be requested to attend . . . a two-day invitational conference to discuss their papers with each other and with members of the research staff and the Health Care Institutions Branch. The planned conference will be a symposium-type gathering, to be held in Ann Arbor. . . . In the interests of productive discussion writers will be requested to send a draft of their paper for distribution to all participants in advance of the conference.

You are free, of course, to approach the topic, problem, or substantive area that you choose to review in whatever manner you deem appropriate and convenient, within the context of the proposal. Naturally your personal professional views would be very helpful to us, as would your observations on the work of others. We would generally hope that each author might find it feasible to focus his attention on some major area and be concerned with such matters as the following:

(a) The current status of organizational (social-psychological, administrative-professional) knowledge in the particular area, and the principal strengths and weaknesses of past hospital organization research in it; recent and present research trends (substantive, theoretical, methodological) in the area, and important unanswered questions, neglected problems, or unresolved issues; and promising directions that future organizational research in the area might take, given the present state of knowledge and existing gaps or inadequacies, in the light of presumed research capabilities in the field.

(b) Indications of some of the most important, more productive, or most imaginative-innovative research—sociological, psychological, administrative, or professional studies focusing on hospital organization—conducted in American hospitals during the 1960's, with selected references to the literature now available.

(c) Major empirical findings from reported and/or ongoing practical or operational innovations that may have been instituted in hospitals to improve the organization, patient care, or administration on a systematic basis, with special attention to efforts utilizing research results or controlled experimentation.

(d) Suggestions as to the kinds of things to look for (concepts, hypotheses, methods, etc.) in the process of our review, evaluation, and integration of the research literature in the focal area, or propositions that you might like us to test on the basis of data extracted in the process, given the objectives of the project.

(e) Any other recommendations or comments pertaining to the above concerns, or related interests and concerns that you may have at this time, and observations which in your view will facilitate the project; e.g. comments regarding the relationship of the area chosen to any of the other areas specified in the proposal, specific analytical categories or variables to be used in the analysis or to characterize reviewed studies, and the like.

These are some of the possibilities which have occurred to me. Needless to say that they are not intended to be exhaustive or mandatory. They are only illustrative and suggestive, and you might well prefer to be guided by other considerations. An alternative approach might be equally appropriate yet preferable . . . . We would very much like to have the benefit of your knowledge and experience, and I hope that you will find it possible to accept the invitation. Your cooperation would be most valuable.

Working papers were produced and submitted as planned. These were all circulated to the contributing authors and selected colleagues, and then discussed at a special two-day research symposium. The conference was organized into four sessions, two per day. During each of the first three sessions, three different papers were discussed, as follows: first, the author made a presentation of his work, not exceeding thirty minutes, with interruptions only for clarification; the participants then raised issues and questions and commented on the paper and presentation, for approximately another half hour; discussion of the next paper followed, in the same manner; and, finally, after the three papers had been considered, general discussion followed for nearly an hour before the session was concluded. The fourth and final session was devoted to hearing some general remarks by three participants (Dr. White, Dr. Christman, and Dr. Pellegrino) and to closing comments by the contributors. These discussions were taped, then edited and condensed, and ultimately incorporated in the book to accompany the formal papers—the original papers, revised and resubmitted by the authors after the conference.